The Complete Book of Stair Climbing

2012 Edition

The Complete Book of Stair Climbing

2012 Edition

John Smiley

John Smiley Publishing
Philadelphia

Published in the United States by John Smiley Publishing
PO Box 2062
Riverton, NJ 08077-2062
U.S.A.

smileypublishing@johnsmiley.com

Cover Photo by Felicia Peretti

http://www.perrettiphotography.com/

The Complete Book of Stair Climbing 2012 Edition

ISBN: 978-1-61274-027-0

Printed in the United States of America.

10 9 8 7 6 5 4 3 2 1

First Edition: February 2012

Dedicated to my wife Linda.
Without you, none of this would be possible.

About the Author

John Smiley, MCP, MCSD, MCT has been programming and teaching for more than 25 years, and has written over 15 books on Computer Programming. He is the President of John Smiley and Associates, a Computer Consulting firm serving clients both large and small in the Philadelphia Metropolitan area. John is also an adjunct professor of Computer Science at Penn State University, Philadelphia University, and Holy Family University, and also teaches in a variety of Internet venue

In his spare time, he runs, plays basketball, and of course climbs stairs!

Acknowledgments

I want to thank the many people, involved in the great sport of Stair Climbing that I've met, corresponded with or read about during the last year. Some of them are quoted in this book, some are written about. All of them are great stories.

Many thanks to my wife for putting up with my athletic activities, particularly my latest one, Stair Climbing. Because I train in the house, I've worn quite a spot in the rug on the stairs.

Thanks to the many people who I have cornered over the last year discussing Stair Climbing and asking for donations to the American Lung Association. Thanks for being interested.

Thanks to the people (Melissa Smiley, Sophorn Smiley, Tim Gradoville, Bob Gauss, Danielle Turner, and Nora McCloskey) who joined Team Smiley and climbed the 50 floors of the Bell Atlantic Tower for the Philadelphia Fight For Air Climb on March 19, 2011. It was great fun, wasn't it? It wouldn't have been nearly as much fun without you.

Thanks to the Team Smiley Support Team: my wife Linda Smiley, Jamie Gradoville, and Jim Smiley who while they didn't climb, gave great encouragement, facilitated practice climbs and gave generously of their time to inspire the team to new heights.

Thanks to Jamie and Tim Gradoville for allowing Team Smiley to use their 25 floor Condominium fire escape to practice. I wish we had it this year.

Thanks to Rachael Pettigrew and the Philadelphia Branch of the American Lung Association for their efforts in arranging the 2011 climb. Rachael spent a lot of time communicating with the various teams and climbers and did a great job.

Thanks to Sherri Fiorentino and the Philadelphia branch of the American Lung Association for their efforts in planning and arranging the 2012 climb. I know it will be great! Thanks Sherri for inviting me to participate in the planning.

Thanks to all of the climbers, first responders and volunteers who made the 2011 Philadelphia Fight For Air climb a big success.

And of course, I would be remiss if I didn't acknowledge why we hold the American Lung Association Climbs to begin with. Although many of us think of these as athletic endeavors, they are primarily fund raising events to combat, and hopefully one day eradicate, the horrible lung diseases and afflictions that affect our world, and the many thousands of people who have lost their lives because of them. God Bless them--let us never forget them.

Table of Contents

How this book came to be

I began this book with the idea of talking about my new love of Stair Climbing, how I started with the sport, how I found my first Stair Climb, how I trained for it, and my experiences with the climb, but it has evolved into much more.

Along the way I discovered, met, and corresponded with a bunch of great people, some of whom are mentioned in this book.

I discovered that, in addition to a great form of exercise, Stair Climbing is indeed a sport. Some of those records and record makers are noted in this book.

If you want to learn more about Stair Climbing as an exercise, as a fun pursuit, or even as a serious event, read on.

CHAPTER ONE

My Timeline

In **late November** of 2010, shortly after completing the Philadelphia Half Marathon, I recalled that Philadelphia had a Stair Climb event that I had thought about entering in early 2010, but I had injured my foot running in a snowstorm, and couldn't do it.

I wasn't sure what organization hosted it, how high it was, or how much it cost to enter, but I had wanted to do it in 2010 and decided to try it for 2011.

On Thanksgiving Day, I 'googled' Stairclimb + Philadelphia and found it.

There actually were two events, one hosted by the Cystic Fibrosis Foundation(CFF) and the other one by the American Lung Association (ALA).

I chose the American Lung Association Climb, and in a matter of minutes I was registered and also 'tweeting' that I had just entered a stair climb.

The location: Three Locust Square, formerly called the Bell Atlantic Tower.

At this point, I had no idea how to prepare for and train for a stair climb--- all I knew is that on a trip to the Philadelphia Art Museum a few weeks earlier, I got winded going up the 'Rocky' steps. By the way, after completing the 2011 Philadelphia Fight For Air Climb in a time of 10 minutes of 37 seconds, good for 9th in my age group, I still get winded going up those steps. The difference now is that I know it's normal.

On **December 8th** of 2010, I started training.

I thought of driving to a high rise, but anything really high is in mid-town Philadelphia (Philadelphia natives refer to that as Center City), with expensive limited parking, I discounted that possibility.

I live in New Jersey and there are limited high rises near me--mostly apartments.

Time was ticking away when I decided to climb up my stairs until I got tired.

Climb up my stairs?

Yes, that's right, the stairs in my house.

It wasn't long before I was tired---7 flights and I stopped.

If you don't believe me, you can check my You Tube video of the 7 flights here...

http://www.youtube.com/watch?v=uaH77zHHul0

If you check out the You Tube video, you can see I did 7 flights of stairs, accompanied by the strange looks of our dog Madison, and the sounds of my wife making a delicious dinner.

7 flights up, 7 flights down. 14 steps up. 14 steps down.

I decided not to count the down steps, so I entered 98 (7 times 14) in my spreadsheet. (Always record your exercise, it's one of my tips that you'll read about later.)

7 flights didn't seem like a lot, but I wanted to make sure I could do 8 the following day.

8? Where did I come up with that number?

Well, somewhere on the stairs, I got the bright idea to add 1 flight of stairs to my training every day until I got to something?

Something being perhaps the number of flights in the building that the actual climb was taking place (50).

Something being perhaps the number of steps in the building that the actual climb was taking place (1,088)

Perhaps some kind of round number like 100 flights of stairs in the house.

And so, on **December 9th**, I did 8 flights of stairs in my house.

On **December 10th**, I did 9 flights. Apparently, I also had time to drive to Drexel University to pick up my son Kevin, and either on the way there, or the way back, I took this beautiful picture of the Bell Atlantic Tower, the building we would be climbing on our Stair Climb on March 19th.

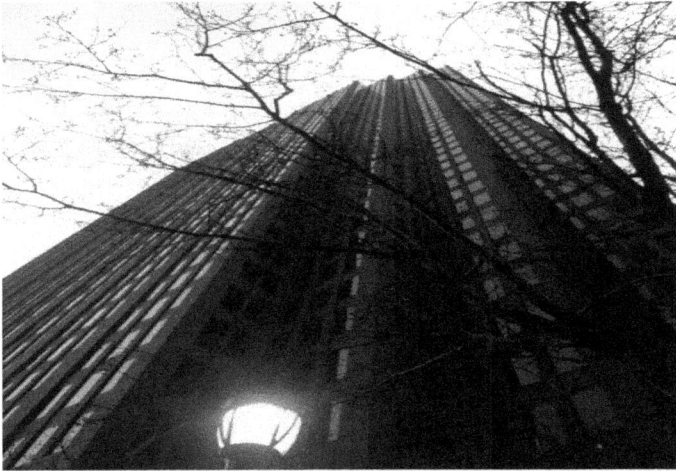

From the sidewalk looking up at the Bell Atlantic Tower. December 10, 2010.

I added 1 flight of stairs every day through **December 13th**, when I did 12 flights of stairs.

Something was bothering me.

I wanted the flights of stairs I was climbing to equal the day of the month---strange I know, but it would make it easier for me to know how many I was doing on a particular day.

Believe me when I say I'm literally just sitting in my chair, reading and answering emails, working on a computer program, teaching an Internet class when suddenly I get up, head to the stairs and start climbing them.

In December of 2010 I didn't put a lot of thought into the process which meant simplifying even the process of knowing how many flights of stairs to climb was a big thing to me.

Therefore, on **December 14th**, instead of doing 13 flights of stairs, I did 14---adding 2 flights instead of 1.

I did 15 flights on **December 15th** and 16 flights on **December 17th**.

Friday, **December 17th** life caught up with me---I worked a full day, and I had a 5K to run the next morning and I promised my wife Olive Garden. I took my first day off from the stairs.

The next day, Saturday, **December 18th**, I ran the 5K race in the morning, and then climbed my stairs in the afternoon.

What to do about the number of flights climbed?

Instead of doing the 17 flights I was scheduled to do the previous day, I did 18 instead.

This started a pattern of 'catching up' on missed days, of which there were few.

I climbed the stairs in the house **December 19th** through **December 22nd**.

Thursday, **December 23rd** was another hectic day. A full day of work, and because of the upcoming Christmas holiday, my wife and I decided to take in a movie on the 23rd, since Christmas Eve and Christmas day were out.

Having skipped **December 23rd**, **December 24th** saw me add 2 flights of stairs to reach 24. **Christmas Day** was no exception. I climbed 25 flights of stairs, one quarter of my way to my half spoken goal of 100 flights.

I finished the year by climbing every day, adding 1 flight each day so that on **December 31st**, I did 31 flights or stairs in the house.

For the year **2010**, I had climbed a total of 422 flights of stairs in my house, 5908 steps in all.

January 1st I celebrated the arrival of 2011 by climbing 32 flights. To remember how many I had to do that day, all I had to do was add the calendar day to the number of days in December and I was set.

This told me that the day before the 2011 Fight For Air Climb (March 18, 2011), I would be climbing 108 flights of stairs (you'll have to read on to see if I did that.)

I climbed every day from **January 1st** through **January 14th**.

While I was climbing (usually in the late afternoons), I was generally doing some kind of running in the morning 3 times a week.

It wasn't always the case, as the January weather in Philadelphia was very snowy in 2011, and I had severely sprained my foot in January of 2010 trying to get a run in before a blizzard arrived. I was in no hurry to hurt myself again, but when the streets outside were relatively dry, you could count on me running about 5 miles three times a week.

For those of you who may be anxious to say that's the reason for my success climbing stairs in the March 19th climb, let me assure you nothing could be farther from the truth.

My runs are more like jogs---what I do on the stairs is much more strenuous, which is why I love Stair Climbing so much. It's really hard to cheat or take it easy on the stairs the way it is when you run. Just walking up stairs can be a great workout.

I see my running in the morning as good cross training for stairs, but I wouldn't cite it as a requirement to climb a tall building. Lots of stair climbers climb stairs, and only climb stairs, as their primary training tool.

I mentioned that I climbed every day from **January 1st** through **January 14th**.

What about **January 15th**?

That was the day we tackled Tim's condo.

Tim (Tim Gradoville) who you will be introduced to later in the book, is a friend of mine who I recruited, along with our daughter Melissa, my nephew Jim Smiley and his wife (my niece) Sophorn, and another friend Bob Gauss to join Team Smiley. (Two others would join Team Smiley later, Danielle Turner and Nora McCloskey.)

Along with being a superb athlete, Tim also possessed something that would make him a formidable climber on **March 19th** at the Fight For Air Climb. He lived in a 25 story high rise Condominium!

To be specific, Tim lived on the 17th floor of a 25 floor condo, and he and his wife Jamie generously offered to let us practice climb in their fire escape, something Tim had been doing since joining Team Smiley in late December.

And so, **on January 15th, 2011**, Bob and I travelled to Tim's Condo to climb the stairs. (Melissa and Sophorn would join us at later practices, Nora and Danielle didn't make our team practices.)

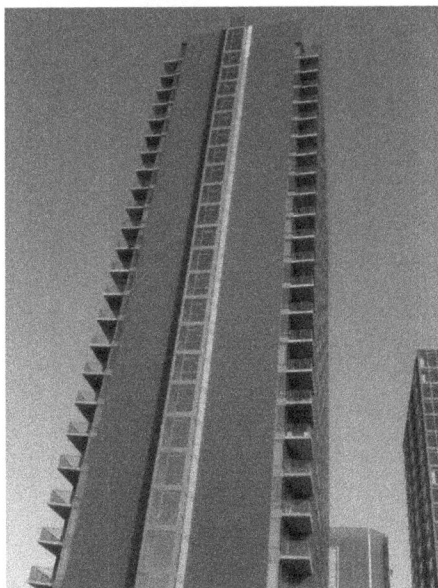

The building looked pretty imposing from the outside, but it's "only" 25 floors, about half as high as the Bell Atlantic Tower's 50 floor height.

As a true native Philadelphian, and team captain, I supplied the soft pretzels for post climb nourishment. Tim and his wife Jamie supplied fruit and water.

Only Tim had climbed more than a few flights of steps at one time--to the rest of us, it was all new.

We left some stuff in Tim's condo, then took the elevator down to the 2nd floor, entered the fire escape, and walked down to the first floor.

We decided to climb separately, about 15 seconds apart.

Tim went first, followed by Bob, followed by me.

I can't speak for them, but I double stepped my way until about the 7th floor. I was getting pretty tired at that point--exhausted might be a better description of how I felt. At that time, I was double stepping up 45 flights of stairs in my home, but that process was 1 flight up, 1 flight down, and there's no doubt that the flight down gives me a chance to rest a bit. In a high rise, its' straight up.

So, after 7 flights, I stopped double stepping, hoping to recover a bit and just started walking up the stairs.

It was around the 13th floor that I felt what I told my team mates at the top was the demon---the air demon, lung demon, whatever you want to call it that seemed to suck the air right out of my lungs.

My heart rate was high, my breathing deep and labored---I really felt that I miss know what it feels like to suffer from a lung disease such as asthma or COPD, unable to catch my breath.

Getting to the top, after floor 13, was just a matter of putting one foot in front of the other and stepping up.

For me, as a runner and a stair climber, there's a point where you're not sure you can make it, and another point where you know you will make it.

For me, the floors between 13 and 22 were the 'not sure' floors.

Once I hit the 22nd floor, I knew I would reach the top.

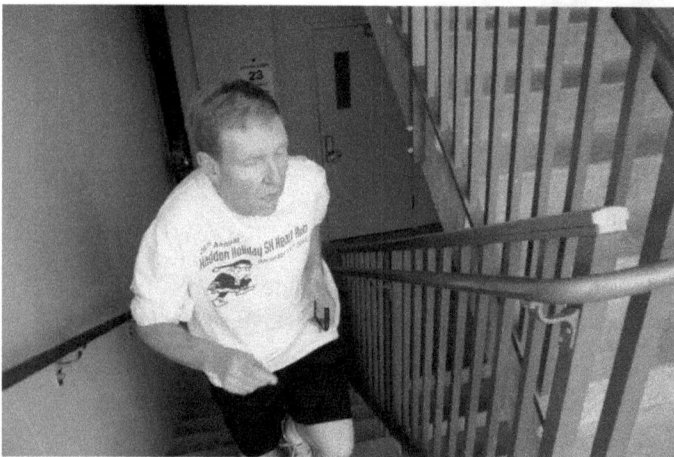

John Smiley reaching floor 22

I could hear Tim and Bob at the top, breathing heavily, but also encouraging me.

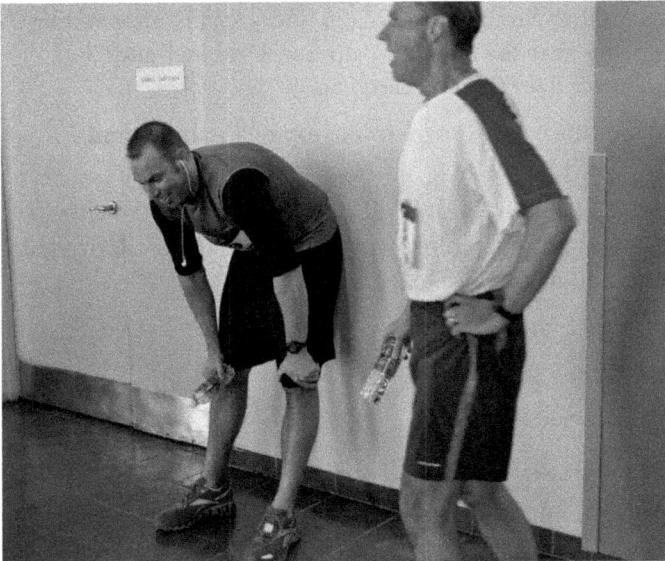

Tim and Bob waiting for John to reach the top after the first climb on January 15, 2011

I reached the top of the stairs, and even though I was pretty tired, I still had the presence of mind to stop my watch and see my time: 4 minutes and 5 seconds. Bob and Tim's times were not that far ahead of mine, so I felt pretty good about that.

We spent about 5 minutes recovering, comparing notes, talking about the demon on the 13th floor, when Bob said, "Ready to do it again."

Amazingly, after a 5 minute rest, all three of us were ready to try it again.

Once again, we took the elevator down to the 2nd floor, entered the fire escape, climbed down the 1st floor, and go ready to do it again.

Tim and Bob went off first, separated by about 10 seconds.

I started off again.

The second set was better--I knew what to expect.

Not better in time (my time was actually slower) but a better experience.

I hardly double stepped the second time---just found a nice comfortable rhythm and basically walked my way up.

I reached the top the 2nd time in 4 minutes and 19 seconds.

My walking time was only 14 seconds slower than the time in which I double stepped.

Once reaching the top, Bob and I agreed that knowing what to expect was a big help.

We ended up doing another climb up the full 25 floors, again, after resting for about 5 minutes. My time for that climb up was 4 minutes and 26 seconds, 7 seconds slower than the 2nd climb up.

I essentially walked the entire way and go to the top in 4 minutes and 7 seconds..

Amazingly, we had the energy to do a 4th climb, but we decided to stop at the 17th floor, which was Tim's Condo floor. I reached the 17th floor tired, in a time of 2 minutes and 34 seconds.

Here are my times for each of the climbs:

First set of 25: 4 minutes, 5 seconds

Second set of 25: 4 minutes, 19 seconds

Third set of 25: 4 minutes, 26 seconds

Fourth set (17 flights): 2 minutes, 34 seconds

Total time for 92 flights: 15 minutes and 14 seconds

Take note that it typically takes me about 6 minutes to do 25 flights of stairs in my house, because in addition to going up, I'm also going down. Extrapolating these times for the Philadelphia Fight For Air climb, you would think I would finish between 8 and 9 minutes.

That the extrapolation doesn't take into account is the way each of us felt when he hit the 25th floor---like we didn't want to go any farther!

Notice that my time was 15 minutes and 14 seconds for 92 flights---no time wasted in climbing down.

I heartily recommend that if you can, you find a high rise like this to practice in at least **once** before your actual climb.

It will prepare you for the real thing.

Some Stair Climbs have 'practice' climbs for their climbers.

As for our team, we wound up doing this condo practice climb twice more (**February 12th** and **March 5th**), each time improving on our times, and gaining some valuable experience.

January 16th was the Sunday after our first practice climb of 25 floors (actually 92 floors in total.) I was curious as to how I would do on my regularly scheduled practice climb in my house.

I had done 45 flights on **January 14th**, and so, decided to do 47 on the 16th. No problem. I felt strong, doing them in 11 minutes and 12 seconds. I had done 45 flights on the 14th in 11 minutes and 16 seconds, so my 'pace' for 2 additional flights was actually faster.

From **January 17th** through **January 27th**, I continued to add 1 flight per day to my total, completing 58 flights (a total of 812 steps) on the 27th.

Following the suggestion of a Facebook friend, Lisa Kinsner Scheer, a stair climber with a lot of experience, on **January 20th**, rather than climb 51 flights with no rest, I broke up my routine by doing 25 flights, resting 5 minutes, then 26 more flights, for a total of 51.

I wasn't sure how I liked doing flights like this. Lisa told me the idea was to push myself harder for the 25 flights, which I definitely did. I'm not sure my body liked the 5 minute resting period. I felt sluggish starting again.

I tried this same approach on **January 21st** (52 flights), **February 9th** (71 flights), **February 10th** (72 flights) and also on **February 11th** (73 flights).

Ultimately, I decided this wasn't for me---I just hate to stop, and when I do stop, I really have a hard time starting again.

On Friday, **January 28th** we had to rush our dog Madison to the University of Pennsylvania Veterinarian Hospital for a life saving blood transfusion (she's fine now.) Obviously, no Stair Climbing that day and the first day I had missed since December 23rd (a total of 34 straight days of Stair Climbing training.)

Saturday, **January 29th**, after some promising news on our dog Madison, I did 60 flights.

I followed that up with consecutive training climbs from **January 30th** (61 flights) through **February 11th**, when I did 73 flights.

Saturday, **February 12th**, was Team Smiley's second practice session at Tim's Condo.

This time, in addition to me, Tim and Bob, Sophorn Smiley joined us for her first practice climb.

Sophorn is a long distance runner. She completed her first Marathon, the Philadelphia Marathon, in November of 2010, along with her husband (my nephew Jim)and after the Philadelphia Fight For Air Climb in March, she and Jim flew to Chicago in October to do the Chicago Marathon (Jim was scratched from the Chicago Marathon with a stress fracture of his foot) and she ended her running year by completing the JFK 50 Ultra Marathon in Hagerstown Maryland.

I mention this here for those long distance runners wondering if you need to climb stairs to train for a stair climb.

Sophorn runs, and also does a lot of Yoga work, and did some machine Stair Climbing in the gym, but for the most part, her preparation involved just her running routine.

Our second practice session at Tim's condo went just about the same as the first.

3 sets of 25 floor climbs, with about a 5 minute rest in between, followed by a 17 floor climb to Tim's floor, and post climb refreshments (Philly soft pretzels, fruit, and water.)

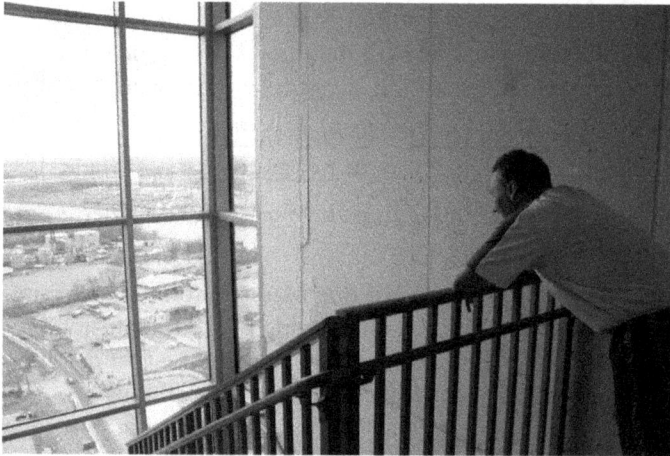

Bob at the top, waiting for Team mates Tim, John and Sophorn on February 12, 2011.

The results were a bit better than the first climb, not only for me, but for Tim and Bob as well. Here are my results for our **2nd Practice Climb.**

First set of 25: 3 minutes, 52 seconds

Second set of 25: 4 minutes, 6 seconds

Third set of 25: 4 minutes, 7 seconds

Fourth set (17 flights): 2 minutes, 31 seconds

Total time for 92 flights: 14 minutes and 36 seconds

Each individual climb was faster than the first practice climb back in January, and overall, my time was 38 seconds faster than the previous one.

In addition to the faster time, each of us who had done the first practice climb in January felt a lot more confident that we could complete the actual Philadelphia Fight For Air climb on March 19th.

We hoped to squeeze in one more practice session in Tim's condo sometime in March (and we did.)

What do you do the day after you climb 92 floors in a Condo?

Practice climb in your house, of course, and that's exactly what I did on Sunday, **February 13th**. I had done 73 flights on February 11th, so naturally on the 13th I did 75 flights., although my legs felt a bit tired and I completed them in 18 minutes and 55 seconds.

At this point, I began a modification to my training program.

I had been running in January and February, but I had yet to find my normal rhythm.

I habitually run 3 times a week, early in the morning, usually Monday, Wednesday and Friday. I average somewhere around 15 miles per week, about 60 miles per month.

On **February 10th of 2010**, trying to beat the arrival of a projected blizzard, I had run early in the morning, and just about a quarter of a mile from my home I severely sprained my foot, and was out of action for about a month (it still hurts today.)

Because of that injury I was very caution in **January** and **February** of 2011.

The Philadelphia weather during the winter of 2011 had been pretty snowy and cold---and the snow that fell wasn't going anywhere.

We had a major snowfall on **December 26th**, another one on **January 10th**. On **January 26-27th**, we were socked with 16 inches of snow.

I had 6 runs in January totalling 26.18 miles.

Through **February 13th**, I had run only twice, totalling 10 miles.

If there was snow or ice on the ground, I wasn't venturing out (certainly not in the dark.)

I was consoled by my work on the stairs. And since in early **February** I was now able to climb up and down the stairs of my house for over 15 minutes, I knew I was still getting a good workout in.

After climbing 75 flights of stairs on **February 13th**, I ran a nicely paced 5 mile run on Monday, **February 14th**, and with no snow or rain in the forecast for the remainder of the week, I looked forward to a week or normal running, which brought me to a crossroads in my training.

Should I run 3 times a week, and continue to do the stairs everyday?

Or should I do the stairs only on the days I didn't run?

I decided to try doing stairs only on the days that I didn't run for a week to gauge the effects.

On the morning of **Monday, February 14th**, I ran 5 miles and didn't climb in the afternoon.

On Tuesday, **February 15th**, I climbed 77 flights of stairs in 19 minutes and 28 seconds. Perhaps more important than the 77 flights was the number of steps: 1,078. That was 10 short of the 1,088 required to get to the top of the Bell Atlantic Tower for the 2011 Philadelphia Fight For Air Climb. My next climb I would pass that number!

Wednesday, **February 16th**, I ran 5 miles in the morning.

Thursday, **February 17th**, I climbed 79 flights of stairs in 19 minutes and 17 seconds. 11 seconds faster, although I climbed 2 more flights of stairs. And, the total number of steps? 1,106. I had surpassed that psychological barrier. I now knew that I could force my legs to climb more than enough steps to get to the top of the Bell Atlantic Tower. How fast I would do that was another story.

But another important point that I don't want to miss.

On February 17th, I climbed 2 more flights of stairs than I did on Feburary 15th, yet I was faster in doing so.

Was I onto something?

That remained to be seen.

Friday, **February 18th**, I ran 5 miles in the morning.

Saturday, **February 19th**, I climbed 81 flights of stairs in 18 minutes and 48 seconds. 29 seconds faster than **February 17th**, with 2 more flights climbed.

I began to think that I had found an ideal training strategy.

Mix my running with my Stair Climbing.

Sunday, **February 20th**, I climbed again, the first time I had climbed two consecutive days in about a week. No problem. 82 flights of stairs, although my time at 20 minutes and 31 seconds was a little on the slow side.

We had bad weather in the Philadelphia area on Monday, **February 21st**, (President's Day) and so I climbed instead of running, doing 83 flights.

Tuesday was a normal Climb Day, and so Tuesday, **February 22nd**, I climbed again, this time doing 84 flights in 20 minutes and 7 seconds.

I ran on Wednesday, **February 23rd**, and because the weather was nice on Thursday, **February 24th** but not forecast to be so nice on Friday, I ran again on Thursday.

I didn't plan to do NOTHING on Friday, **February 25th**, but that's exactly what happened.

After working a full day, we had a family birthday celebration, and Stair Climbing was now taking over 20 minutes, plus a cool down period of about 10 minutes and a shower. There just wasn't time.

I was concerned what this would do to my next climbing session, but also a bit curious.

I hadn't gone more than 2 days not climbing since I started in December of 2010.

Saturday, **February 26th,** I climbed the stairs in my house, doing 88 flights of stairs in 20 minutes and 41 seconds. a good pace. I had last done 84 flights 4 days earlier in 20 minutes and 7 seconds, so I was pleased that I hadn't 'lost anything.' I also passed the mythical 86 number---the number of flights in the Empire State Building Run Up (although far short of the number of steps.)

Sunday, **February 27th** I climbed 89 flights of stairs.

The weather was bad on Monday, **February 28th**, and so I climbed 90 flights of stairs instead of running.

Tuesday, **March 1st**, I ran 5 miles.

Wednesday, **March 2nd,** I climbed 92 flights of stairs. I looked forward to reaching the 100 flight mark within the next 10 days.

On Thursday, **March 3rd**, I ran 5 miles.

On Friday, **March 4th**, I climbed 94 flights of stairs in the house in 22 minutes and 52 seconds.

On Saturday, **March 5th**, Team Smiley had its 3rd and final climb at Tim's condo. In addition to me, Bob, Tim and Sophorn, this time my wife Linda and our daughter Melissa took part.

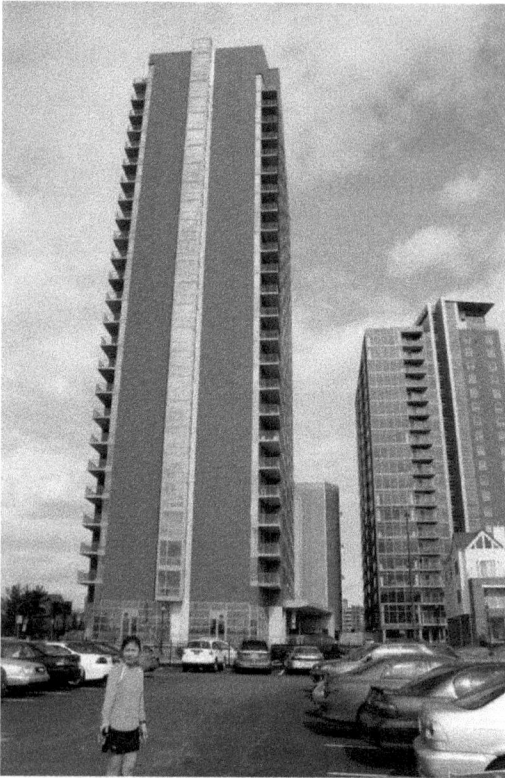

Having a tall building to practice in gives you a big psychological lift for the actual climb

Linda was sitting out the 2011 Philadelphia Fight For Air Climb, but Melissa was ready for it, fresh from a successful season of High School Winter track.

Once again, we set out to do multiple sets of 25 floor climbs, but to more accurately simulate the 50 floor climb we would be doing in exactly two weeks on March 19th, Bob, Tim, Sophorn and I decided that the first person up the stairs would immediately head to the elevator in the hallway, and once inside, hold it for the rest of the team. That meant me going first, followed by the faster members of the team who would arrive roughly at the top of the stairs at the same time. Melissa we more or less left on her own, since it was her first time up the stairs (she had done zero Stair Climbing practice.)

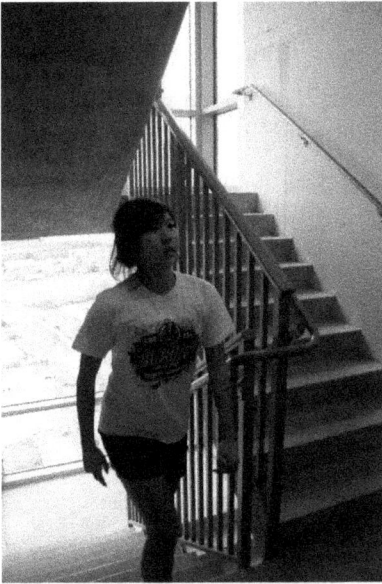

Melissa approaching the top during her only practice climbing session on March 5, 2011. She would go on to finish 2nd in her age group two weeks later at the 2011 Philadelphia Fight For Air Climb. So much for Stair Climbing practice!

The simulation strategy worked well as we were all in the elevator within 30 seconds of finishing our first climb up the stairs---no rest at the top this time---and down to the first floor starting point in just about 90 seconds, ready to do a full second climb, which we all did roughly the same time as our first climb up.

This was an important psychological, confidence building step for us.

What it meant was that we felt we could climb the first 25 floors of the Bell Atlantic Tower, if necessary rest for 90 seconds, then finish the final 25 floors.

I say if necessary, because no one on the team wanted to do that.---stop or rest. But it was important to know that the option was on the table to rest for 90 seconds, and still finish the actual climb with a decent time for the climb.

My first time up the 25 floors was 3 minutes and 41 seconds. My second time up was 4 minutes and 11 seconds. Counting the 90 second 'rest period' for the elevator ride down and walk to the starting point on the first floor, my total time for 50 floors was 9 minutes and 22 seconds. Based on those totals, I was hopeful to complete the actual climb somewhere between 9 and 10 minutes (my actual time was 10 minutes and 37 seconds.)

Up until that 50 floor simulation, all of us on Team Smiley had been wondering what it would feel like to go past the 25th floor for the first time.

The simulation, even with a 90 second rest period (not much we could do about that) for the most part answered that question.

We did our 3rd time up the fire escape, and most of us that with a 17 story climb up to Tim's condo.

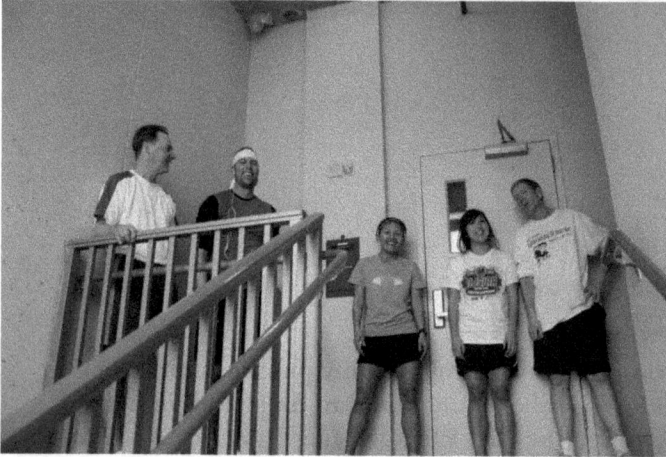

Team Smiley: (Left to right) Bob Gauss, Tim Gradoville, Sophorn Smiley, Melissa Smiley, John Smiley after our 3rd set of 25 floors. We all felt pretty good.

All in all, here are my results from the 3rd practice climb at Tim's condo:

First set of 25: 3 minutes, 41 seconds

Second set of 25: 4 minutes, 11 seconds

Third set of 25: 4 minutes, 7 seconds

Fourth set (17 flights): 2 minutes, 31 seconds

Total time for 92 flights: 14 minutes and 31 seconds

My total time was 5 seconds less than the previous practice climb on **February 12th**.

Melissa didn't say much about her practice experience, other than to pronounce it "intense". I was a bit worried about her, but with little reason. She would go on to beat me by one second in the actual climb on March 19th (despite climbing in the Family Climber category) and finish 2nd in her age group.

We all left Tim's condo that day pretty confident in our ability to finish, and do well, on the actual Climb Day.

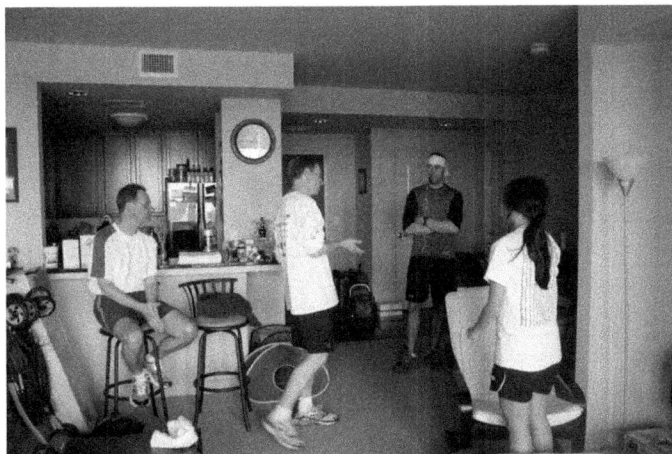

Team Smiley after their practice climb on March 5, 2011, discussing snacks and strategy.

That confident feeling, for me, was a product of daily Stair Climbing in my house, and several practice sessions in a high rise.

The high rise practice sessions were important to give us a feeling for the Oxygen Debt that we would encounter on Climb Day.

I believe without the high rise practice climbs, I probably would have done about as well, but I wouldn't have been nearly as confident and relaxed on Climb Day.

As you'll see, when I describe the actual Climb Day for the 2011 Philadelphia Fight For Air Climb, there were still some surprises that we encountered.

Did you notice that there were two members of Team Smiley who weren't able to join us for our practice sessions.

Nora McCloskey and Danielle Turner were former athletes, in their early 20's, who both regularly worked out and exercised. When you read through the rest of the book and see my tips on finding and using the restroom, think of Nora and Danielle, whose potential for excellent times were derailed by an unscheduled bathroom break somewhere between the 10th and 15th floors. But that won't happen in 2012, I know :)

Sunday, **March 6th** was my 56th birthday. Naturally, I climbed stairs, 96 flights, 1344 steps. That was more than the number of flights in the Hustle Up The Hancock Tower in Chicago. which has 94 flights, but 1632 steps.

Monday, **March 7th** I ran 5 miles.

Tuesday, **March 8th**, I climbed 98 flights. I knew the next time I hit the stairs in my house I would hit the long awaited 100 flight mark.

Wednesday, **March 9th**, I ran 5 miles.

Thursday, **March 10th**, I climbed 100 flights in my house, finishing in 24 minutes and 20 seconds, a time I know now to be an excellent pace.

I don't remember if I celebrated or not (I doubt it,) but I'm sure I tweeted about it, and probably no one raised an eyebrow. Most people, aside from the ones reading this book, either don't understand or don't care :)

The 100 flights also meant I did 1400 steps in the workout, and that number brought my total steps climbed since beginning training on **December 7th** to 58,588.

Friday, **March 11th**, I ran 5 miles.

Saturday, **March 12th**, one week until the actual climb, I approached the stairs in my house and wondered what to do? By climbing 100 flights in my previous workout, I had hit the mark I really wanted to achieve. Would I go past 100 and do 102, or stop at 100?.

 I decided to wait and see how I felt on the stairs, and when I hit 100, I turned at the landing at the bottom of our stairs and ran right up the stairs twice more to finish with 102 flights climbed in 24 minutes and 22 seconds.

Sunday, **March 13th**. I climbed 103 flights in exactly 25 minutes. How long, I wondered, would I continue to keep adding 1 flight?

Monday, **March 14th**, I ran 5 miles.

Tuesday, **March 15th**, I climbed 105 flights.

Wednesday, **March 16th**, Bad weather outside. Instead of running in the morning, I climbed 106 flights. This would be my final practice climb on the house stairs before the real thing on Saturday. In total, I had climbed 4,944 flights preparing for the actual climb, a total of 70,320 steps.

Thursday, **March 17th**, I ran 5 miles.

On that day, I also received an email from the American Lung Association informing me of my start time for the 2011 Philadelphia Fight For Air Climb.

I had registered as an Elite climber, which for the Philadelphia climb meant that I thought I could reach the top of the Bell Atlantic Tower between 8 and 12 minutes.

The email said that Elite climbers would be going up the fire escape between 8:30 and 8:45am,

A big benefit of being an Elite climber was that we had a staggered start, meaning that I would start 15 seconds after the climber in front of me, and 15 seconds in front of the climber behind me. (My teammates Tim, Bob, and Sophorn would be the 3 climbers immediately in front me.)

According to the rest of the schedule in the email, the Opening Ceremony would begin at 8am.

Elite Climbers would go up between 8:30 and 8:45am.

Members of the First Responder Challenge would go up between 8:50 and 9:10am.

Open Climbers would go up between 9:12 and 9:30am.

Team Climbers between 9:30 and 10:30am.

And finally, First Responder Teams, 10:30 to 11:15am.

Awards would follow at 11:30am.

Finally, the email said, the schedule was subject to variations :).

On Climb Day, everything pretty much followed the schedule laid out in the email.

From Thursday to Saturday, I couldn't wait.

Climbers were asked to be at the event one hour prior to our estimated starting time of 8:30. That would mean leaving our house at around 7am.

Registration for the climb would begin at 7am. That would include picking up our Climb Packet.

I'm getting a bit ahead of myself here.

Friday, **March 18th**, I ran 5 miles.

In the late afternoon on Friday, from 4 to 6pm, climbers in the Philadelphia Fight For Air Climb had the option of picking up their Climb Packet at the Bell Atlantic Tower (now known as Three Logan Square) in Philadelphia, or, waiting until Saturday morning to do it.

Rush hour traffic in Philadelphia can be horrendous, so it was an easy choice to wait until Saturday morning to pick up our Climb Packets.

What exactly is in a Climb Packet?

A bib number, a timing chip, and some advertisements for local races. No real need to pick it up earlier, although some climbs (and races) also give you your t-shirt if you pick up your packet early. That allows you to wear in on Climb Day if you wish.

On Friday evening, my wife Linda and I had dinner at Red Lobster, talked about the Stair Climb with some of our friends there, tried (unsuccessfully) to get more team members for Team Smiley, and then headed home.

No, I didn't Carbo-load. No need to do that. I wasn't going to be running a Marathon the next day, just an 8 to 12 minute sprint up a fire escape.

And of course, I avoided drinking any alcohol, which is notorious for dehydrating you.

Speaking of hydration, I had been aware of the need to properly hydrate myself for the event. I typically do this by drinking plenty of water for 3 days prior to the event.

One rule of thumb I've seen is to take your body weight, divide it by 2, and drink that amount of water (in ounces) per day. A 160 pound person would then need to drink 80 ounces of water per day.

One of my Stair Climbing buddies swears that if you aren't properly hydrated, it can cost you a 10% 'hit' on your performance for a running or Stair Climbing event.

For someone like me, hoping to get to the top in 10 minutes (600 seconds), dehydration could cost me an additional full minute in time(600 & 10% = 60 seconds).

Therefore, no alcohol!

Saturday, **March 19th**, Climb Day! The Philadelphia Fight For Air Climb.

I'm accustomed to getting up early for running events, so getting up at **6am** for a Stair Climb was nothing new to me.

I showered, and dressed in a pair of running shorts and a running shirt.

Now, what to eat?

Just as I don't drink alcohol the night before a race or a climb, I don't like a big breakfast.

Ordinarily, I go with a bagel perhaps with a bit of jelly.

I'm a big coffee fan. Like it or not, I can drink a pot a day, but on race or Climb Day, I try to restrict it to 2 cups.

Depending upon how I feel when I wake up, I may also pop in 2 Advil , and that's exactly what I did around **6:45am** on **March 19th**.

After this, it was a matter of waiting for my daughter Melissa to get ready, and at approximately **7am** we were on our way to 1717 Arch Street in Philadelphia., otherwise known as Three Logan Square, formerly known as the Bell Atlantic Tower Building.

We crossed from New Jersey into Philadelphia via the Betsy Ross Bridge, and headed down Interstate 95 to 476, the Vine Street Expressway.

I pointed out the Bell Atlantic Tower to my daughter, and she groaned at the height of it. She had yet to see it, although she had climbed it's height and total number of stairs at Tim's Condo :)

As for me, I had driven by the building at least 10 times since registering for the climb, so I knew my way there, although I wasn't absolutely sure about where to park.

In the email we received on Thursday, we had been told that there was a Parking Garage located in the back of the building off of Cherry Street right after 17th Street.

I didn't have to look very hard for the Parking Garage because a group of very enthusiastic volunteers from the Sanford-Brown School were standing on 17th street with banners literally leading us into the Parking Garage.

Melissa and I entered the Parking Garage around **7:20am**, and parked our car in a lower level space. I can't be sure, but I think that the Parking Garage was getting close to 'full,' even at that relatively early hour. For those of you considering doing the climb in 2012, you may want to bear that in mind, although there are plenty of other Parking Garages and spaces nearby.

After parking, Melissa and I ensured we had everything we needed (for me, really just my iPhone, for Melissa her iPod for Climb music) and then started walking toward the elevator. The Parking Garage is connected to the Bell Atlantic Building.

Before we reached the elevator, we almost bumped into Tim Gradoville and his wife Jamie, and together we headed up the elevator to the lobby of the Bell Atlantic Tower.

When the elevator opened, we exited to the lobby and it was already pretty crowded.

The four of us (me, Melissa, Tim and Jamie) looked for a Registration Desk and quickly found one, where, after identifying ourselves, we were given a Climb Packet containing a bib (a piece of paper with a number on it) and a timing chip which we were given along with some instructions for attaching the timing chip to our shoes. It didn't take long to figure out how to attach it to the running shoes I was wearing.

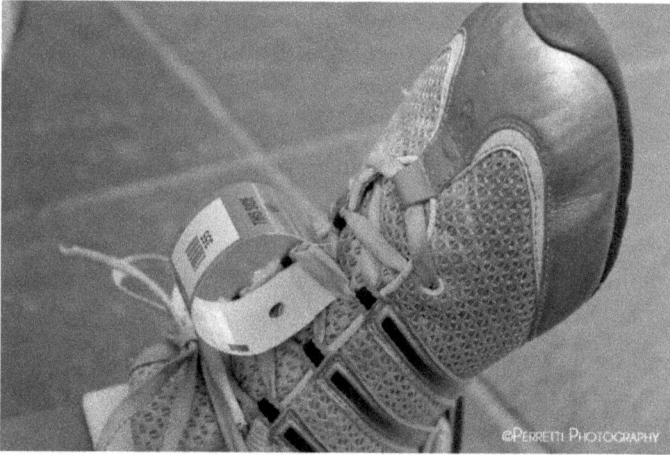

Sneaker and the Timing Chip

Really, the only difficulty in attaching the timing chips to our shoes was to find some available space in the lobby where we could sit on the floor to do that. The lobby was pretty much packed with some of the 600 climbers who would participate in the climb that day.

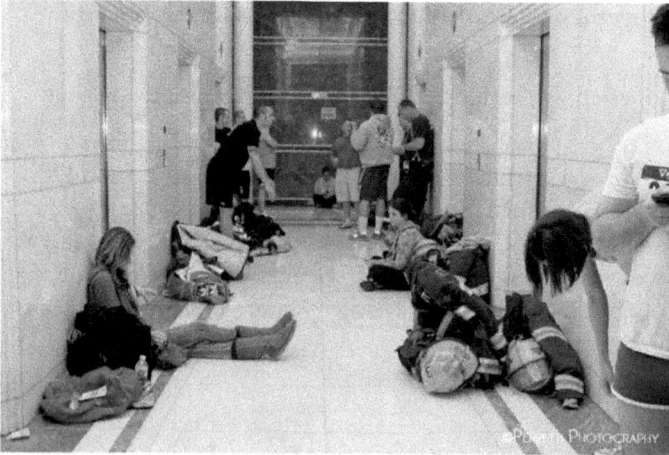

Finding some empty space in the lobby can be tough

With the benefit of hindsight, for the 2012 Philadelphia Fight For Air Climb, I might try to pick up our Climbing Packet the Friday before the climb. It would save us some time on Climb Day morning, and we could attach the timing chips to our shoes/sneakers at home.

With the timing chips attached, you would think it was now just a matter of waiting for the climb to officially begin, but as the captain of Team Smiley, I still had some work to do. I had to find the rest of Team Smiley! Bob, Sophorn, Nora and Danielle.

As I went looking for them, I heard some remarks over the loudspeaker from Rachael Pettigrove, of the American Lung Association, who organized the 2011 Philadelphia Fight For Air Climb. She did a great job!

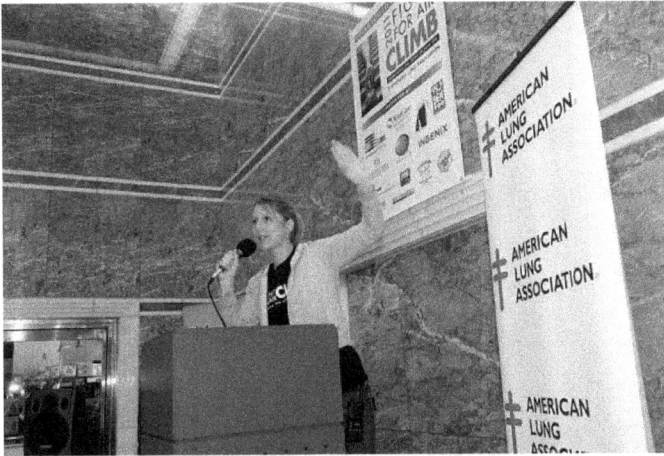

Rachael Pettigrove speaking to the climbers

We were expecting the Mayor of Philadelphia, Michael Nutter, but he wasn't able to make it for 2011. I then heard, and caught part of, the singing of the United States National Anthem.

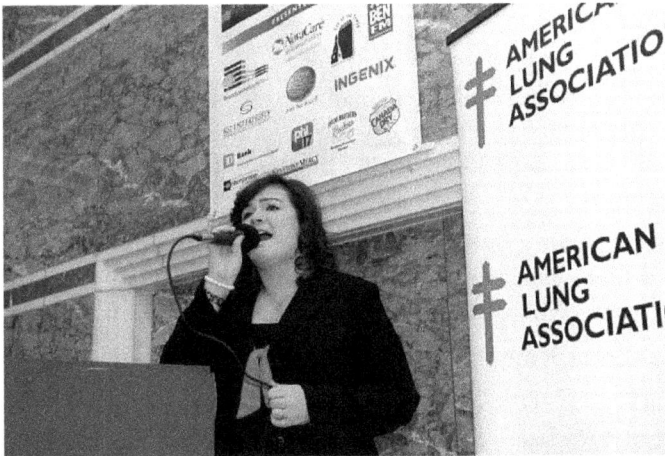

Singing of the National Anthem

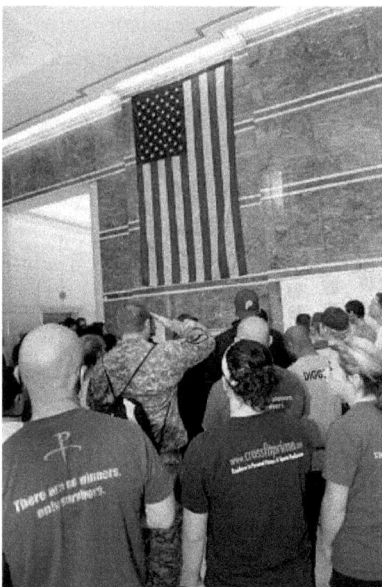

Standing at attention for the National Anthem

It was now about **7:45**.

In addition to my missing team mates, there were some other people I was looking for before I had to line up to begin the climb.

First, as a Team Captain for the event, via email and telephone, I had spent a lot of time dealing with <u>Rachael Pettigrove</u>, the organizer for the 2011 Fight For Air Climb, and I wanted to meet her in person to thank her for all of her help with the event.

Team Smiley had raised quite a bit of money for the climb, and Rachael had helped us numerous times when some of our donors had failed to name either Team Smiley or individual team members with their donation.

Rachael was always very accommodating and willing to help us in any way she could.

Interestingly, I had met Rachael's mother and father at the Registration Desk when I picked up my Climber Packet.

I kept asking climb officials where Rachael was, and all they could really tell me was that she was walking around with a walkie talkie.

I eventually found Rachael, introduced myself, thanked her for all of her help, and let her get back to running the climb. It's a lot of work.

I would guess it was now around **7:55am**.

I was also looking for Felicia Perretti, a local photographer whom I had met via Twitter, who was there to take some photographs of Team Smiley and the overall event and wound up taking pictures so beautiful that she was asked, by the American Lung Association, to come back in 2012 to take photographs of this year's climb. Many of her photographs appear, with her permission, in this book, and you can check out more of her photographs and her work at her website

http://www.perrettiphotography.com/

I eventually met up with Felicia, introduced myself, found Rachael Pettigrove (again) introduced her to Rachael, and then turned around to see Bob Gauss standing there.

Right behind him were my niece and nephew---Sophorn and Jim Smiley.

I assisted Sophorn in getting her Climbing Packet. Jim was not climbing, but in addition to being a superb athlete, he's an excellent photographer and immediately starting taking pictures. Some of his photographs, with his permission, also appear in this book.

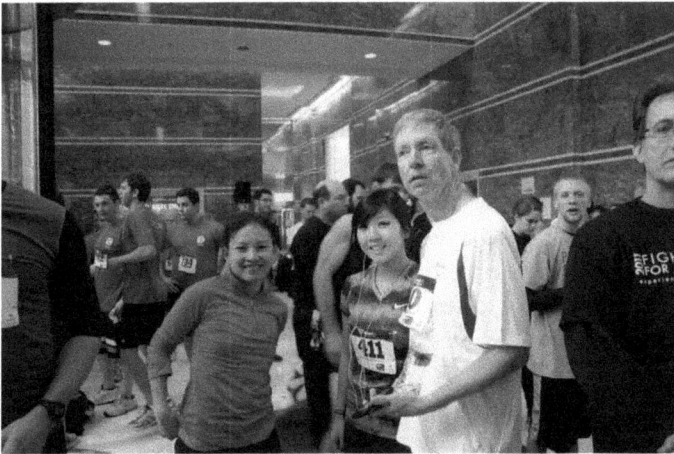

Sophorn and Melissa at the Registration Desk

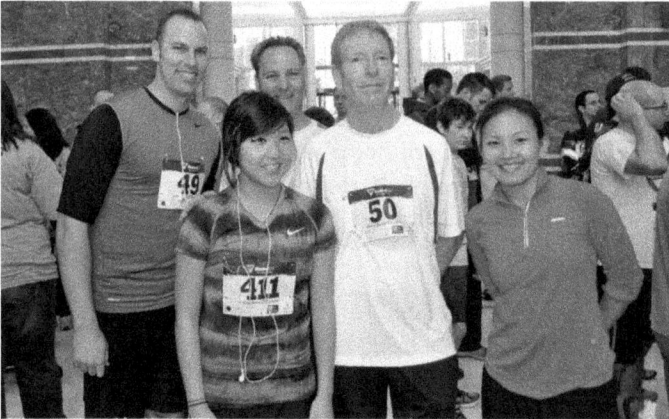

Most of Team Smiley. Tim, Melissa, Bob, John and Sophorn

It must have been **8am** by now. Only Nora and Danielle hadn't shown up yet.

In a big lobby like this, it's possible to be on the 'wrong' side of the lobby, We managed to miss the opening remarks and the National Anthem, which were on the opposite side of the building from us. Nora and Danielle might have been on that side.

For those of you thinking about doing the climb in 2012, have specific ideas in place in terms of meeting up with your team before hand. We will for 2012.

While waiting for Nora and Danielle, we took a moment to sign what I call the Memorial Scroll, and to check the Inspiration Wall, which has tributes to people who have died from Lung disease. They are honored there.

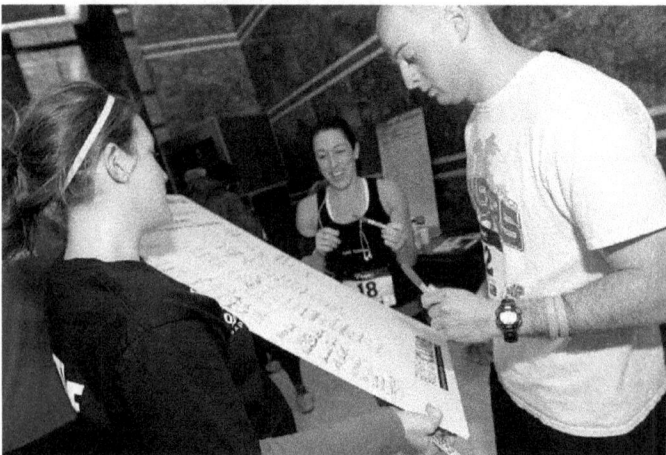

Climbers signing the American Lung Association Memorial Scroll

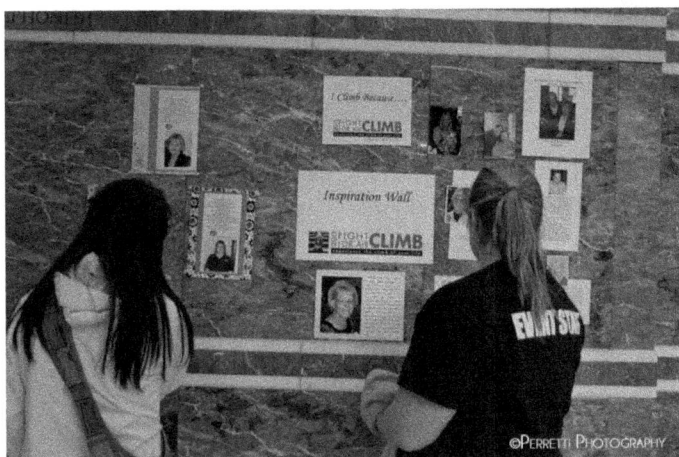

Climbers checking the Inspiration Wall

Still no Nora and Danielle.

Danielle is the sister of one of Melissa's friends, and she had taken me up on the challenge of doing the climb when I posed the idea to her when I saw her at a basketball game we both attended. I hadn't seen Danielle since she said 'yes', although we had sent some emails and Facebook messages back and forth.

Nora is Danielle's cousin (interesting that both Nora and I share a common family last name, causing me to habitually call her 'Cousin Nora'). Nora and I had never met, and I wouldn't have known her if I bumped into her.

I had both of their cell phone numbers, and for the last 30 minutes, I had been texting both of them, hoping to learn that they were somewhere in the building. When I checked my iPhone, I discovered that with all the noise in the lobby, I had been missing their texts and calls. And, as I said before, it's possible to be on the same floor with someone, yet with all of the crowd and noise, not know where they are.

Eventually we finally connected, probably around **8:15am**.

I assisted both of them in getting to the Registration Desk to pick up their Climb Packets. They had no trouble attaching their timing chips to their sneakers, and since they, along with Melissa, were climbing in the Team portion of the climb, and we (me, Tim, Bob and Sophorn) were climbing in the Elite portion of the climb, we separated.

Melissa, Nora and Danielle would be going up together starting around **9:30**.

Our turn to climb would be in about 15 minutes, around **8:30am**.

I suddenly realized that I had forgotten to follow my own Cardinal Rule-- always use the bathroom! But where was it?

I asked a volunteer who told us that Restrooms were on the 7th floor, and that we would have to take one of the elevators in the lobby up to use them. Not any elevator, mind you, but a particular elevator, which she directed us to.

That seemed like a long way to travel to use the restroom, but that's what we did. Bob, Tim and I took it up, used it and were back down in about 5 minutes. By the way, it was very crowded. Almost everyone seemed to be heeding my advice.

It was now around **8:20am**.

We all seemed to have a lot of nervous energy, just waiting around, and we were aware that the climb would start shortly.

Bob and Sophorn, both experienced Marathon runners, wanted to warm up. Tim, a former professional baseball player, was antsy also.

Without giving it a lot of thought, I went through the one of the lobby doors and started running around the block. The other members of the Elite Division of Team Smiley also followed me. Tim and I circled the block about three times. I think Bob and Sophorn did it about 10 times.

We got back into the lobby around **8:30am**, and it wasn't long before an announcement was made that the Elite climbers should begin to line up.

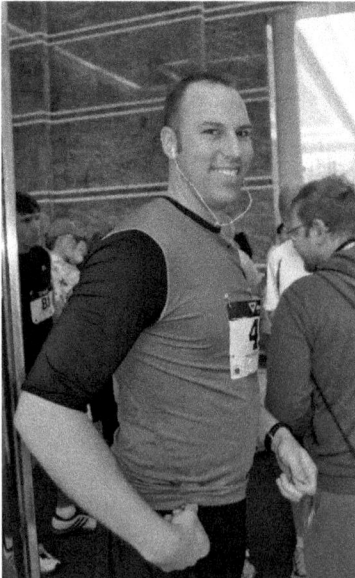

Tim in the lobby as the Elite Climbers start to line up. Jim Smiley is to his right.

I had expected that the climb would begin inside the building. Guess what.? The fire escape entrance is on the <u>OUTSIDE</u> of the building, so we had to line up and work our way outside.

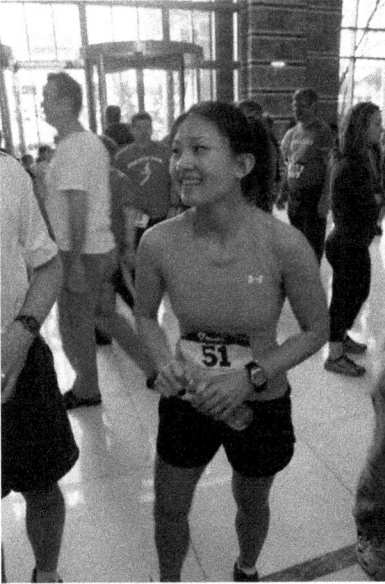

Sophorn looks confident, doesn't she?

We had given this climb a lot of thought, each of us realizing that we belonged in the Elite Climbing Division based on our projected finish, but now the question: Where to line up in the Elite Division?

Anticipated finish times for Elite Climbers were between 6 and 12 minutes.

I realized that lining up in the front of the Elite group would be a foolish thing to do, since I was hoping for a climb time between 9 and 10 minutes. I positioned myself towards the back end of the line, which was well inside the lobby doors. The first climbers in the Elite group were outside---in the cold :) Thankfully, it was a balmy 45 degrees. In March in Philadelphia, it could have been colder.

The time was now about **8:35am**, and the line began to move---obviously, climbers were going up. Perhaps the eventual winner had already reached the top?

Still inside the lobby, Tim, Bob, Sophorn and I started to make our way toward the lobby doors, and now we could see climbers lined up on the pavement, in a line that was heading to the corner of the building, the now obvious entrance to the fire escape. At the fire escape entrance we could see that there was a door that was propped open, and on the ground, a reddish colored timing mat. Note to all future climbers: Don't trip over it :)

In addition to the climbers, we could see well-wishers and spectators lining the pavement, which added to the festive air of anticipation.

There was a gentleman at the front of the line with a stopwatch, who was giving the climbers the signal, every 15 seconds or so to head up the stairs,.

Tim, Bob, Sophorn and I stood together, still inside the lobby, as we awaited our turn. Eventually the line moved again, and Bob and Tim were the first members of Team Smiley to move outside.

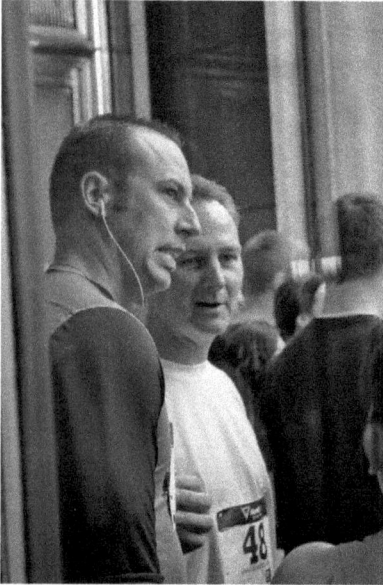

Bob and Tim just outside the lobby doors, John and Sophorn still inside

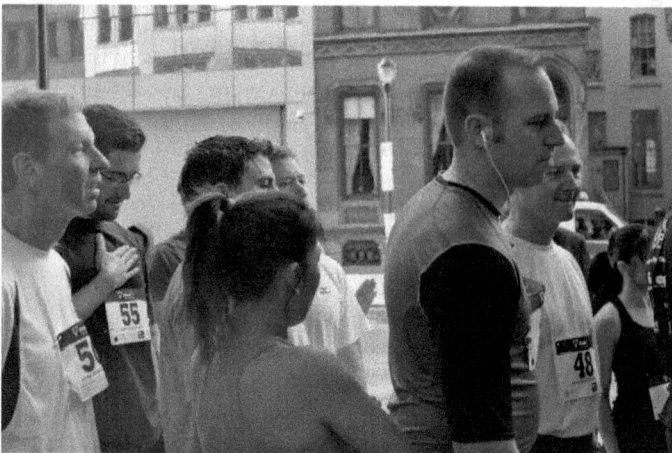

A few moments later all of Team Smiley's Elite Climbers were outside.

It was a bit chilly, as I said about 45 degrees, but all in all we were only outside for about 5 minutes. I estimated that about 30 climbers were ahead of us in line, and they were going up the stairs in 15 second increments. That's about 4 climbers per minute.

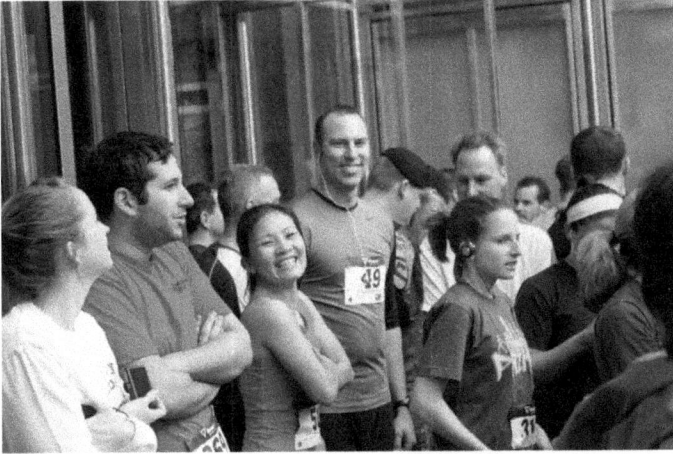

Assembled outside. As you can see, we're a bit chilly.

As we got closer, Bob moved to the front of our team--he would be going up first, followed by Tim, followed by Sophorn, followed by me.

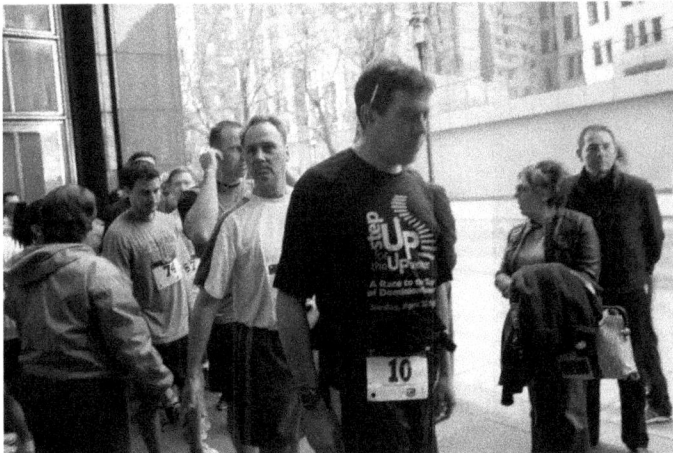

Bob Gauss lining up for his chance at the stairs. He would be the first of Team Smiley to go up.

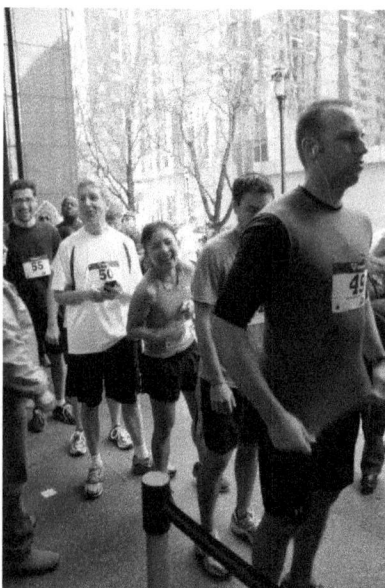

Team Smiley captain John Smiley keeps things loose, amusing his team and the assembled crowd with some words of wisdom.

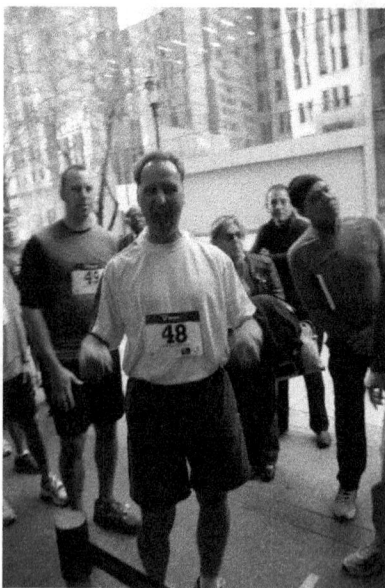

Bob Gauss confident as he approaches the starting line

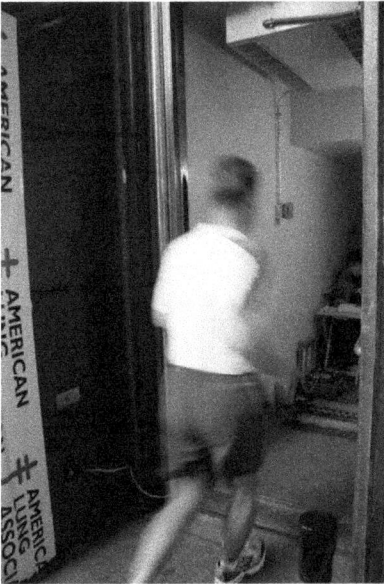

Bob Gauss got the signal to go, and he was off in a blur. It was now 8:46am.

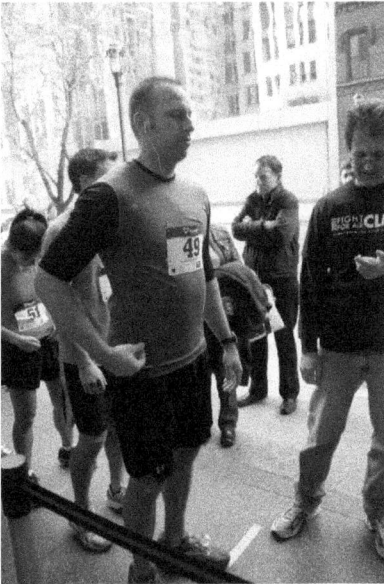

Tim Gradoville approaches the starting line. Notice the tape on the ground

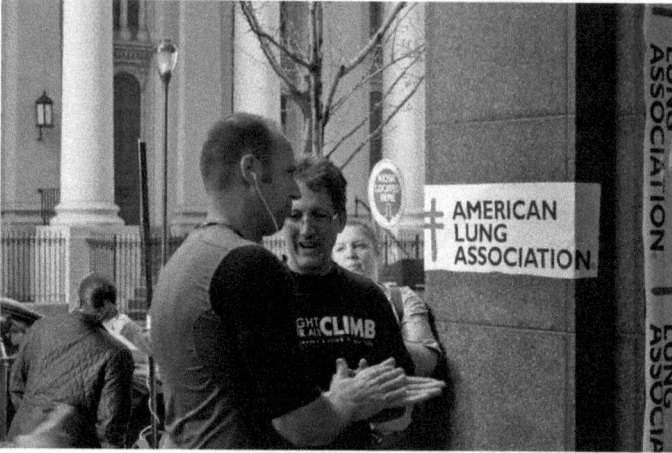

Tim Gradoville waiting for the signal to go up the fire escape

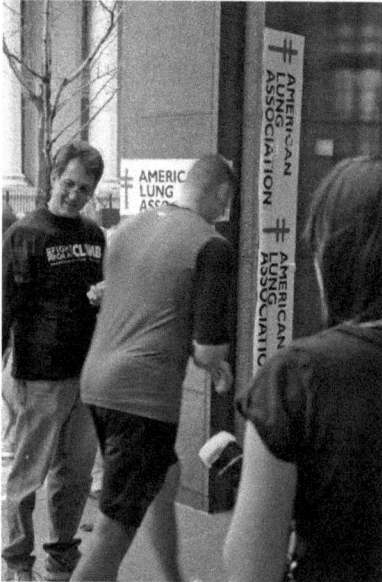

There he goes

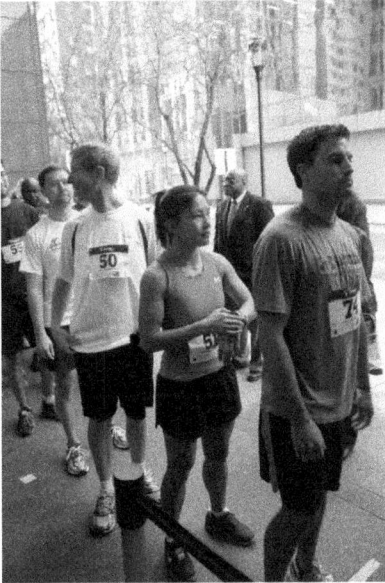

Sophorn approaches the starting line, Garmin watch ready.

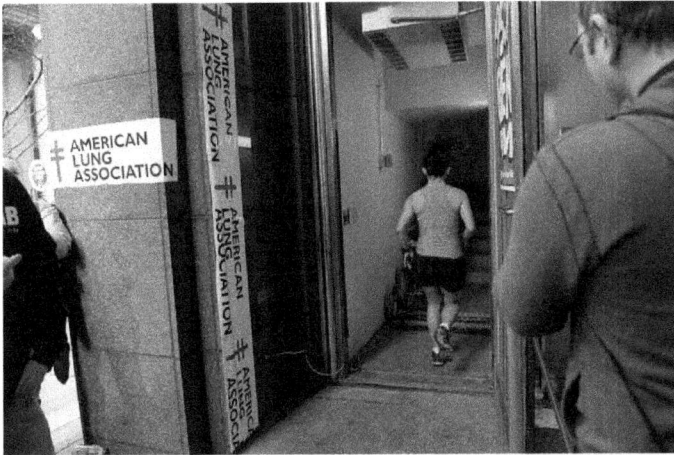

And there she goes...

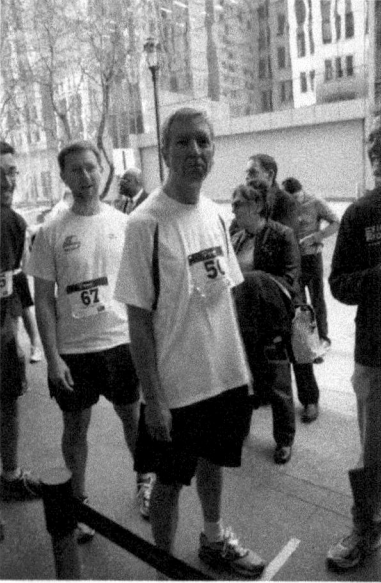

Now it's John's turn. It's now 8:47am

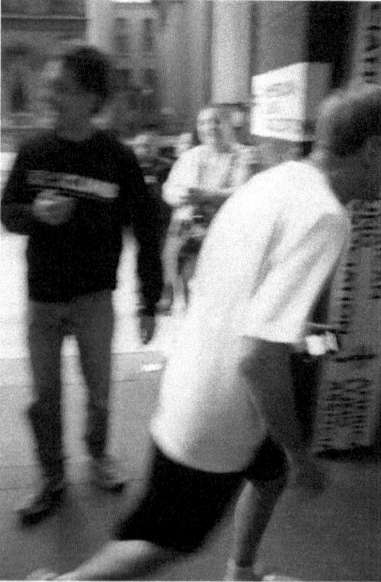

Signal given, and training completed (4,944 Flights of Stairs and 70,320 steps) it's time to tackle the real thing.

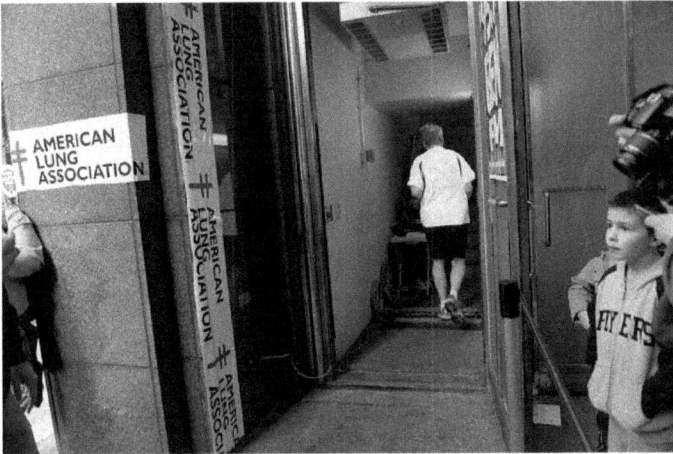

Like a blur, Team Smiley's captain is off and running, carrying his iPhone in his left hand.

Immediately upon crossing the starting mat, there was one flight of steps to climb, which I did running, double stepping all of them and then...

A hallway!

As I recall, it was a T. Go left? Go right?

I hesitated.

I wish someone had put a sign on the wall saying "Go left". You really don't want to have a lot to think about during a climb, and already I had a decision to make.

Because of the staggered start, I couldn't see anyone in front of me, to give me a clue as to whether to go right or left..

A quick look to the right seem to reveal a dead-end, so I went left. (The 2012 Philadelphia Fight For Air climb will have a sign, believe me, I'm on the Planning Committee.)

I ran about 30 feet to the left, and at the end of the hallway, there was an opening on the right side leading to the actual fire escape for the building.

I was on my way.

Each floor had 10 steps, followed by a landing, followed by 10 more steps. Each step 7 inches in height.

The stairway 'turned' to the left.

On the left hand side was a 3 foot high railing, on the right hand side a hand rail was attached to the wall. Width of the stairs was about 3 feet.

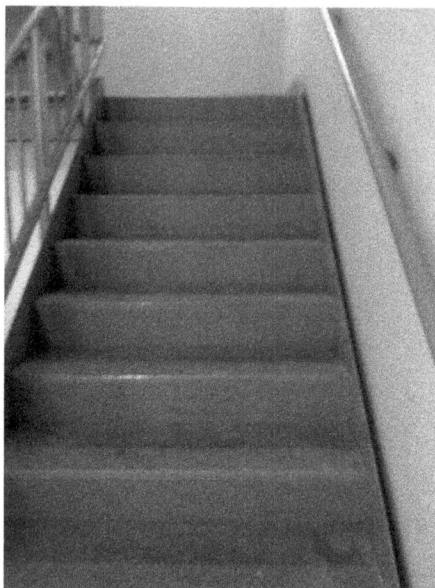

It would be possible to use a one handed rail technique, or a two handed technique (one hand on each side,) if you wished. Unfortunately for me, I hadn't practiced using handrails, so it would be a "no rails" climb for me. Using handrails is faster, if you practice that way.

As for the fire escape itself, it was well lit, not hot, not dry, just comfortably cool.

It was pretty noisy.

Every five floors or so, there was a large ventilator fan, so there was plenty of air flowing.

As a team, we had all agreed we wouldn't look at floor numbers. The only floor number I remember seeing clearly was 50 :) But it's hard not to know were you are in the building.

Volunteers manned water stations every 10 floors, so we would know when we were at 10-20-30-40 and the final destination of 50 would be an obvious one.

I would say I double stepped up to about the 3rd floor.

In terms of steps, step height, and width, the stair way was very similar to Tim's condo, it even turned in the same direction..

But I have to admit, I missed the beautiful view that Tim's fire escape afforded.

The Bell Atlantic Tower fire escape had <u>no</u> windows, and you almost had the feeling you were traveling in a tunnel going under a river.

Bright lights, noise, ventilation fans, and not a single person to be seen.

You could hear, in the distance, the faint sounds of sneakers squeaking their way up the stairs. But that was it.

I really had trouble getting my rhythm. I think I was thrown off a bit by the start.

One of my first thoughts was that this climb was a lot different than the practice sessions I had been doing at home or in Tim's condo.

But I didn't panic. I remembered that, almost without fail, it takes me about 13 floors to get into a good rhythm.

And that's exactly what happened.

Around the **13th floor**, after saying hello to the pleasant volunteers on the 10th floor handing out water, I began to feel pretty good. My legs felt warmed up. I was sweating a bit. My heart was racing.

I still didn't know how I would feel passing the 25th floor, or if I would need to rest, but at this point, I was just walking up the steps, feeling the rhythm of my body as it carried me up, farther and farther.

I passed the **20th floor** water station, said hello to the volunteers, and kept walking.

I had brought my iPhone with me to use as a stop watch. I started it as I crossed the timing mat at ground level.

I had intended to hit the lap button on the stop watch app as I passed the 10th, 20th, 30th and 40th floors.

However, I got into such a comfort zone that I entirely forgot. In fact, I didn't look at my watch until about 5 minutes <u>after</u> I reached the top--but I'm getting ahead of myself.

Somewhere between the **20th** and **30th** floors, I recall being passed by two people who looked like they were climbing Mt. Everest.

It was a man and a woman---they were double stepping past me as if I were standing still, each one holding onto a handrail.

I moved to the right to permit them to pass.

I believe at least one of them grabbed both handrails as they made their way to the top.

In every race I've done, there's always a point of doubt, when you're not sure that you'll finish.

There's also a point where you know you will.

I expected that point of knowing that I would finish to be somewhere between the **40th** and **50th** floors, but it actually occurred much sooner.

I realized I would finish when I got to the **30th floor** water station and realized I hadn't blinked when I passed the halfway mark at the **25th floor**, the maximum number of floors any of Team Smiley had ever climbed without a break. Without realizing it, I had gone right past the **25th floor** now I was now at the **30th floor**, and feeling good.

Somewhere around the **40th floor**, someone else passed me.

Around the **44th floor**, I passed him.

I began to realize, with 6 floors remaining, that the rest of Team Smiley who had started before me were probably at the top of the building.

That was true for Tim, who made it to the top in 9 minutes and 9 seconds, and Bob, who got there in 9 minutes and 24 seconds. Because of the staggered start, Bob left started up 15 seconds earlier than Tim. Bob and Tim arrived at the top almost at the same time.

Sophorn, an experienced Marathon runner, inexplicably suffered from legs cramps around the **47th floor** and as I approached her, she told me to pass her.

When I got to the **48th floor**, I started sprinting and double stepping up the stairs.

I arrived at the top and crossed the timing mat in 10 minutes and 37 seconds.

My arrival was met with some hooting and hollering on the part of the volunteers, who obviously were impressed with my sprinting---they probably thought I maintained that pace the entire time :)

Sophorn got there in 11 minutes and 10 seconds.

I felt great as I passed the **50th Floor** sign

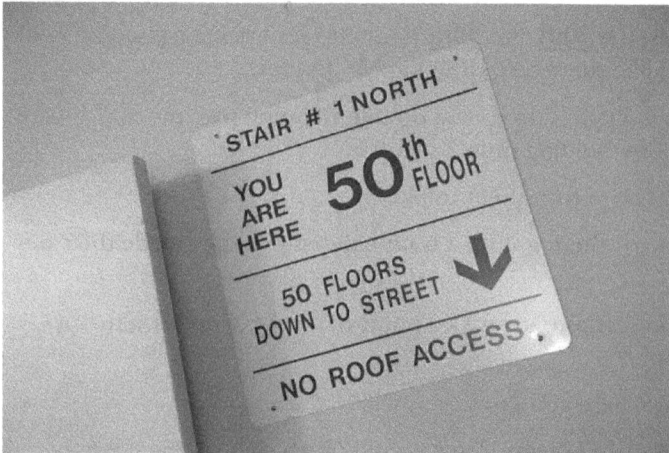

and crossed over the timing mat It was now **8:57am)**. Sophorn arrived at the top about a minute later, her time 11:10.

As I write this, I'm looking at my Timing chip which I have hanging proudly on the wall in my office. It was quite a climb.

In addition to that moment of truth in a race or a climb when you realize that you will finish because either you have trained properly to finish, or you simply won't quit, there's also some self reflection at the end.

Did I give my all?

Many runners and climbers aren't content unless they collapse at the finish.

Others are content if we just finish.

I'm somewhere in between.

I suspect I could have gone faster.

The confusion at the start of the climb probably cost me a few seconds.

The fact that I was able to fairly easily double step the last two floors tells me I could probably have double stepped the last 4 or 5.

I might have gone faster if I had trained using handrails.

But that's what next year is for. Shaving seconds, even minutes, off of this year's time.

Now it was time for a quiet celebration.

After crossing the timing mat, I was handed a bottle of water by one of the volunteers, and I could see almost immediately that climbers were being asked to head down the elevator to the ground floor.

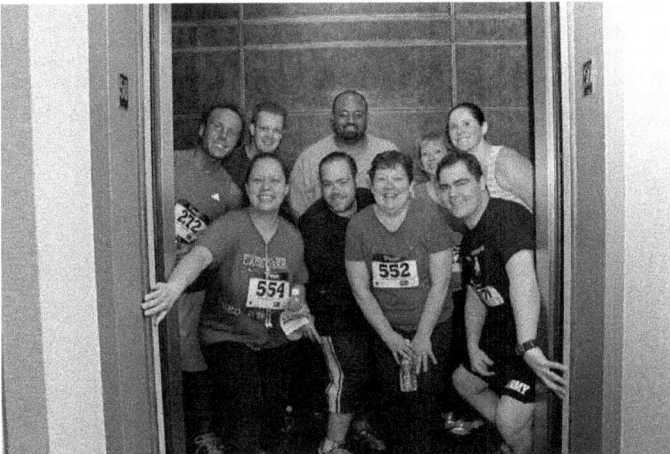

Rob Gurtcheff of the Blank Stairs Team is on the right

Sometimes, after crossing the final timing mat in a race or climb, climbers are asked to return their timing chip. This was not the case with the Philadelphia Fight For Air Climb. These timing chips were disposables-- that's why mine is hanging on my wall of my office.

Sophorn and I did our best to avoid being ushered down the elevator without spending some time with the other members of our team at the top of the building. First we had to find them.

I looked around for the rest of the team, and I saw Bob and Tim not far from us.

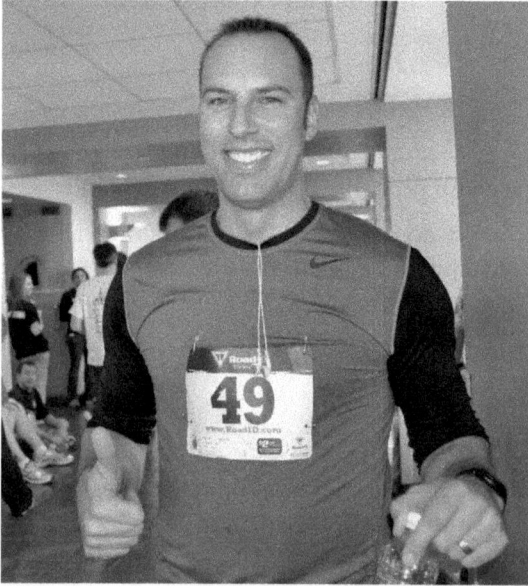

Tim looking fresh after reaching the top

To my surprise Tim's wife Jamie was also there (pregnant with their first child, she didn't climb, she took the elevator.) Jamie took this photograph.

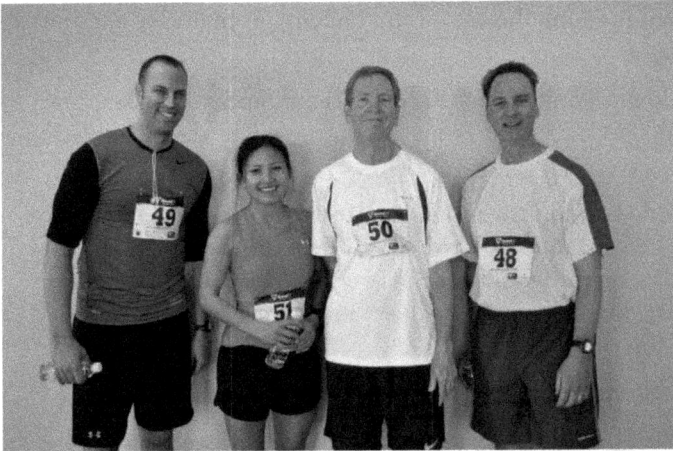

Team Smiley's Elite Climbers at the top. Tim, Sophorn, John and Bob. No problem!

We started to discuss the climb and our experiences with it.

As you can see from the photograph above, everyone, each and every one of us, was thrilled with the event, and immediately vowed to do it again next year.

To quote Sproule Love, one of the greatest Stair Climbers in history:

"It's a great conversation piece. I'll tell people I cross-country ski, run in marathons, do mountain races, and the only thing they'll remember is the Stair Climbing."

And Terry Purcell, also one of the greatest Stair Climbers in history:

"Tell people you ran a marathon and they say, 'Oh, OK. If I say I ran up the Hancock, people are gob smacked."

To quote John Smiley, the training was well worth it. Even for an old guy like me, people are impressed when you say you can run up 50 flights of stairs. We all had a lot of fun, and a wonderful time.

Speaking of time, when I glanced down at my iPhone to check my elapsed time I realized that not only had I forgotten to hit the lap button on my iPhone at floors 10-20-30 and 40, but I had forgotten to stop the stop watch app when I crossed the timing mat.

As a result, I had no idea what my final Climb time was until the official results were posted on the Internet later in the day. (After examining Climb Day pictures, I realized that unofficial results were also posted on a wall in the lobby.)

Maybe I was more tired than I thought.

Other climbers were reaching the top of the building in bunches, and it was now about **9:15am.**

I wanted to head downstairs to see the rest of Team Smiley (Melissa, Danielle and Nora) start off in the Team Division, which was scheduled to begin at **9:30am.**

We decided we needed just a little more time at the top to have a few more photos taken, and I also wanted to say hello to Felicia Perretti who by now had taken hundreds of photographs of the event, and was literally being mobbed by climbers (and teams) asking her to take their picture after they emerged from the top of the stairs.

I managed to say hello to her--but that was about it.

At the far end of the **50th floor**, we noticed a private banquet room, where we thought we could hang out for a while. One of us took this picture of Jamie and Tim, looking out over the Philadelphia Skyline.

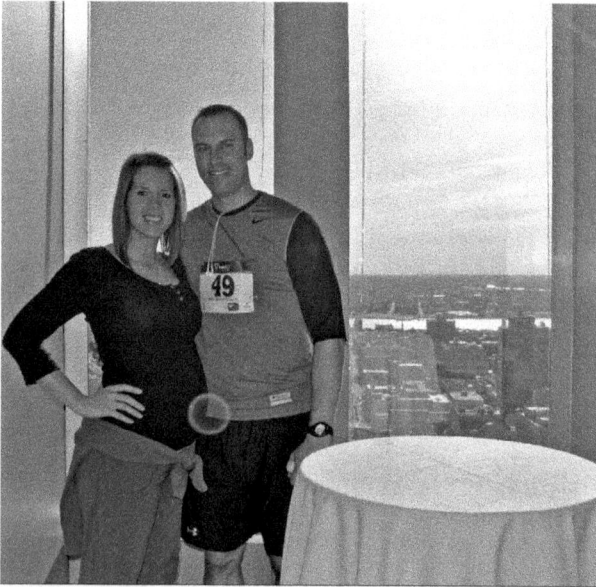

Jamie and Tim, with Baby Johnathan (born on June 7th) marked by the orange circle.

A security guard came in and politely asked us to clear the room, as there was an event scheduled for the room and they needed to set up.

No problem, we told him, but before we headed down, he permitted my nephew Jim to take this final photo of the four of us at the top.

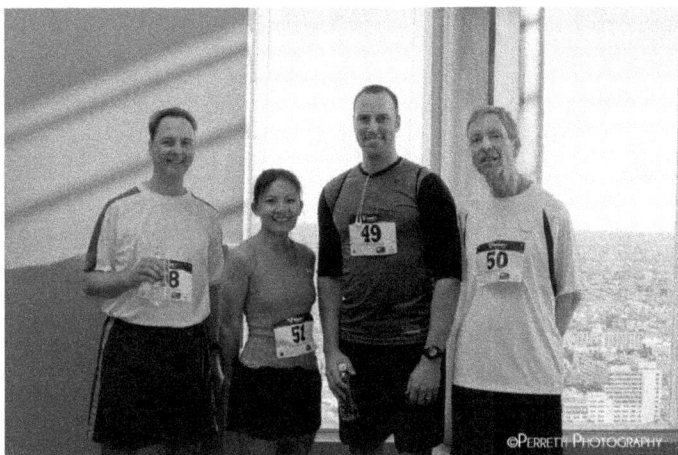

Team Smiley's Elite Climbers (Bob, Sophorn, Tim and John) overlooking the Philadelphia skyline.

We got into the elevator and took it down to the first floor. Believe me, it's a lot faster going down than going up!

Bob, Tim, Jamie, Sophorn and Jim headed to the after event party at Tír na nÓg, an Irish Bar & Grill about a block away.

I told them I would join them after seeing the rest of Team Smiley off on their 50 flight journey.

It wasn't hard to find the rest of Team Smiley---I just headed to the outdoor area where climbers were waiting to head up. I took this picture of Melissa, Danielle and Nora just as they were about to head up the stairs. It was **9:46am**.

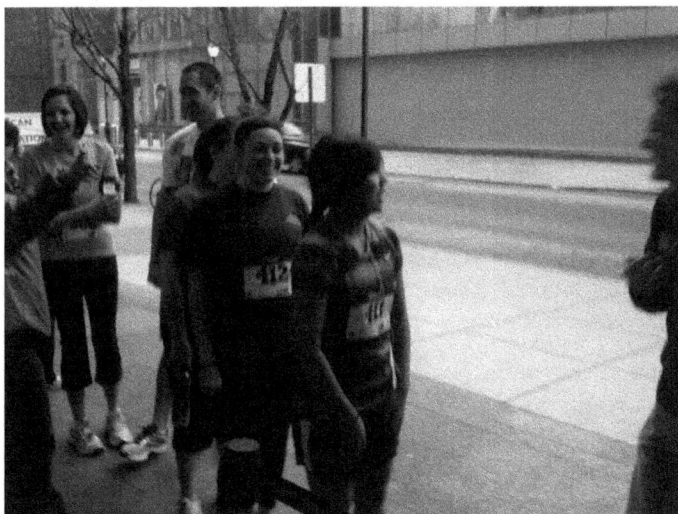

Melissa went up first, followed by Danielle and then Nora.

As soon as they were off, I ran down the street to Tír na nÓg to meet up with Tim, Jamie, Bob, Sophorn and Jim.

I also wanted to pick up my commemorative 2011 Philadelphia Fight For Air Climb t-shirt, which was being distributed at the bar/restaurant, and to check out the food that awaited us there.

I didn't stay long.

The place was mobbed (there was an Irish soccer match on television and the bar was packed.)

I did manage to pick up my t-shirt, and grab a genuine Philly soft pretzel.

I put the t-shirt on (it appears in some of my later pictures) and headed back to the Bell Atlantic Tower. It was now **10:01am**, and I decided I would try to get to the top of the building to meet up with Melissa, Danielle and Nora.

It had been about 15 minutes so I saw them head up the stairs. so I figured there was a good chance they would still be there when I got there.

Elevators to the top were restricted to volunteers, photographers, and staff, but after I explained to the elevator attendant that I was the Team Captain for 3 climbers who were now making their way to the top, she kindly agreed to give me a ride to the 50th floor.

When I got there, I looked around and almost immediately found them.

Melissa, Danielle and Nora had plenty of stories to tell about their adventure to the top.

Melissa reached the top in 10 minutes and 36 seconds, and for those of you really paying attention, that was exactly 1 second faster than me :) In addition to coming in 2nd for her age group, Melissa acquired family bragging rights for the year., which I hope to win back in 2012.

As for Nora, she got to the top in 22 minutes and 44 seconds.

Danielle made it in 22 minutes and 50 seconds.

From what Melissa told me, Nora and Danielle were alternating sprinting up the stairs and walking, and doing a good job at it, right on her heels when all of a sudden, she no longer heard them.

What happened?

A bathroom break.

Danielle needed to use a rest room, and she hadn't followed my advice about visiting the rest room prior to the climb beginning. Actually, I don't think I ever got the chance to tell her, but she'll be well prepared for 2012.

Of course, it would probably have helped if the rest room hadn't been located on the 7th floor.

Be that as it may, Danielle needed to stop somewhere between the **10th** and **15th floor**, and because of security regulations, she had to wait for a volunteer to page Security, who then escorted her (and Nora) to a restroom, waited for them to finish, and redirected them to the staircase.

All in all, this probably cost them 10 minutes. I suspected they both would have finished the climb in about 12 minutes.

Both Danielle and Nora are looking forward to improving upon their time for the 2012 Philadelphia Fight For Air Climb.

Shortly after hearing their story, Felicia Perretti took this photograph. Notice my 2011 Fight For Air Climb t-shirt in the picture.

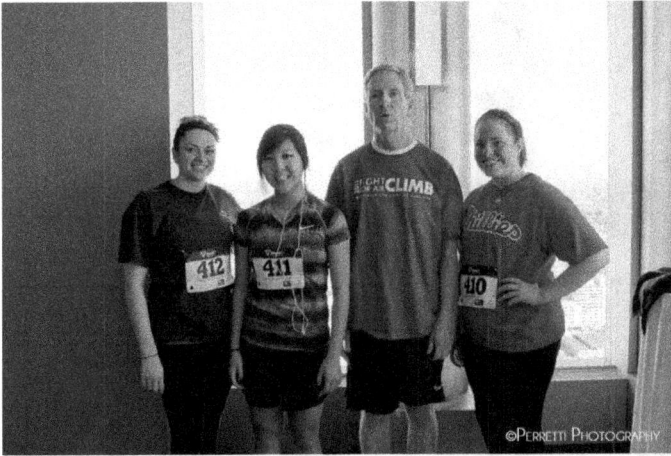

The rest of Team Smiley (Danielle, Melissa, John and Nora) at the top of the Bell Atlantic Building.

With not a lot to do at the top of the building, we all took the elevator down to the first floor.

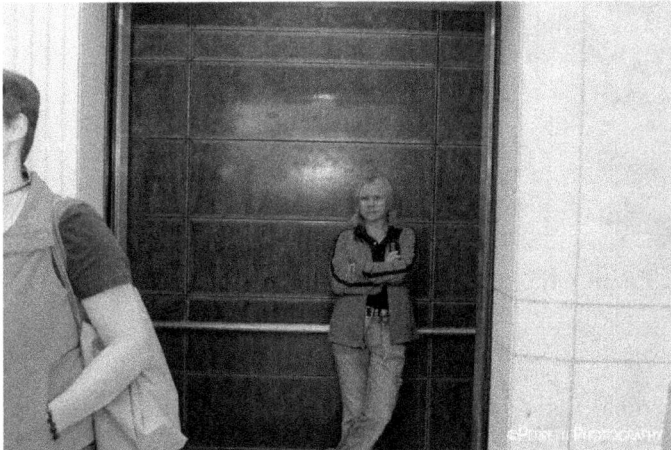

Friendly Elevator Operator who gave us a ride down to the lobby

Danielle and Nora decided to stick around the lobby area to watch the First Responder Team Challenge in process.

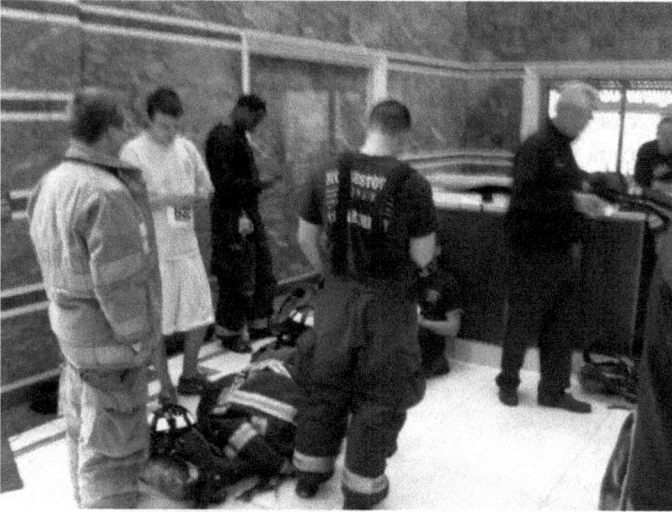

First Responders Team Challenge

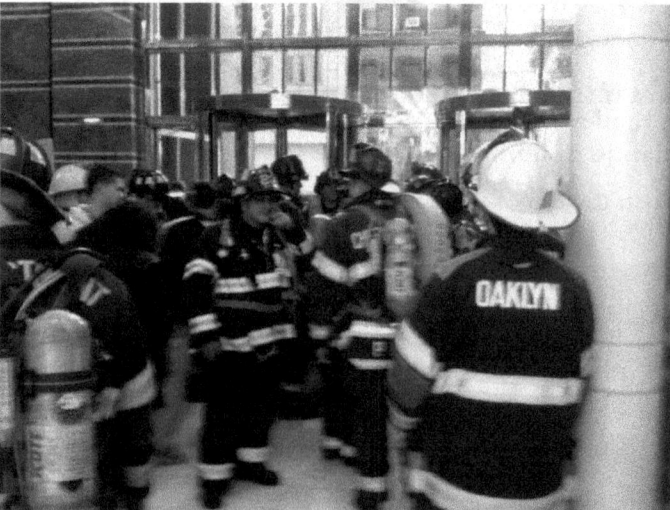

First Responders Team Challenge

Melissa and I watched a bit of it, then the two of us headed to Tír na nÓg to pick up Melissa's t-shirt.

By this time, Bob, Sophorn and Jim had already left, and Tim and Jamie had stayed long enough to congratulate Melissa on her finish.

Melissa and I took a few minutes to check out the festivities and free food, and then decided to head home.

Formal awards were probably about an hour away, and we didn't anticipate winning anything anyway. (I finished 9th in my age group and Melissa finished 2nd in hers.)

We headed to the Parking Garage, found our car, handed the cashier the Parking Voucher that we had received in our Climb packet ($5 discounted parking) and drove home.

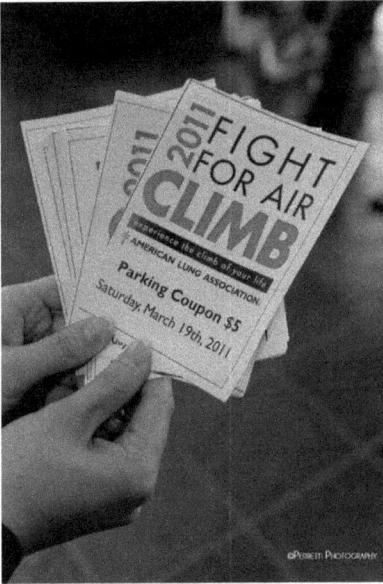

Parking Voucher for Parking in the Bell Atlantic Tower

Except for the final results, for us anyway, the Philadelphia 2011 Fight For Air Climb was history.

Sometime around **4pm**, the Official Results were posted via this link

http://www.compuscore.com/cs2011/march/phlstair.htm

Here they are: (Name, Age, Gender, Tim in minutes, seconds, hundredths)

Tim Gradoville	31 M	9:09.86
Bob Gauss	48 M	9:24.99
Melissa Smiley	14 F	10:36.15 (2nd in Age Group)
John Smiley	56 M	10:37.82 (9th in Age Group)
Sophorn Smiley	31 F	11:10.97
Nora Mccloskey	25 F	22:44.55
Danielle Turner	22 F	22:50.88

The actual climb was over, now what? What, you might ask, does one do the day after their first organized Stair Climb of 50 flights of stairs?

Climb more, of course.

And that's exactly what I did.

On Sunday, **March 20th**, I climbed 110 flights of stairs in the house (in 26 minutes and 24 seconds,)which was 1 second faster than I had climbed 106 flights on **March 16th**, the last time I climbed stairs in the house.

People were asking me why was I still climbing? How much longer did I intend to do this?

My short answer was this: I was preparing for the 2012 Philadelphia Fight For Air Climb. Surely I wasn't finished with 1 stair climb.

As for how long I could continue to add 1 flight to my Stair Climbing regimen each day, I wasn't sure---I figured my body would tell me when to stop adding flights.

On Monday, **March 21st**, my body said to keep going, and I climbed 111 flights of stairs in the house.

I ran 5 miles on the morning of Tuesday, **March 22nd**, so no stairs for me that day.

I climbed 113 flights on **March 23rd**.

I ran 5 miles on **March 24th** and **March 25th**.

On **March 26th** I climbed 116 flights of stairs in the house, followed by 117 flights on **March 27th**. Still no end to the 1 flight progression in sight.

I ran 5 miles on **March 28th**.

March 29th, I climbed 119 flights of stairs in the house.

March 30th, I ran 5 miles.

I closed out the month of **March** by climbing 121 flights of stairs in the house, which took me 30 minutes and 42 seconds. I had passed the 30 minute threshold on the stairs. That's a long time to go up and down stairs in the house.

I started **April** by climbing 122 flights of stairs in the house on **April 1ˢᵗ**. I followed that up by climbing 123 flights on **April 2ⁿᵈ**, and 124 flights on **April 3ʳᵈ**. Still no end in sight, and my body felt fine.

On **April 4ᵗʰ**, I ran 5 miles, then ran my 5K course on **April 5ᵗʰ**.

On **April 6th**, I climbed 127 flights of stairs in the house. To be honest, at this point, although my body and legs felt OK, I was getting pretty mentally bored.

April 7ᵗʰ, I ran 5 miles and on **April 8ᵗʰ** I ran my 5K course.

On **April 9ᵗʰ**, I climbed 130 flights of stairs in the house, and on **April 10ᵗʰ** I climbed 131 flights, which took me 32 minutes and 53 seconds.

I had no way of knowing at the time, but this would be the end of me adding 1 flight of stairs each day. 131 flights was the most I would ever do.

Why?

My body felt good, and I really didn't know when I would stop, but after running 5 miles on April 11ᵗʰ, I woke up on the morning of April 12ᵗʰ with a sore knee.

I've had aches and pains during my training sessions.

I've started climbing stairs in the house with a slight twinge in my knee or leg, but they always went away.

I'm one of those people who always tells his running and climbing friends to listen to their bodies.

If someone tells me that something hurts, I tell them to rest it, and it's advice I generally take myself. In this case I did.

When I work up on April 12th and had trouble coming down the stairs to get my morning coffee, I knew something was wrong.

I made several routine trips up the stairs during the day (something you will do in a two story house) but each time I did I limped up.

Listening to my body, I did no running or climbing from **April 12ᵗʰ** through **April 14ᵗʰ**.

I felt a bit better the morning of **April 15ᵗʰ**, and ran my 5K course.

On **April 16ᵗʰ**, I got ready to do my stairs.

I had been off the stairs for 4 days, which meant I was 'scheduled' to do 135 flights of stairs.

With no organized Stair Climb on the horizon for 11 months, and with no end in sight to adding 1 flight of stairs each day (at this rate, I would be doing 500 flights of stairs prior to the 2012 Philadelphia Fight For Air Climb,) I decided to end it there.

At this point, 30 minutes on the stairs seemed to be more than enough to stay in shape for Stair Climbing. I decided to go into 'maintenance mode' and climb 'only' 100 floors.

Starting **April 16<u>th</u>** and extending through **May 19<u>th</u>**, whenever I didn't run in the morning, I climbed 100 flights of stairs in the afternoon.

The time it was taking me to complete the 100 flights was consistently in the range of 24 or 25 minutes, which experience has taught me is a good pace for the stairs.

On **May 20<u>th</u>** I ran my 5K course, and the next morning woke up once again with a <u>sore knee</u>. It felt the same as it had in April, but the effects would linger longer.

I'm not sure what I did, but I wasn't able to do anything again until the morning of **May 31<u>st</u>**, when I ran 5 miles. That was 11 days with no running or climbing.

To make a long story short, I really wasn't able to do anything (running or stairs) until **June 20<u>th</u>**.

Effectively, I was shut down for about 6 weeks, with the exception of a few 'test' runs to see how my knee felt.

The only Stair Climbing I did in our house between **May 19<u>th</u>** and **June 25<u>th</u>** was a 20 floor 'test' climb in my house on **June 13<u>th</u>**. My knee still hurt.

My wife and I visited Chicago on a mini-vacation from June 21st until June 24th. We stayed in the Raffaelo Hotel, a hotel with 20 floors, and we were on the 17th floor.

I'm happy to say we walked down and up the stairs many times, avoiding the elevator whenever possible. One time, thinking we were going into the internal fire escape, I accidentally opened a door to the outside fire escape (at 17 floors up, this isn't something I would recommend to everyone.)

The Raffaelo was a block away from the 94 floor Hancock Building, the sight of the annual Hustle Up The Hancock which is held in February every year. I vowed to return one year to do it, but it won't be in 2012.

We walked quite a bit in Chicago, it's a great walking town.

On **June 25<u>th</u>**, the day after our return from Chicago, I did 100 flights of stairs in the house in about 25 minutes. I repeated 100 floors on **June 26<u>th</u>**, and pronounced my knee fit again.

It hasn't bothered me since, and I'm really not sure what I did to it, although it may have had something to do with the 35 an over Men's Basketball League I joined in mid May of 2011.

In hindsight, I probably should have seen a sports doctor, but I didn't have a race or climb to prepare for, so I took a cautious wait and see approach.

In **July**, I went back to the pattern of doing 100 flights of stairs in my house on days when I didn't run, but in **August** I went into even more of a 'maintenance mode" by doing the stairs only on Sunday afternoons---a pattern that I followed for the remainder of the year.

After completing my final set of 100 stairs on **Christmas Day** (which was a Sunday), I added up my total and found that in the year 2011, I had climbed 10,969 flights of stairs (all but 326 of those in my house), a total of 154,918 steps. It's safe to say that my stairs and I developed quite a relationship.

As far as the year 2012, you'll need to pick up the 2013 Edition of this book to see, but I can tell you that in order to prepare for the 2012 Philadelphia Fight For Air climb, I plan on going back to doing 100 flights of stairs in the house 4 days a week, on the days I don't run.

I hope you have enjoyed my story, that it inspires you to try a Stair Climb of your own, and that you enjoy the rest of the book.

Remember, Team Smiley always needs members!

CHAPTER TWO

The ABC'S of Stair Climbing

AMA Recommendations.

Buy Nothing. Just start running up the Stairs

Celebrities Who Do Stair Climbing. Stair Climbing is a **C**ompetitive Sport.

Down the Stairs--a bad idea

Every Day. Do something. It doesn't need to be Stair Climbing, but do something physical every day.

Find a Stair Climbing Event Near You and Register. Look for a climb to enter.

Great! What's so great about Stair Climbing.

Hills are your friend.

How many stairs today? This week? This Month? This Year?

Impact Sport? Not Stair Climbing.

Just start your training by doing one flight of stairs, then adding one flight of stairs each day until you reach 100 flights.

Keep a Daily Diary of your efforts.

Lactic Acid means your legs may burn.

Make it fun.

New. Stair Climbing is a new way to run. Almost straight up.

Oz says. Dr. Oz weighs in on Stair Climbing.

Promises. I can't guarantee you anything but you will improve.

Quit? Please don't. For many of you, it's your last chance.

Running is a good form of Cross Training for Stair Climbing.

Start your training by doing one flight of stairs, then adding one flight of stairs each day until you reach 100 flights. Scientific Evidence.

Stop? I hate to stop.

Training? Do I really need to train for a Stair Climb?

Unless you're a mountain goat, Stair Climbing will be strenuous.

Visualize your way to the top of the stairs. I visualize that my body is a locomotive and that I'm powering my way up the stairs.

What is Stair Climbing? Why Stair Climbing? Who is Stair Climbing for? Who is Stair Climbing Not for? Who does Stair Climbing.

X-Ray's are the only conclusive way to diagnose knee or ankle arthritis

Your doctor is a person you should check with before you begin an exercise program.

Zen. One of my buddies is into Zen. While on the stairs, he contemplate.s I find great peace there also.

AMA Recommendations.

The American Heart Association has a goal for every American:

Moderate Aerobic Activity such as walking for 30 minutes 5 or more days a week

--- or ---

vigorous activity like jogging for 20 minutes or more at least 3 times a week.

Stair Climbing meets the test for 'vigorous' activity.

I find it more 'vigorous' than the jogging I do.

I don't know about you, but I like to get my exercise over and done with.

I'd rather climb stairs for 25 minutes 3 times a week than walk 5 or 6 times a week for 30 minutes.

I have some neighbors who walk by my house early in the morning, at noon time and then again in the evening. They probably walk about 6 miles a day (a good thing,), but they're taking about 2 hours to do so.

I see another man walking all the time who I'm told walks over 10 miles a day, and he comes from a neighboring town.

All of these neighbors look to be in pretty good shape.

I've been tempted to ask them to join my Philadelphia ALA Climb Team.

In fact, I have my 2012 Philadelphia Fight For Air Climb poster hanging in my window right now.

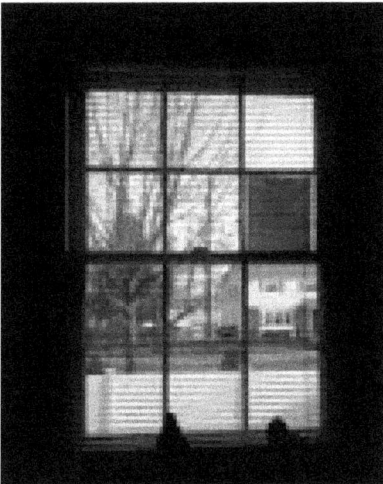

Buy Nothing. Just start climbing up the Stairs

That's the beauty of Stair Climbing.

You don't need to buy a thing.

All you need to do is get up out of your chair or off your couch, and walk or run or climb up and down the stairs of your house.

No expensive equipment.

No expensive workout clothes.

No gym membership required.

Simple.

Celebrities Who Do Stair Climbing

Just a few that I've been able to find...

- **Maddona**: Rumor has it that fitness buff, Madonna, would climb stairs (50 flights according to one unconfirmed report!) when she would be on tour and would not be able to do her usual workout. (Cited by UltimateStairClimbing.com)

- **Miranda Lambert**: According to **Shape Magazine** (December 2011 issue), Country Singer Miranda Lambert, when on tour, climbs up and down stairs in the arena for her cardio and lower body workouts.

- **Jennifer Lopez**: The singer and actress uses an intense routine of weights and cardio that includes her climbing up stairs with a weighted vest. (Cited by UltimateStairClimbing.com)

- **Tom Brokow**: According to **Pyschology Today**, the NBC News Anchorman climbs the stairs at hotels for 15 minutes whenever he's on the road.

- **Alex Rodriguez**: The New York Yankee All-Star third basemen gets up at 6AM in the off-season to climb stairs. (Cited by UltimateStairClimbing.com)

- **Tom Brady**: The New England Patriot and Super Bowl MVP use stair sprints as part of his off-season workout regimen. (Cited by UltimateStairClimbing.com)

- **Curtis Martin:** The future hall of fame running back of the New York Jets travels to the famous Santa Monica steps: A 200 step climb! (Cited by UltimateStairClimbing.com)

- **Dante Cullpepper**: The Quarterback of the Minnesota Vikings uses stair exercises to improve his speed and quickness. Many of his NFL counterparts do so as well.. (Cited by UltimateStairClimbing.com)

- **Padma Lakshmi**, According to the New York Daily News, the Top Chef host - who gave birth to daughter Krisha earlier this year - said that prior to working out the gym, she first ran up and down 70 flights of stairs, then ate breakfast and headed off to the gym to life weights for an hour---then walked home!

Ok, so celebrities love Stair Climbing.

We all know celebrities have it easier than the rest of us. They have more money, personal trainers, etc. But what about the rest of us?

Hang on a minute. What did you notice about the celebrity Stair Climbing mentioned above?

For one, it didn't require a gym. For many of them, that was the beauty of it.

It didn't require expensive equipment.

It could be performed virtually anywhere, and at any time.

It could be performed alone.

Just like you and me.

Down the Stairs--a bad idea

Repeat after me.

Walking down stairs is a bad idea.

Running down stairs is a bad idea.

Climbing down stairs is a bad idea.

Going down stairs is a bad idea.

It's been said that going down stairs exerts stress on your knees that is 5 times your body weight.

Going up stairs exerts stress on your knees that is 2 times your body weight.

Therefore, going down stairs is twice as stressful as going up stairs.

'PJ Glassey, noted United States Stair Climber, in his series of You Tube videos on Stair Climbing, explains in detail why going down stairs will make your legs sore. I have links to his excellent videos in Chapter 16 of this book.

Climbing down stairs is one of the worst things you can do, and you should avoid it at all costs. I also don't like running down hills for the same reason---I can feel the Patellar tendon in my right knee about to explode.

Many people ask me if you have to take the stairs down after you complete your organized climbs.

Of course not, we ride the elevators!

In 1994, my family and I climbed up to the top of the **Statue of Liberty**, which is 354 steps up a circular staircase. No problem climbing up, but during the climb down I could feel my calf muscles tightening up.

Chris Solarz, who set the Guinness Book of World Records record for the greatest vertical climb in a 12 hour period (he climbed the 50 story building 55 times, a total of 33,000 feet, over 6 miles). Chris smartly took the elevator down after each 50 story trek. In fact, if you check out this You Tube video, you can see that Chris used the elevator ride down to the 1st floor as an opportunity to rest and strategize.

www.youtube.com/watch?v=b-DeG_N5Twk

If you practice climbing up a 25 floor high rise, as Team Smiley did in its training climbs, take the elevator back down. We did it as quickly as possible, and were able to get down in about a minute, which kept our heart rate going.

In the meantime, repeat once again after me.

Walking down stairs is a bad idea.

Running down stairs is a bad idea.

Climbing down stairs is a bad idea.

Going down stairs is a bad idea.

Every Day.

Do something.

It doesn't need to be Stair Climbing, but do something physical every day.

I try to do something physical every day.

From January 1st until the Philadelphia Fight For Air Climb, which is typically the 3rd Saturday in March, I follow this schedule

Monday. 5 mile run

Tuesday. Lift weights, 100 Flights of Stairs in the house.

Wednesday. 5 mile run.

Thursday. Lift weights, 100 Fliights of Stairs in the house.

Friday. 5K run (3.1 miles)

Saturday. Life weights. 100 Flights of Stairs in the house.

Sunday. 100 Flights of Stairs in the house.

Once my annual competitive Stair Climb is complete in March, I go into maintenance mode, doing 100 Flights of Stairs in the house only on Sunday afternoons.

All else remains the same.

Either running, weights, or stairs.

And...

If you are in training mode, and following my training program, every day increase the number of flights you climb by 1.

On December 8, 2010, I started with 8 flights of stairs and every day added 1 flight until I was well over 100 flights of stairs in my house by actual Climb Day.

There is more on my Training Plan in Chapters 1 and 4 of this book..

Find a Stair Climbing Event Near You and Register.

One of the most important things you need to do if you are going to Stair Climb is to actually enter a Stair Climbing event.

Finding a Stair Climbing event used to be tough.

In comparison to running events, there aren't that many Stair Climbing events (89 major ones in the United States that I've cataloged in this book,) and I don't find that they are that well advertised.

Stair Climbing events aren't nearly as popular as running events, such as 5K's, and are a lot more difficult for the organizers to put together.

The best place to find the nearest Stair Climbing event to you (in the United State that is) is probably in this book :) I have 95 from the year 2011 listed, and most likely all of them (and some more) will be done again in 2012.

Another great resource is this web site, run by Sebastian Wurster and Michael Reichetzeder

http://www.TowerRunning.com

TowerRunning.com has an excellent calendar of Stair Climb events, and is updated frequently.

If you are in Canada, be sure to check out this excellent Website, run by Trevor Flogering (more on him later in a Spotlight section.)

http://www.StairClimbCanada.com

Great! What's so great about Stair Climbing?

Stair Climbing is great!

I love it because I get a great workout in less time, and unlike other activities, it's really hard to give less than 100% on the stairs.

What I mean by that is unless you stop, your heart rate will really be churning.

I also love the fact that you can do it anywhere---I do it in my house----and it costs me nothing. No gym membership required.

Also, if you are trying to lose weight, Stair Climbing burns twice as many calories as other sports and activities. Stair Climbing burns 8 to 11 calors per minute.

Hills are your friend.

My friend Ed, an accomplished Marathon runner, used to say that when training, hills are your best friend. I wonder what he would say about stairs?

How many stairs today? This week? This Month? This Year?

I advise starting your program on the first of the month—it helps keep the number of flights you need to do that day fresh in your mind. On the 1st, do 1. On the 5th, do 5. On the 21st, do 21. You get the idea.

If you don't need to start with 1 flight, then coordinate your efforts with the number of flights you think you can handle.

Do a test climb.

Comfortably climb up the stairs of your house, climb down, then repeat until you feel either out of breath, or your legs are burning. (This shouldn't take long.)

That number of flights should be your starting point.

Impact Sport? Not Stair Climbing.

When people tell me they can't climb steps because it's hard on their knees, they frequently tell me that Stair Climbing is an impact sport or activity. I beg to differ.

Certainly, Stair Climbing is an impact sport when compared to sitting on your couch and watching television.

There's also more impact on your knees when you compare Stair Climbing to walking. However, in comparison to running, it's a lot less.

According to Orthopedic studies done comparing Stair Climbing to running

The pressure on the patella is 1.8 times your body weight with each step when walking on a level surface. When climbing up stairs, the force is 3.5 times body weight and when going down stairs it is 5 times body weight. When running or landing from a jump the patellofemoral force can exceed 10 or 12 times body weight.

This means that Stair Climbing is about one-half the impact of running, and I can attest to that from my own training.

However, with half the impact of running, I get the same workout in half the time.

The bottom line: You can get a great workout with Stair Climbing in less the time than running with about half the impact on your knees.

And some of my Stair Climbing buddies claim the impact is even less if you exhibit good posture and technique, and use stair or handrails to pull yourself up.

More on that later in the book..

Just start your training by doing one flight of stairs in your house, then adding one flight of stairs each day until you reach 100 flights.

Slow and easy.

Add 1 flight each day.

Check out my training plan in Chapter 1 and 4.

Keep a Daily Diary of your efforts.

I'm big on diaries---I've maintained a weight diary since 1998 (actually, I just use an index card to record my weight and body fat. I have 4 columns on the card, so I can record about 2 months of weight data on each card.)

Diaries can really help you track your progress.

Progress isn't necessarily a daily thing---look for trends, but maintain a steady goal.

For instance, I add one flight of stairs to my training sessions each day.

On December 9th, I started with 9 flights of steps.

On December 31st, I climbed 31.

On Januay 15th, I climbed 46.

On January 31st, I climbed 62.

On February 15th, I climbed 77.

On February 28th, I climbed 90.

On March 6th, I climbed 96.

I think you get the idea.

On days where you can't do a stair session, the next day do the number of flights you were "scheduled" for.

For instance, on March 5th, I was "scheduled" to do 95 flights.

I ran 5 miles in the morning, and opted to skip climbing the stairs that evening.

The next day, March 6th, I climbed 96 flights---my scheduled number for that day.

Lactic Acid means your legs may burn.

Lactic acid builds up in your muscles during Anaerobic exercising, such as sprinting and Stair Climbing.

It's normal.

It won't kill you.

It does burn a bit.

When you are finished your climb, continue with moderate activity, such as walking, and make sure you drink plenty of water, and the burning and soreness will pass.

Make it fun.

Exercise doesn't have to be painful.

It bothers me to see the way exercise is portrayed by some popular television shows (Such as 'The Biggest Loser') in which contestants are tortured by 'trainers' who take delight in their vomiting.

Exercise can be fun.

Don't get me wrong, exercise can be a challenge if you are woefully out of shape, but the journey of a thousand miles begins with the first step.

Take that first step (no need to vomit doing so,)

Tomorrow, take 2 steps.

The day after, 3 steps.

Slow and easy.

It's the essence of the program.

New.

Stair Climbing is a new way to run. Almost straight up.

Trevor Folgering (more on him in the book later) says that Stair Climbing is a new way to run.

Trevor, who is a Personal Trainer and workout fanatic, observes that at the gym treadmills and elliptical trainers fill up faster than any other apparatus. According to Trevor, who has made a study of Stair Climbing, virtually nothing is as hard as climbing stairs (hard is not a bad thing.)

For every minute that you walk at 4.0 mph (that's a 15 minute mile pace,) you burn 6.8 calories whereas you burn 8.8 calories on the stairs.

That may not sound like a big difference but the effort expended Stair Climbing is greater and burns more calories.

Stair Climbing targets the body's large muscles such as the glutes and quads.

The more muscle you have, the more calories you can burn.

Stair Climbing is a great way to get in shape and lose weight.

Oz says. Dr. Oz weighs in on Stair Climbing.

A lot of people love Dr. Oz, and through his Television show, make him a daily part of their lives.

Dr. Oz is a big believer in exercise, and in January of 2011, during a trip to Chicago to promote a health and fitness challenge, and speaking at the Navy Pier said...

Take these high rises behind me," Dr. Oz said at Navy Pier last January during a visit to Chicago. "How many of you work in high rises or buildings like that?"

A few health and fitness challenge participants raised their hands.

"Good!" said the doctor. "Perfect! So instead of taking the elevator, you take the steps to work and you've got your steps in. You actually haven't put it off until the end of the day. You've incorporated it into your life."

Chicago, as it turns out, has more organized Stair Climbs than any other city in the United States. Five of them in fact. Check out Chapter 17 for more information on them.

Dr. Oz also says:

"The fitness gains from doing 11 minutes of daily Stair Climbing for eight weeks rival those of walking 36 minutes a day for six months."
— Dr. Oz report, *Las Vegas Review Journal,* **2008**

Promises. I can't guarantee you anything.

The world is full of false promises.

Look around you---how many organizations make money on the repeated failures of their members?

Weight loss clinics, Gyms, Health Clubs.

They are full of members who fail.

These organizations get rich on the failures of their members who continue to re-up.

I make no false promises---all I can do is tell you what I've done, and believe me, I'm no Lance Armstrong.

Check out my climbing-running diary in Chapter 1 and 4 and see for yourself.

The human body adapts and grows stronger.

If you give my program an honest effort, I can guarantee that you will see improvement.

Quit? Please don't. For many of you, it's your last chance.

I'm not joking.

I tell my friends that if I ever quit running, at my age (56), I doubt that I would ever be able to start again. It's just too hard.

If you embark on my program to get off the couch, give it your best effort, and whatever you do, don't quit!

At least get to the point of registering for a stair climb.

See if doing a Stair Climb isn't one of the best things you've ever done.

But please, please, please, don't quit.

It could save your life.

Running is a good form of Cross Training for Stair Climbing.

When I started Stair Climbing, I noticed almost immediately that my running improved.

Generally, I'm a jogger, pretty slow, medium distances (3 to 7 miles,)

Stair Climbing, as an exercise, is more of a sprint (speed work as the runners call it,) and that is something I really don't do enough of.

So you see, Stair Climbing complements my running.

In the same way, running complements my Stair Climbing, the mileage I do each week contributing to my overall stamina and fitness.

I should also mention Weight Training.

Lifting weights is great for building strength in your core.

When I climb stairs, I visualize myself as a Steam Locomotive barreling along the tracks.

This requires a strong core, and I'm getting there thanks to my weight training.

Start your training by doing one flight of stairs, then adding one flight of stairs each day until you reach 100 flights.

What more can I say?

It's the essence of my training plan. I'm the 'tortoise' in the race between the tortoise and the hare. And I beat many hares on March 19, 2011.

Slow and steady works.

Scientific Evidence.

Quoted in a New York Times article on March 10, 2011, Paul M. Juris, a kinesiologist and executive director of the Cybex Institute for Exercise Science, in Medway, Mass., the research arm of the maker of Cybex exercise equipment. says:

"There's good scientific evidence that the activity itself is quite beneficial,"

Mr. Juris, a former researcher at Beth Israel Medical Center in Manhattan and a past consultant to professional sports teams, including the Dallas Mavericks of the N.B.A., pointed to stair-climbing scholarship. It concludes that a few brisk climbs a day, like my modest regimen, can increase aerobic capacity and reduce cholesterol.

A 2000 study published in Preventive Medicine monitored the health of 22 sedentary college-age women who began climbing stairs progressively over seven weeks.

By the end of the study, these women were found to have reduced heart rates, oxygen uptake and blood lactate levels uptake while climbing. Their HDL ("good") cholesterol levels had also increased.

Stair Climbing is a Competitive Sport

Stair Climbing has developed into an organized sport.

According to Michael Reichetzeder and Sebastian Wurster, every year several Stair Climbing races are held around the world with the competitors climbing/running up the stairs of some of the world's tallest buildings and towers (e.g., the Empire State Building, Gran Hotel Bali), or on outside stairs such as the Niesenbahn Stairway.

World class athletes from the running and cycling worlds regularly compete in such events. Some have specialized exclusively in Stair Climbing races. Prizes, awards, and other accolades are given for the top performers by gender and age group.

Stair Climbing is one of the most grueling of sports, requiring competitors to move their entire body weight vertically, as well as horizontally.

The results of more than 160 races on all continents are evaluated each year for the Towerrunning World Cup.

The most important - about 15 so called "Masters Races" - have a predefined factor of 1.5 to 4, whereas all other races are given 0.5 or 1 depending on class and internationality of the participants.

2010 World Cup winners were Melissa Moon (NZL) and Thomas Dold (GER).

2011 World Cup winners were Cristina Bonacina (ITA) and Thomas Dold (GER).

Skyscrapers? Do you really need one?

It's nice to get some practice in once a while on more than a single set of stairs, but that can be difficult to find.

I do most of my training in my 2 story house.

My stairs have 14 carpeted steps.

I run up the steps, skipping each one, get to the top then walk down. I repeat this over and over again until I hit my target for the day.

When I first started training, on December 8th, 2010, I started with 7 flights of steps, and I was pretty winded by the time I finished. My first time was 1 minute and 19 seconds.

On March 6th, I did 96 flights of steps in 23 minutes and 13 seconds, and although climbing stairs in your home can be pretty boring, I was never really winded. My heart rate climbed to about 120 beats per second, and I perspired a lot, particularly towards the end of the session. You'll definitely need a shower when you're done, but first, plan on enjoying a runner or climber's high.

If you live in, or near, a big city, even if you can find a skyscraper or high rise, you may find that Security regulations prohibit you from being permitted to enter or use its fire escape for your training.

Even while preparing for the 2011 Philadelphia Fight For Air Climb in the Bell Atlantic Tower, my teammates and I found that we couldn't get permission to practice in the fire escape (even on weekends.) The Building Manager was understanding, but he couldn't give us access.

If you try hard, you may be able to find some location where you can practice, particularly if you know someone who lives in a high rise in a large city.

Some large city hospitals are very tall---and if you find one, and can gain access, you'll probably see a lot of activity in the stair well. I know I've seen doctors running up and down the stair wells of some hospitals I've visited.

Parking Garages can be another source of training. Some are quite high.

Be careful though---you may attract some attention if you dress like Rocky and start running up and down fire escapes.

Stop? I hate to stop.

Some people, when they run, can stop, walk a bit and start right up.

Some people when they climb stairs have no problem climbing for a while, stopping, and then starting again.

As for me, I have problems stopping and starting again---whether it's running or climbing.

I just hate to stop.

My body starts to go into a cool down mode and it feels awful to start up again.

Training? Do I really need to train for a Stair Climb?

Yes you do.

Just about every organized Stair Climbing event is going to be 30+ floors.

Even if you are a well conditioned athlete, you will want to do some training, and if you are like most of us, you will need to properly train for this event.

Last year, on Team Smiley, we had two Marathon runners, and the first time they did a 25 floor practice climb, they realized they would need to do a few more to get ready.

The good news is that there are a number of good training programs available (including mine,), and just about all of them will have you completing a 30+ floor Stair Climb event by training for just about 8 weeks.

Unless you're a mountain goat, Stair Climbing will be strenuous.

I don't want to lie to you.

I've cited many reasons why I love Stair Climbing, and one is that the workout achievable in <u>25 minutes</u> is equal to about <u>50 minutes</u> of running and <u>2 hours</u> of walking.

Let's do that again:

Stair Climbing: 25 minutes

Running: 50 minutes

Walking: 2 hours

Results like this don't come because it's easy.

And that's just practice.

If you participate in an Organized Stair Climb, it will be even more strenuous (well, it doesn't have to be, but most people give a little bit 'more' in an actual event.)

Your legs will get tired and burn.

Your lungs will burn.

But it's over in 10 minutes (15 or 20, anyway.)

And when you're done, you'll love the fact that you've done something that many people could do, but because they won't get off the couch, won't ever do..

Visualize your way to the top of the stairs.

I'm a big believer in the power of positive thinking, and I like to use visuals as a way of putting myself in the positive mode.

When I climb, I visualize that my body is a Steam Locomotive, using my legs to power my way up the stairs (sadly, this visualization doesn't work nearly as well for me when I run.)

My friend Bernie Parent is a big believer in the power of positive thinking.

It worked well for him.

He's in the National Hockey League Hall of Fame, and he was the starting goalie for 2 Stanley Cup Winners (1974 and 1975 Philadelphia Flyers.)

What is Stair Climbing?

I know, why wait until now to answer this question?

I've really already addressed this question.

The basic act of Stair Climbing is something we've all been doing for a long time, almost since we learned to walk: moving our legs and feet to climb a set of stairs.

Stair Climbing has also been formalized, as many of the things we human beings do is formalized, into an organized activity. (Please read Sebastian Wurster's account of creating the World Cup System later on in the book. It all started with his formalization of recording climbing times of his classmates after lunch recess was over.).

Stair Climbing is many things:

It's a necessity, it's an activity, it's a sport, it's a charitable event, it's good exercise, it's a way of meeting interesting people, it's a way to challenge yourself. I can go on and on.

Some would note that those descriptions pertain to other formalized activities, such as walking, running and bike riding.

Absolutely true.

In fact, Stair Climbing reminds me a lot of running, which is something I've done for a number of years.

How is it different?

It's as different from running as running is from walking or bike riding. Totally different activities.

In the mid 90's, I took up bike riding for exercise.

In the last 90's, I gave up bike riding and took up jogging/running.

One reason I gave up bike riding for running was that with 30 to 40 minutes of running, I could get the same benefit I got from 2 hours of biking, perhaps more.

Same thing with Stair Climbing.

Some people have described Stair Climbing as a Vertical 5K---running straight up.

That's a pretty good description.

Running or climbing straight up (well almost straight) to the top of a tall building.

The distance travelled is only 500 feet for a 40 to 50 floor building, more like a thousand for the Chicago Hustle Up The Hancock, at most that's only about 1/5th of a mile.

I've heard some long distance runners, once they do their first Stair Climb event, swear they'll never run long distances again.

Why run a 3 hour marathon when you can get the same intensity from a 6 minute stair climb?

Kevin Crossman, the #10 ranked man in the world for 2011, says:

"I don't get why people do marathons. They take forever. I don't want to run for three hours."

Exactly the way I feel.

Stair Climbing's popularity is growing.

In the United States, I've cataloged over **89** official Stair Climbing events. In 2008, there were only 40.

World wide, in 2011, there were 170 World Cup Stair Climbing events. In 2008, there were 109.

You might say there are thousand's of running events in the United States alone, and you would be correct.

Stair Climbs are more complicated to arrange and coordinate than running races, which is why there are less of them.

And, unless you're a professional, or live in Chicago which has 5 events of its own, most of us will do just one Stair Climb event per year, and raise money for a charity to be able to do so.

Boston, Dallas, Los Angeles, New York, Philadelphia and Seattle each have 3 annual Stair Climb events. People living nearby can possibly do multiple events.

If you are lucky enough to live in Chicago (a great city full of high rises), you can choose among 5 climbs, or even do them all of them.

Stair Climbing is becoming more and more popular as an event because many large institutions (the American Lung Association(ALA), the Cystic Fibrosis Foundation(CFF), the Multiple Sclerosis Society) have discovered that there are great fundraising opportunity.

The American Lung Association hosted **60** Stair Climbing events in 2011.

The Cystic Fibrosis Society hosted **17** events in 2011.

The other **12** United States Stair Climbs I've cataloged benefit a number of other fine, for the most part, independent institutions and hospitals.

Why Stair Climbing?

After completing the Philadelphia Half Marathon in November of 2010, I announced (no one really cared) that I was ending my competitive running career. I'm old (relatively anyway at age 56) my best days as a runner are behind me and I really have no inclination to do anything more than a Half Marathon again (maybe with one of our kids.)

I decided to remain a recreational runner---I still run three times a week in the early morning hours, and I thought I would continue to do one 5K every year, the Haddon Holiday Heart Run 5K, which has become sort of a family tradition.

However, about a week after the Half Marathon, I decided to do something else---Stair Climbing.

I'm not sure if I was looking for another challenge, but perhaps I was.

The year before, in 2009, I had seen an advertisement for some kind of Stair Climb.

I wasn't sure what organization hosted it, how high it was, or how much it cost to enter, but I had wanted to do it in 2010 and decided to try it for 2011.

On Thanksgiving Day, I 'googled' Stairclimb + Philadelphia and found it.

There actually were two events, one hosted by the Cystic Fibrosis Society (CFF) and the other one by the American Lung Association (ALA).

I elected to go with the American Lung Association Climb and in a matter of minutes I was registered and also 'tweeting' that I had just entered a stair climb.

Climbing, walking, running to the top of a 50 floor building sounded like quite a challenge. I was ready!

Ironically, another reason I decided to do the Stair Climb was an 'out of breath' walk up the Philadelphia Art Museum Steps, otherwise known as the Rocky Steps, that I had in April of 2010.

Many people are familiar with the scene from the movie Rocky where Rocky Balboa punctuates a strenuous workout by running up the steps of the Philadelphia Art Museum (accompanied, of course, by the Rocky Theme song.) The steps are pretty high, and long, not terrifically steep.

In April of 2010 (April 16th to be exact,) my wife Linda and I were visiting the Philadelphia Art Museum to see an Art Exhibit, Picasso In His Early Years, and after parking at Eakins Oval, I found myself huffing and puffing to get all the way to the top of the steps.

"Wait a minute," I thought to myself, "I run 5 to 7 miles at a time, 3 times a week, why am I huffing and puffing?"

I thought about it for a bit, and I came to the conclusion that there must be something missing in my running training. (My friend Ed would say hills, I'm sure.)

"Too much long distance running," I thought to myself. "I need to do more speed work, track work, hills."

But I really hate those things. It's hard to get up early in the morning and do sprints and track work in the dark.

However, one thing I've always liked doing is climbing stairs.

I'm one of those people who avoid elevators.

I use stairs everywhere I go.

If there's a staircase or a fire escape, I'll use it.

"Maybe this is something I would enjoy," I thought.

I completed my first Stair Climb on March 19th of 2011, and afterwards, continued to train for my next stair climb.

I am already registered for the 2012 Philadelphia Fight For Air Climb.

It's a form of exercise that I simply love.

What I love about Stair Climbing is that it's much more intense than anything else I do, and I can get a lot more benefit from doing it in a shorter amount of time than I can with walking, biking or running.

According to noted Cardiologist and TV Personality Dr. Oz,

"Fitness gains from doing 11 minutes of daily Stair Climbing for eight weeks rival those of walking 36 minutes a day for six months."

I can tell you from my own experience that is definitely true. 25 minutes of Stair Climbing has my heart beating as fast as a 50 minute run.

In addition to the greater intensity, I love the fact that since I train in my house, all I need to do is put on my sneakers and running shoes, and head up and down the stairs of my house.

I don't need to drive anywhere. I don't need to worry if it's cold or hot, or raining or snowing outside.

It's a perfect exercise, and a worthwhile pursuit.

Who does Stair Climbing.

People who gravitate to Stair Climbing cite a number of reasons why.

I've already mentioned that some celebrities incorporate Stair Climbing into their personal workouts.

Many Stair Climbers are finely tuned athletes who have turned to Stair Climbing as another challenge to tackle, another mountain to climb.

Some people who tackle stairs do it for a charity that they support. They're not what you would describe as athletes. They huff and puff their way to the top. Many of the people who do the Philadelphia Fight For Air Climb would probably describe themselves in that way.

Some people who do Stair Climbs are First Responders---EMT's, Fireman, Policemen, who tackle the stairs as a way to test their training, and to build camaraderie. Most organized Stair Climbs have a First Responder Challenge, where Fire Responders hit the stairs---in full gear. Talk about a challenge!

Who is Stair Climbing for?

Just about everyone.

Old people.

Young people.

People with artificial legs.

However, before you begin, be sure to get your doctor's OK.

Who is Stair Climbing Not for?

Well, I think it's for just about everyone, but there are some obvious exceptions, and there are people who MOST DEFINITELY need to check with their doctor first.

Check with your doctor.

If your doctor believes you can't climb 30+ floors of a high rise, ask him or her why not.

If your doctor tells you that your health condition would most likely mean dying on the stairs, that's a GOOD REASON **not** to climb.

If your doctor tells you that you shouldn't climb because you're too old, refer to Chapter 15 of the book, which is devoted to older climbs. Also consider finding a new doctor. Old age, or what people perceive to be old age, is not an impediment to exercise, and it should never be used as an excuse not to exercise.

As I always say, use it or lose it---and by lose it, I mean lose your life.

Live.

Also, don't accept a diagnosis of arthritis in your knees or feet as a reason not to climb unless you have your joints xrayed.

I had a friend in his 40's whose doctor told him he had arthritis based on his description of knee pain. He didn't.

According to the Arthritis Foundation website,

In order to make a diagnosis of osteoarthritis, your doctor will ask about your medical history and symptoms, then conduct a physical exam, paying special attention to your joints and how they move. Traditionally, an OA diagnosis is made only after joint pain and stiffness becomes persistent and an X-ray shows loss of cartilage and resulting damage to bones.

Don't permit your doctor to make a diagnosis of arthritis without an X-ray that shows loss of cartilage and damage to your bones.

I can't tell you the number of people who tell me their knees are 'bone on bone." When I ask these people what their X-ray's revealed, they look at me as if I asked them how they enjoyed their trip to the moon.

Let's face it, as you age, you get aches and pains, even more so if your weight is not properly maintained.

Don't let your age be a death sentence.

Too many people these days are looking for an excuse to stay in that easy chair or couch.

Get off that couch and do something.

Of course, I'd like it to be Stair Climbing, but if not, join my neighbors and start walking around your neighborhood.

X-Ray's are the only conclusive way to diagnose knee or ankle arthritis

Accept nothing less than an X-Ray diagnosis of an Arthritic condition in your joints.

Too many people self-diagnose their joint pain as arthritis, and use it as an excuse to stay on the couch.

Your doctor is the person you should check with before you begin an exercise program.

According to the Mayo Clinic...

Regular exercise can help you control your weight, reduce your risk of heart disease, and strengthen your bones and muscles. But if you haven't exercised for some time and you have health concerns, you may want to talk to your doctor before starting a new exercise routine.

I advise **everyone** to check with their doctor before embarking on any exercise program, regardless of your age, background and health condition.

The Mayo Clinic isn't quite as strict. According to the Mayo Clinic, you should use these guidelines:

Although moderate physical activity, such as brisk walking, is safe for most people, health experts suggest that you talk to your doctor before you start an exercise program if any of the following apply:

- You have <u>heart disease</u>.
- You have <u>asthma</u> or <u>lung disease</u>.
- You have <u>diabetes</u>, or <u>liver</u> <u>or kidney disease</u>.
- You have <u>arthritis</u>.

You should also check with your doctor if you have symptoms suggestive of heart, lung or other serious disease, such as:

- Pain or discomfort in your <u>chest</u>, <u>neck</u>, <u>jaw</u> or <u>arms</u> during physical activity
- <u>Dizziness</u> or loss of consciousness
- <u>Shortness of breath</u> with mild exertion or at rest, or when lying down or going to bed
- <u>Ankle swelling</u>, especially at night
- A <u>heart murmur</u> or a <u>rapid</u> or <u>pronounced heartbeat</u>
- <u>Muscle pain</u> when walking upstairs or up a hill that goes away when you rest

Finally, the American College of Sports Medicine recommends that you see your doctor before engaging in vigorous exercise if two or more of the following apply:

- You're a man older than <u>age 45</u> or a woman older than age 55.
- You have a family history of <u>heart disease</u> before age 55.

106

- You <u>smoke</u> or you quit smoking in the past six months.

- You haven't exercised for three months or more.

- You're <u>overweight</u> or <u>obese</u>.

- You have <u>high blood pressure</u> or high <u>cholesterol</u>.

- You have <u>impaired glucose tolerance</u>, also called <u>prediabetes</u>.

Again, my feeling is that, regardless of your age, you should see your doctor before beginning any training or exercise program. I recommend that everyone see their doctor at least once a year---young and old alike. I know I do.

Stair Climbing for me has been a lot of fun<u>. **I don't want anyone reading this book to die or hurt themselves training for, or doing, a Stair Climb.**</u>

There are stories in the news almost every week about young people who die while either in training for an athletic event or during one. These are usually the result of a hidden health problem that they (or their family) didn't know they have.

<u>The bottom line:</u> See your doctor before you begin.

I end with the official disclaimer from the <u>Stair Climbing Association</u> website:

DISCLAIMER: Stair Climbing is a grueling, strenuous sport and such a sport should not be embarked upon without first consulting your physician. If such a strenuous activity as this is started without being ready or fit, physically and/or emotionally, serious health consequences could result, including death. Consult your physician.

Zen.

One of my buddies is into Zen.

While on the stairs, he contemplates. I'm not sure what he is contemplating, but he tells me he does.

As for me, I find great peace on the stairs also.

It relaxes me.

It gives me time to think.

One of the great Stair Climbers in the United State, <u>David Snyder</u> can tell you even more about Zen and Stair Climbing than I can. There is more about David later on in the book.

CHAPTER THREE

Numbers and Things

As I was going through the book, I found myself making lists and recording numbers. I decided they all belonged in the same place.

70,320. Number of steps I climbed preparing for the 2011 Philadelphia Fight For Air Climb.

39,700. Number of steps in the Radebeul, Germany clmb, designed to approximate an ascent of Mount Everest from sea level to the summit.

11.674. Number of steps in the longest single-staircase race, the Niesen Treppenlauf, in Switzerland.

5847. Number of High rises in New York

4944. Number of flights of stairs I climbed preparing for the 2011 Philadelphia Fight For Air climb

2058.steps in the world's tallest building, the KL Towerthon in Kuala Lumpur.

2046. Number of steps up the Taipei 101, the second-tallest building in the world.

1978. First year for the Empire State Building Run Up in New York City

1855. Number of High rises in Toronto

1632. Number of Steps in the 94 story Hancock Building Climb

1169. Number of High rises in Shanghai

1156. Number of High rises in Tokyo

1130. Number of High rises in Chicago

746. Number of High rises in Hong Kong

644. Number of High rises in Mexico

638. Number of High rises in Vancouver

604. Number of High rises in Montreal

539. Number of High rises in Los Angeles

737. Members of the Facebook group Stairclimbing Sport

422. Total number of Flights of stairs, in my house, that I climbed in the year 2010.

5908. Total number of steps, in my house, that I climbed in the year 2011.

354. Number of steps to the top of the Statue of Liberty. It's a circular staircase.

168. Number of stories in the world's tallest building, the Burj Duba.

108. Equivalent floors in the country's tallest observation tower, The Stratosphere in Las Vegas, NV.

103. Number of floors in the country's tallest skyscraper, the Willis Tower, formerly known as the Sears Tower, in Chicago.

102. Number of floors in New York's Empire State Building. The Empire State Building Run Up ends at the Observation Level, which is floor 86.

101. Number of floors in the world's second tallest building, the Taipei 101 in Taipei, Taiwan, the Republic of China.

94. Number of floors in the Chicago Hancock Building Climb.

95. Number of organized Stair Climbs covered in this book.

10 Tallest Buildings In The World

	Name	Year Built	Height Feet	Floors
1	Burj Khalifa, Dubai	2010	2,723	163
2	Abraj Al Bait, Mecca, Saudi Arabia	2011	1,972	120
3	Taipei 101, Taipei, Taiwan	2004	1,670	101
4	Shanghai World Financial Center	2008	1,614	101
5	Intn'l Commerce Centre, Hong Kong	2010	1,588	118
6	Petronas Towers, Malaysia	1998	1,483	88
7	Nanjing Greenland Financial Center China	2009	1,480	89
8	Willis (Sears) Tower, Chicago 108	1974	1,450	
9	Jin Mao Building, Shanghai, China	1998	1,381	88
10	Two International Finance Centre Hong Kong	2003	1,362	88

Source: Emporis

10 Tallest Buildings in the United States

	Name	Year Built	Height Feet	Floors
1	Willis (Sears) Tower, Chicago 108	1974	1,450	
2	Empire State Building, New York	1931	1,250	102
3	Bank of America Tower, New York	2008	1,201	54
4	Aon Center, Chicago	1973	1,135	83
5	John Hancock Center, Chicago	1969	1,129	100
6	Chrysler Building, New York City	1930	1,047	77
7	New York Times Building, New York	2007	1,047	52
8	Bank of America Plaza, Atlanta	1992	1,024	55
9	U.S. Bank Tower, Los Angeles	1989	1,020	73
10	AT&T Corporate Center, Chicago	1989	1,007	60

Source: Emporis

10 Oldest Male Stair Climbers in the United States in 2011

Anders Jacobsen(86),25:25 25th Big Climb Seattle (69 floors) and 14:59 ALS Seattle (51 floors)

James Devenney(86),40:14 14th Hustle Up The Hancock, Chicago (94 floors)

Bob Terry(83),14:36 28th Bop To The Top, Indianapolis (36 floors)

Charles Coleman(82),10:47 ALA Oakbrook Terrace (31 floors)

Tony Yacek(81),32:08 ALA San Francisco (52 floors)

John Troy(80),36:28 ALA Boston (41 floors)

John Schultz(78),16:14 CFF Philadelphia (53 floors)

Kenneth Ryan(78),12:41 ALA Denver (56 floors)

Mike Mollo(76),7:22 ALA Providence (28 floors)

Tom Kutrosky(76),8:19 18th Stair Climb for Los Angeles (75

Robert Grouche(76),44:28:15 2nd Step-Up for the Up Center, Norfolk (100 Floors)

10 Oldest Female Stair Climbers in the United States in 2011

Gloria Schiffler(83),1:00:33 3rd Sky Rise Chicago (103 floors)

Marilyn Olen(83),20:47 ALA Denver (56 floors)

Shirley Lansing(81),36:49 25th Big Climb Seattle (69 floors)

Joanne Keaton(78),10:46 ALA Indianapolis (30 floors) and 8:49 ALA Oakbrook Terrace (31 floors)

Cathi Watson(77),18:24 ALA Chicago (45 floors)

Ginette Bedard(77),22:15 34th Empire State Building Run Up (86 floors)

Jean Toth(74),9:39:10 9th Tackle The Tower, Cleveland (38 floors)

Hallie Simmins(74),23:49 ALA Little Rock (39 floors)

Charlotte Prozan(74),29:21 ALA San Francisco (52 floors)

Judy Hess(73),17:45 5th Trek up the Tower Omaha (40 floors)

Judy Cheng(73),28:41:67 ALA Philadelphia (50 floors)

10 Top Stair Climbers Of All Time

According to TowerRunning.com, these are the top 10 Stair Climbers of all time (the Top 50 appear in Chapter 14.)

Based on performances in an age/gender group from year 1987 to present for the Empire State Building Run Up (NYC) and from year 2002 to present for the Willis (Sears) Tower (Sears Tower) race (ST) and from year 2003 to present for the US Bank Tower Race (LA) and from 2005 to present for the Taipei 101 race (TP). These races are chosen because they are major events and get a good International turnout.

Highest rankings go to the athletes with the most points. 3 points for first place finishes, 2 points for second place, 1 point for third place. If two or more athletes are tied, then the faster time. Overall win among male or female counts as an additional win (3 points).

Name	1st-2nd-3rd	Home	Total Points
1. Cindy Harris	32-3-0	Indiana	102 points
2. Thomas Dold	16-1-2	Germany	62 points
3. Piero Dettin	16-3-0	Italy	54 points
4. Chico Scimone	15-0-0	Italy	45 points
5. Terry Purcell	13-1-1	Australia	42 points
6. Paul Crake	12-0-0	Australia	42 points
7. Syd Arak	10-4-2	Indiana	40 points
8. Andrea Mayr	9-0-0	Austria	36 points
9. Hal Carlson	8-4-3	Illinois	35 points
10. Tim Van Orden	10-1-1	Vermont	33 points

Top 10 2011 World Cup Men

Name	Country	World Cup Points
Thomas Dold	GER	1000
Jesse Berg	USA	838
Tomas Celko	SVK	814
Piotr Lobodzinski	POL	804
Omar Bekkali	BEL	724
Matthias Jahn	GER	692
Fabio Ruga	ITA	680
Pavel Holek	CZE	638
Justin Stewart	USA	627
Kevin Crossman	USA	619

Top 10 2011 World Cup Women

Name	Country	World Cup Points
Cristina Bonacina	ITA	840
Cindy Harris	USA	780
Kristin Frey	USA	774
Kourtney Dexter	USA	700
Kerstin Sewczyk	GER	649
Julia Evangelist	AUT	614
Valentina Belotti	ITA	550
Melissa Moon	NZL	497
Sandra Nunez Castillo	MEX	403
Marie Fee-Breyer	GER	382

10 things you probably don't know about Steps, Stairs and Risers

Are all steps and stairs the same size?.

The answer is no.

Stan Schwartz, a noted Stair Climber and member of the Facebook Stair Climbing group has done a lot of thinking about stairs. Stan maintains a great blog called Stan's Obligatory Blog

http://www.1134.org/blog

Here are Stan's thoughts on the subject of steps, stairs, and sliders, which fits in quite nicely with this chapter's theme on numbers. Be sure to check his blog for even more fascinating facts, figures and numbers.

For what it's worth, I got some hard numbers on step height in some of our favorite staircases.

The standard stamped-steel stairs like at Wells Fargo and Wilshire-Figueroa are 7 inches per step.

The Los Angeles Aon stairs are 7.5 inches.

So it's not your imagination that those stairs are harder than most.

And the stairs at Willis are 7.7, so yes, they're even steeper than Aon. But no matter how you slice it, it still just plain hurts.

The number of steps per floor is generally consistent in any given building.

The only exceptions are the mechanical floors at the top of each bank of elevators. Those floors tend to be bigger.

For instance, the Los Angeles Aon building has them (mechanical floors) at about 21 and 43 or so. So the main stairway has sort of three main 'verses'.

From 4-20 it's the left-hand double stairway.

Then from 20-24 is the mechanical floors and the stairs turn right.

Then it goes back to left-hand double stairway from 24 to 43.

There's another little break and right-hand turns up to 45.

Then it's back to left-hand turns and a double stairway.

The other side of the double stairway ends at 52, and then it's just a single the rest of the way.

It's 22 steps per floor, aside from the mechanical floors.

I've done a little research on steps and stairs myself.

Since most organized Stair Climbs are done in building fire escapes, naturally those are what most interest me.

Building Codes dictate the steepness of stairs in a Commercial Fire Escape.

Residential buildings can be much steeper. Bear this in mind if you practice climb in the stairway of an old apartment building or condo.

The steepness (or slope) of a stairway is dependent on the height of the steps (referred to as riser height) and the tread depth, or how deep the step is.

Commercial Building Codes in the United States dictate a Riser Height of between 5 and 8.5 inches. This, in combination with the tread depth, would tell you how steep the stairs are.

Building Codes also dictate the variance permitted in a stairway.

Did you know that the slope of a stairway is not permitted to change within a floor?

This make sense, as stair climbers get 'used to' the slope of a stairway, and changing it suddenly could cause them to trip.

As you make your way to the top of a building, particularly in a very tall building, expect the slope of the stairs to change.

I'm told that there are great variations in the Empire State Building (I was hoping to find out myself in 2012, but I wasn't chosen in the lottery, and since I'm not a World ranked climber, I didn't receive an invitation.)

For the 2011 Philadelphia Fight For Air Climb, we climbed 50 floors with 1,088 steps.

That's about 20 steps per floor, 10 steps plus a landing plus 10 more.

I didn't notice any variation in the slope during my 50 floor ascent to the top.

10 Things You Definitely Should Do

1. Do some form of exercise <u>almost</u> every day

2. Vary the exercise that you do. Make it <u>fun</u>.

3. Have a <u>day of rest</u>--it will refresh your body and mind

4. <u>Eat well</u>

5. Get enough <u>sleep</u>

6. Maintain an <u>Exercise Diary</u>

7. Maintain a <u>Food Diary</u>

8. Get <u>weighed every day</u> in the morning but don't obsess about daily fluctuations Pick the day of the week when you are consistently the lightest (for me, it's Friday) and use that as a trend point for weekly analysis. In other words, if your Friday morning weight is consistently going up, that's a bad trend.

9. Maintain a <u>Weight Log</u>

10. Properly <u>Hydrate</u>. Drink lots of water. If you must drink diet drinks, watch your sodium intake. Most diet drinks contain lots of sodium. I prefer the Safeway 'refresh' Sparkling Water Beverage which contains 0 calories and 0 sodium.

10 Things You Definitely Should NOT Do

1. Don't give up after one day

2. Don't give up after one week.

3. Don't over do it--easy does it

4. Don't get discouraged if your training doesn't result in straight line improvement. Look for trends, week over week, month over month.

5. Don't get discouraged if your muscles ache or burn. This is normal. It's the way your body rebuilds itself---stronger.

6. Don't get discouraged if your bones ache. Ligaments and tendons will get stronger. Bones will get stronger and denser. Just don't over do it.

7. Don't compare yourself to others. You're improving yourself---in comparison to yourself, not to others.

8. Don't eat in your automobile. It's mindless eating.

9. Don't eat standing up. It shows a lack of respect for your body. Take the time to eat sitting down.

10. Don't eat or snack after 9pm

10 excuses people give me for not Stair Climbing

Since starting Stair Climbing last December, I've heard a bunch of excuses that people give me for not joining Team Smiley in their next ascent of the Bell Atlantic Tower. Here they are:

1. It hurts to Climb Stairs.

Comment: Most people who say this to me haven't even tried it.

I'm not sure what's hurting, but most likely they're not talking about climbing some stairs.

If it's real pain, they should see a doctor, and I hear excuses all the time as to why people won't visit a doctor once a year.

Exercise, of course, shouldn't hurt, but that doesn't mean you won't feel tired when you're done. The next day, you may feel a bit sore. This is your body's way of telling you that something good is happening.

So, most likely, the 'hurt' that you feel are the aches and pains associated with getting up off the couch.

You'll just need to suffer through it a bit until you achieve some conditioning.

2. My knees are bad

Comment: If your doctor has diagnosed you with arthritic knees, that is a valid excuse for not Stair Climbing., and you should definitely be treated by a doctor, perhaps even consider a knee replacement. By all means, do some sort of exercise program, perhaps water based.

However, as I've stated elsewhere in this book, do not self diagnose arthritis in your joints or permit your doctor to do so without the benefit of an X-Ray.

The Arthritis Foundation says that the definitive diagnosis for Arthritis of the joints is the X-Ray.

3. I don't have the time

Comment: I guess it's possible, however most people I know have 25 minutes to devote to themselves 3 times a week. That's a little over an hour.

Frequently the people who tell me this have plenty of time to do activities that would be considered by some to be fairly non productive.

Why not take some time for yourself to make yourself healthier?

Some suggestions I have: Borrow time from the following activities for your Stair Climbing: Watching Television, Surfing the Internet, Facebook, YouTube, Twitter, and Texting.

4. I have no place to train

Comment: Just about everyone can find a place to train.

If you live in a 2 story house, you have stairs you can use.

If you have a basement, you have stairs you can use.

If you live in or work in a high rise, you're in business.

If you belong to a gym that has a StairMaster, Stair Mill or Jacob's Ladder, you're all set.

5. I can't get motivated to start

Comment: That's understandable. If you're out of shape, it's tough to get started.

All I can is this: Believe me when I tell you that in 90 days you can complete an organized Stair Climb and feel better than you have in years.

As I say all the time, the journey of a thousand miles begins with the first step.

Take it :)

6. I'm already in good shape

Comment: I know a lot of very fit people (mostly runners,) and I can't get them to consider doing an organized Stair Climb. They really don't know what they're missing.

However, there's always room for improvement, and as some of the world class Stair Climbers will tell you, Stair Climbing will get you into even better shape than you are now.

Unless you can climb to the top of a 50 story building tomorrow in 6 minutes or less, there's always room for improvement.

 I was in good shape when I started training for our staim climb and I didn't realize how much better I would be in 90 days.

7. I can't find a Stair Climb to do

Comment: Sure you can. There are over 100 each year in the United States alone.

That's not to say that you may need to travel a few hundred miles to find one, but most people should be able to find one nearer to them than that.

8. I don't like to sweat

Comment: Yes, believe it or not, I've heard this one. It's probably their way of telling yours truly to get lost and stop bothering them.

As for me, I love to sweat---it lets me know I'm alive.

9. I'll die on the stairs

Comment: Sadly, this is possible.

I'm not aware of anyone dying in a Stair Climbing event, but it may have happened, and it probably will happen sometime in the future.

Deaths occur at all sorts of athletic events---that's why we sign a waiver before entering.

Most likely, it won't happen to you, particularly if you first seek the advice and approval of a doctor before beginning an exercise program, and once approved, that you properly train and use common sense on Climb Day.

10. I'm too old

Comment: Age should not be a barrier to anything.

You'll read further on in the book about Stair Climbers in their 90's who climbed, and climbed well.

In fact, I have an entire chapter (Chapter 15) devoted to older Stair Climbers.

If they can do it, you can also.

10 reasons "it" must be the stairs..

1. My legs feel like steel pistons…it must be the stairs.

2. People say I look young…it must be the stairs.

3. People marvel at the energy I have…it must be the stairs.

4. My morning 5 mile run is faster…it must be the stairs.

5. My morning 5K run is much faster than it used to be…it must be the stairs.

6. My annual 5K time December of 2011 was 4 minutes faster than last year.

7. I lost 10 pounds in 3 months…it must be the stairs.

8. I now have a better idea what it feels like to have asthma or COPD and fight for a breath…it must be the stairs.

9. I have a new found respect for First Responders…it must be the stairs.

10. When I make vacation plans, I look for a city with high rises…it must be the stairs.

10 reasons why Stair Climbing is better than jogging

1. There are no dogs on the stairs to chase and attack you.

2. You can still climb stairs in your house even when there's a blizzard outside.

3. There is no ice on the stairs to make you slip and hurt your foot.

4. You won't get wet on the stairs if it's raining outside

5. You don't need to bundle up in the cold.

6. You shouldn't overheat. Stairs are warm in the winter, cool in the summer.

7. There's no wind in your face on the stairs.

8. Provided you keep your practice stairs clear of shoes and roller skates, you shouldn't trip over anything.

9. You're less likely to be mugged on the stairs (but heed my warning about practicing alone in lonely fire escapes and Parking Garages.).

10. Stair Climbing provides better bragging rights. Just about everyone jogs these days---very few people climb stairs.

10 best things you can do to prepare for an organized Stair Climb

1. Register for a climb---this is a great first step! This is the problem with most people. They never register.

2. Join a team. It will make preparing easier. If you can, join a team that has members on it who have done a Stair Climb before.

3. Raise money (and a bunch of it) for the event and the charity it supports. This will give you positive vibes as you practice and train for the event. If you can, aspire to be a top fund raiser.

4. Find a high rise to practice in. If you can't find a high rise, at least practice on stairs.

5. Train Properly. Don't try to wing it on Climb Day. Try to climb the height of the building or the number of stairs of the actual climb before you do the actual climb.

6. Lose some weight prior to the climb. If you can't lose weight, at least don't gain any. The great thing is that the training you do in order to prepare for the climb should result in some weight loss.

7. Pick up your packet the day before the climb. If you can't pick up your packet the day before, get to the climb early enough on Climb Day that you are not rushed

8. Don't party the night before the climb. In particular, DON'T drink alcohol. There's also no need to Carbo-Load the night before Climb Day.

9. On the morning of the climb, eat a good breakfast, but keep it light, nothing that will make you bail out at floor 23 of the 50 story climb.

10. Recognize that the climb will be strenuous, but it will be over quickly, and you will feel as though you've really accomplished something.

CHAPTER FOUR

My Training Plan/Diary

In this chapter, I present two views (one brief, and one more detailed) of my Training Plan along with my 2010-2011 Personal Diary.

Brief Version: Start with 1 flight of stairs in your house on Day 1. On Day 2, add 1 flight and do 2. On Day 3, do 3 flights, etc. 100 days later, on Day 100, you'll be able to do what I do--climb 100 flights of stairs in about 25 minutes, and you're ready for every major Stair Climb in the world!

Longer Version:

It's a very simple plan.

Start with one flight of stairs (up and down) in your house, increase your flights 'climbed' by 1 each day until you've reached 100.

If necessary, break up the 100 flights climbed into intervals, for instance, do 20, rest 5 minutes, do 20 more, rest 5 minutes, repeat until you're done 100.

Using this technique, in 100 days and you'll be ready for your first stair climb.

Here's my Training Diary for the 2011 Philadelphia Fight For Air Climb as proof.

Thursday, November 25, 2010

Wow, it's Thanksgiving and for some reason I just signed up for the American Lung Association 2011 Philadelphia Fight For Air Climb to be held on Saturday, March 19th, 2010.

It's something I thought I might do last year, but I hurt my foot jogging in February of 2009 and I just couldn't commit to it.

I don't know much about it, except that you walk-run to the top of the Bell Atlantic Tower in Philadelphia. It's 50 floors, and 1,023 steps.

As a runner, I figure it shouldn't be a big problem, however, when I visited the Philadelphia Art Museum in April, I still got a bit tired just walking up the 40 or so steps to the top of the Art Museum.

Preparing for this climb will be good for me—and will also raise money for charity.

Wednesday, December 8, 2010 (Day 001—7 Flights, 98 steps, 1:19)

I started my program with 7 flights of stairs. Didn't much know what I was doing, but I did 7 flights up and 7 flights down in 1 minute and 19 seconds. I doubled up—skipped one stair each on the way up, just walked down. I was pretty winded by the time I was finished. With 14 steps on our stairs, I figured I did a total of 98 steps. The Bell Atlantic Tower has 1,088 steps to the top.

Thursday, December 9, 2010 (Day 002---8 Flights, 112 steps, 1:25)

I figured that the tortoise wins the race between the tortoise and the hare (at least I think it did.) so I decided each day I would add 1 flight of stairs to my training. I did 8 flights of stairs (112 steps) in 1 minute and 25 seconds. If you're following along at home, I know you can do this. 8 flights up (I'm doubling the steps, but you can do them single), and then 8 flights down. I'm doing my training in a two story house, so that means I run up (doubling the steps) then walk down, then run up, then walk down, etc. The walk down gives you a chance to catch your breath.

It's amazing how little things can really derail your exercise.

My mother, Rita Smiley died on October 28th, and one of the nuns at her Nursing Home arranged a mass in her memory for today at 11am.

I try not to get depressed, but it's not always easy.

I used to talk to my mother at the Nursing Home a lot about my exercise. She worried about me running in the dark at 5 in the morning, and as I did my 9 flights up the stairs, I thought that she would probably be happy I was climbing them.

Friday, December 10, 2010 (Day 003---9 Flights, 126 steps, 2:02)

Once again, I'm adding 1 more flight to yesterday's total.

Yesterday I did 8, today I did 9 flights of stairs, 126 steps, in 2 minutes and 2 seconds. I just cracked the 2 minute mark. My goal, for the Philadelphia Fight For Air Climb on March 19th, is to climb it in less than 11 minutes.

For those of you who say you don't have time to do this kind of training, it's really not a problem.

You don't need any equipment, just put on a pair of sneakers and climb your stairs.

Time? Right now, 2 minutes a day. You can certainly afford that amount of time, and you can do it whenever you want, day or night, even during a commercial break in your favorite television show.

Saturday, December 11, 2010 (Day 004----10 Flights, 140 steps, 2:36)

I regularly spend most of Saturday catching up on my work---writing computer programs, teaching computer programming classes, writing books on computer programming, answering fan mail about my books. After that, I and my wife attend 4:30 Mass, and then we go to a movie and out to a late dinner.

Finding time to do stairs isn't a problem---I can take 2 minutes to do them around 4pm, and then it's off to Church.

Today I did 10 flights of stairs in 2 minutes and 36 seconds (let's abbreviate that as 2:36 from now on.)

My heart rate climbs, but for now, I wouldn't say I'm working up a sweat.

For you who are following along with me, that might be different.

It may be tougher for you to get up and down the stairs 10 times—but keep at it. And you might find yourself sweating a bit. That's OK too. As you read on, you'll see that the most stairs I climbed, the more intense the workout became. Not surprisingly, this meant more time on the stairs, more recovery time and a much needed shower afterwards!

A friend of mine just said that no one who is overweight would be interested in reading my book on Stair Climbing. I disagree. There are many overweight people who want to lose weight, and getting up and down stairs is a great way to do it.

Sunday, December 12, 2010 (Day 005---11 Flights, 154 steps, 2:13)

Today is my first Sunday climb. It's not something I was looking forward to, and I had to work around today's Philadelphia Eagles game (great game, the Eagles defeated the Cowboys 30-27) but it took me only 2 minutes and 13 seconds to do the 11 Flights. I was pretty tired after the 11 Flights, but I've got to keep at it.

Today's time of 2 minutes and 13 seconds beat yesterday's time of 2 minutes and 36 seconds by 23 seconds---and with one additional flight of stairs. I'm making progress.

Monday, December 13, 2010 (Day 006---12 Flights, 154 steps, 2:30)

I had a full day's work today, and when I got in around 5pm, I really didn't feel like running up and down the steps 12 times, but I really wanted to get my workout in, and dinner was going to be ready in 15 minutes, so I pushed it.

A funny thing happened though.

I feel like I finally got 'warmed up' after 11 flights, and the 12 flight felt like nothing.

It's possible I've made some kind of breakthrough.

Reminds me of the second wind I got in 1978 when I was biking the first day of the Cape May 200 from Philadelphia to Cape May.

Around mile 15, I was just about out of gas, but I found a nice rhythm which lasted me until mile 87.

The last 13 were very tough, but that's a story for another day.

For now, I'm wondering how I'll feel tomorrow.

Tuesday, December 14, 2010 (Day 007---14 Flights, 196 steps, 3:11)

How I felt on Tuesday you can gather from the fact that I didn't do my regularly scheduled 13 Flights (1 more than Monday), but I added 2 Flights to the workout.!

Once again, after 11 flights of stairs, my legs felt great. I probably could have gone even farther.

By doing 14 Flights today, this now 'syncs' my stairs climbed to the date--- 14 flights on December 14th. Now, at least for the duration of the month, I don't need to think about how many times to go up and down the steps--- provided I know the date, I'll just do that number of flights.

Wednesday, December 15, 2010 (Day 008---15 Flights, 210 steps, 3:21)

15 Flights, and it's the 15th day of the month. See how easy that is? Once again, it seems like after 11 flights or so, my legs warm up, and that achy feeling goes away. I'm still breathing pretty hard by the time I'm done, and don't forget, I'm 'doubling' (two steps at a time) the stairs up, and single stepping the stairs down.

3 minutes and 21 seconds doesn't seem like a long time to run up and down stairs, does it? I think the part that makes it challenging is the double stepping up. I'm still not sure if I'll be doing that on Climb Day (March 19th)

Thursday, December 16, 2010 (Day 009---16 Flights, 224 steps, 3:42)

Another flight added, another 21 seconds added to the workout.

In general, I've noted that it seems to take about 15 seconds to do a complete up and down circuit. Probably about 5 seconds to run up the steps (doubling them) and then about 10 seconds to carefully walk down, make the turnaround at the bottom of the steps, and do another set.

At this rate, when I get to 100 Flights of Stairs (my goal prior to the actual Climb Day) I'll be running up and down the stairs for about 25 minutes. We'll see how close I come to that prediction.

Friday, December 17, 2010 (Day 010---0 Flights, 0 steps, 0:00)

Oops, what happened. No climb?

Life caught up with me---I worked a full day, and I had the Haddon Holiday Heart Run 5K to run the next morning and I promised my wife Olive Garden for dinner. I took my first day off from the stairs since starting my program.

I don't think I've mentioned this, but I do some recreational running in addition to my new found zeal for Stair Climbing.

In general, I run 3 times a week, almost exclusively in the morning before the sun rises. Usually either 3 or 5 miles.

Stair Climbing I hold off until the end of the day.

Tomorrow I have the 5K race to run, so I decided to give myself a day off from Stair Climbing.

Saturday, December 18, 2010 (Day 011---18 Flights, 252 steps, 4:11)

I started the day with a pretty lackluster Haddon Holiday Heart Run 5K in the morning.

Our 14 year old daughter Melissa beat me, which was great, although (making an obvious excuse here) I was not at my healthiest---although I hope to be by March 19th.

Since I skipped stairs yesterday, I decided that instead of incrementing my Flights by the normal one set of stairs, I would 'catch up' by incrementing two flights to 18.

I'm now over 4 minutes of Stair Climbing, feeling good.

Sunday, December 19, 2010 (Day 012---19 Flights, 266 steps, 4:10)

Our daughter Melissa did well in her track meet earlier in the day and ...I watched a phenomenal Eagles-New York Giants game highlighted this Sunday evening by the

Miracle of the Meadowlands II, as Desean Jackson ran back a punt with no time left to give the Eagles the win, 38-31 after training 24-3. That win pushed the Eagles record to 11-4.

Sadly, the Eagles wouldn't win another game all season, losing in the playoffs to the eventual Super bowl winner Green Bay Packers.

As far as Stair Climbing, earlier in the day, I did 19 Flights in 4 minutes and 10 seconds.

Interestingly, I added 1 flight of stairs, but was one second faster than the previous day.

Monday, December 20, 2010 (Day 013---20 Flights, 280 steps, 4:45)

20 Flights in 4 minutes and 45 seconds means that I'm one fifth of the way to my goal of 100 Flights of Stairs.

I was doing some math in my head on the stairs, and the Philadelphia Fight For Air Climb (previously known as the Bell Atlantic Tower Climb) has 50 flights of stairs, so 100 may be overkill. However, it has 1,088 steps.

My home stairs have 14 steps per flight, so if you count just the number of steps to go up one flight in my house, and multiply by 100, if I reach my goal, I'll have climbed 1,400 steps.

In actuality, 1,088 steps in my house would be roughly 77 flights of stairs.

I'll celebrate that day when I get to it!

Have you noticed? I'm one-fifth of the way there!

It's psychological, I know, but it is significant.

In fact, flights of 20 will become very significant to me in the future as I train.

Even today, I measure my Stair Climbing workout in splits of 20, and I know a good time (sub 5 minute time) versus a bad time (5 minute plus) based on the split.

Earlier in the day, my wife and I went to see an old friend of the family in the neighborhood where I grew up

I talk about Stair Climbing now wherever I go---I think my former neighbor thought I was crazy, but she wished me well!

Tuesday, December 21, 2010 (Day 014---21 Flights, 294 steps, 4:53)

Some days, you just don't know how well you'll do on the stairs.

Sometimes, you can feel lousy all day long, and then find yourself energized on the stairs. This is what happened today.

Amazing what the body can do.

Wednesday, December 22, 2010 (Day 015---22 Flights, 308 steps, 5:07)

I had a Dentist appointment earlier in the day, but after receiving a clean bill of Dental Health, on the steps I went!

22 Flights in 5 minutes and 7 seconds. I crossed the 5 minute threshold!

Thursday, December 23, 2010 (Day 016---0 Flights, 0 steps, 0:00)

I don't like to make excuses for not climbing stairs but December 23rd was another hectic day.

A full day of work, and because of the upcoming Christmas Holy Day, my wife and I decided to take in a movie on the 23rd, since Christmas Eve and Christmas Day were out for a movie.

I was off from work today, and spent a lot of the day working on a new Computer Programming book.

Earlier in the day, I had run 5 miles, as tomorrow is Christmas Eve, and I wouldn't be running..

And then, in the back of my mind, a "little voice" was wondering what would happen if I took a day off? Would I be stronger tomorrow?

We'll see.

Friday, December 24, 2010 (Day 017---24 Flights, 336 steps, 5:33)

Christmas Eve! My family and I knew we were going to 4pm Mass, so I needed to get up and down the stairs a bit earlier than usual.

Yesterday I skipped my workout. I was scheduled for 23 Flights, but things happened, and I didn't do any.

No problem today. 24 Flights in about 5 and a half minutes.

There's some talk about the possibility of a White Christmas, but most likely the snow is going to start late Christmas night before pounding us with a blizzard on Sunday, December 26th.

Saturday, December 25, 2010 (Day 018---25 Flights, 350 steps, 5:52)

Merry Christmas! My wife thinks I'm crazy doing this on Christmas day, but I am on the steps. I'm **one quarter** of the way there. 25 Flights, 350 steps.

Sunday, December 26, 2010 (Day 019---26 Flights, 364 steps, 5:54)

A blizzard is raging outside in the Philadelphia area, but inside, it's nice and toasty, and I'm on my steps.

Sad to say, there's no football in Philadelphia today.

The Eagles-Minnesota Vikings final regular season game has been postponed.

The Eagles are a heavy favorite in this game, hoping to further solidify a playoff position, and a possible #1 NFC seed.

Sadly, I can tell you that when the game is played on Tuesday (the first time in NFL History that a game will be played on a Tuesday night.), the Eagles will lose to a rookie quarterback. In fact, sadly, they will not win another game this season!

Monday, December 27, 2010 (Day 020---27 Flights, 378 steps, 6:06)

Total climb time is now over the 6 minute mark.

Monday climbs are tough for me---they are usually done after a long day of work.

I'm also beginning to perspire so much after the workout that I need a shower, which is adding another 10 minutes to the total workout time.

Tuesday, December 28, 2010 (Day 021---28 Flights, 392 steps, 6:43)

Bummer. My Eagles lost to the Minnesota Vikings on Tuesday Night Football.

The game was originally scheduled to be played on Sunday, December 26th, but Philadelphia had a blizzard, and the game had to be postponed.

I'm glad I ran the stairs earlier in the day.

If I had waited until after the game, I don't think I would have had the motivation to finish.

Wednesday, December 29, 2010 (Day 022---29 Flights, 406 steps, 6:35)

29 Flights climbed, and overall, 8 seconds faster than yesterday. Not bad!

I've mentioned to some people that I've been climbing stairs, and most people don't understand, particularly when I tell them I'm doing the flights inside of my house. I suspect they think I'm either crazy or live in a high rise.

Thursday, December 30, 2010 (Day 023---30 Flights, 420 steps, 7:04)

There's still a lot of snow on the ground, so Stair Climbing is about the only exercise I've been able to do. No running outside for me. The last two years I've had foot injuries due to slipping on ice in the dark during my morning run. So far, I haven't been injured on the steps.

I did 30 Flights today, and I'm now over the 7 minute mark for continuous Stair Climbing. I don't yet know how long it will take for me to reach the top of the Bell Atlantic Tower, which is making me nervous.

Whenever I prepare for any athletic endeavor, I train mainly for time.

For instance, if I'm training for a Half Marathon, I estimate my finish time and shoot for that (plus a little bit more) in training.

I figure that when I finally reach 100 Flights of stairs in my house, it will take me about 25 minutes to complete them.

For the actual Stair Climb on March 19th, at this point I have no idea what my time will be.

Friday, December 31, 2010 (Day 024---31 Flights, 434 steps, 7:14)

It's New Years Eve. Guess what I'm doing?

That's correct. I'm running on the stairs!

And really, if you think about it, what's the big deal, really?

I can spare 7 minutes and 14 seconds, although I'm now so winded after doing the stairs that I need to rest 5 minutes and shower.

Saturday, January 1, 2011 (Day 025---32 Flights, 448 steps, 7:23)

Yes, it's New Years Day, but after watching the Philadelphia Mummers Parade, I'm set to do the stairs. 32 Flights(one more than yesterday) and 9 extra seconds.

I can't believe the workout I'm getting on the stairs.

Anymore, when I'm done, I'm really tired, and need some recovery time. I'm also perspiring pretty heavily.

Sunday, January 2, 2011 (Day 026---33 Flights, 462 steps, 7:45)

Argh. My Philadelphia Eagles lose to the Dallas Cowboys 14-13 in their regular season finale.

Although my football team was not a success, I'm a success on the stairs.

33 Flights (one third of the way to 100) in 7 minutes and 45 seconds. Good job!

Monday, January 3, 2011 (Day 027---34 Flights, 476 steps, 7:55)

In addition to a 5 mile run this morning, .I did 34 flights on the stairs this afternoon. Just short of 8 minutes of duration on the stairs. Double exercise, cross training for each.

Tuesday, January 4, 2011 (Day 028---35 Flights, 490 steps, 8:52)

35 flights, 490 steps, just short of 500 steps on the stairs.

Almost a full minute longer than yesterday though. I felt very tired.

Wednesday, January 5, 2011 (Day 029---36 Flights, 504 steps, 8:32)

In addition to a 5 mile run this morning, I did 36 flights of stairs this afternoon. 20 seconds quicker than yesterday with an additional flight. I'm finally over the 500 step mark, which is just about half-way to the 1,088 steps I'll need on March 19th.

Thursday, January 6, 2011 (Day 030---37 Flights, 518 steps, 8:55)

In addition to a 3 mile run this morning...I did 37 flights of stairs this afternoon.

Friday, January 7, 2011 (Day 031---38 Flights, 532 steps, 9:12)

38 Flights climbed and over 9 minutes in total climbing time.

For me, reaching 10 minutes in total climbing time is my next goal.

Saturday, January 8, 2011 (Day 032---39 Flights, 546 steps, 9:27)

Getting close to 40 flights. I'm on a roll now.

Sunday, January 9, 2011 (Day 033---40 Flights, 560 steps, 9:36)

The Philadelphia Eagles are hosting the Green Bay Packers in an NFL Playoff game. It's a close game that they will lose.

Our daughter is also participating in a New Jersey track meet. I'll need to pick her up later.

Both of these events necessitate that I get my 'climb' in early.

That's the beauty of Stair Climbing.

It's really an easy sport to participate in.

You don't need to leave your house, and there's little prep time. I put on my running shoes, ready my stop watch, and go!

Today's practice climb, 40 flights, means I'm **40%** percent of the way to my goal of 100 flights climbed, and I'm also approaching 10 minutes of Stair Climbing.

I also realized today that since I started training, I have now climbed a total of 746 Flights, a total of 10,444 steps!

Monday, January 10, 2011 (Day 034---41 Flights, 574 steps, 10:22)

41 Flights climbed, but even more importantly, 10 minutes of continuous Stair Climbing!

Some of my friends have asked me what I think about while I'm Stair Climbing. In general, I try not to think about anything.

Stair Climbing isn't like running outside---there are no trees or nature to take in.

Even on a treadmill, you can flip on the television.

In my home stairwell, there's nothing to break up the monotony of the stairs, although I guess I could always listen to some music. But I've never been a music kind of guy.

Before I start, I do open the front door (which is what I run toward when I'm coming down the steps.) I can see people walking by, and I have a view of some trees (and snow) outside, so it doesn't feel quite as claustrophobic.

When I do open the front door, our dog Madison takes it as a signal that someone is coming home, and she lies down at the front door and waits with anticipation for their arrival.

Sometimes Madison interferes with my 'turnaround' at the bottom of the stairs--but this is a small price to pay for her company.

I often think that Madison must think I'm crazy, seeing me run up the steps, and then walk down---over and over again.

Tuesday, January 11, 2011 (Day 035---42 Flights, 588 steps, 11:31)

I was tired today, struggling today to do 42 Flights. I finished them, but I did them a full minute longer than yesterday's climb.

In fact, today was probably the first time that I seriously considered stopping and taking a rest.

To combat feelings like this, I have started mentally breaking my climbs into segments of 20 flights climbed. Today, I did 2 sets of 20, plus 2 more flights.

My 20 flight 'splits' are around 5 minutes, so I concentrate getting to the 20 flights.

This will come in handy as I approach 100 flights of stairs climbed which will be 5 sets of 20.

Wednesday, January 12, 2011 (Day 036---43 Flights, 602 steps, 10:42)

43 Flights climbed. 1 more flight than yesterday, but nearly a full minute less in time!

Exercise is funny that way.

Some days you know you're going to struggle. You can just feel it when you start out. Other days you feel lousy, you may even put off exercising, but when you start, all of that goes away.

Regardless, one thing is true regardless of the type of day I'm having.

I still feel an initial period of leg fatigue, This tends to go away after 10 flights or so.

After that, it's a matter of waiting for real fatigue to set in, and yesterday that was around Flight 38.

That means Flights 11 to 37 were a breeze! If only they all could feel that way.

A lot of people ask me how this process of adding one flight a day to my training is working out.

For the most part, the additional flight is pretty easy to handle--but some days, it feels like I should be doing one flight less not one flight more!

Thursday, January 13, 2011 (Day 037---44 Flights, 616 steps, 10:51)

I mentioned a few posts earlier that my total exercise time is now the time it takes me to actually climb the stairs plus time for a shower afterwards.

I need to amend that.

My flights up and down are leaving me drenched in sweat by the time I'm done.

In addition to the shower afterward, I now need to have a cool off period of 5 to 10 minutes before getting into the shower.

I don't know if you've ever heard of a 'runners high', but I'm definitely beginning to experience it. I should call it a "climbers high."

For me, it's that period of time after I've really pushed myself on the stairs that I'm cooling down, feeling me heart beat almost out of my chest, and being ever so grateful to be alive---and no longer climbing!

Friday, January 14, 2011 (Day 038---45 Flights, 630 steps, 11:16)

Today felt great, just a little nervous tension awaiting tomorrow's practice session which is going to take place at Tim's 25 floor condo!

Saturday, January 15, 2011 (Day 039---92 Flights, 1,656 steps, 15:14)

My team and I did some steps at our teammate Tim's 25 floor condo.

Tim had warned us the climbing the steps in his fire escape would be intense, and he wasn't kidding.

We each did 3 sets of 25 flights, and 1 set of 17 flights (his condo is on the 17th floor), with about a 5 minute rest in between.

It was the first time any of us had gone multiple flights---as you know, my training has all been single flights of stairs.

The fire escape was hot and dry. (My Facebook friend Lisa Kinsner Scheer recommends cough lozenges for this.)

I started out double stepping the stairs---I was able to do that for about 7 flights, then single stepped my way to the top.

After about 10 flights, it felt like something had sucked all of the air out of my lungs. Is this the climber's equivalent of the Runner's Wall?

After hitting that imaginary wall, it was a matter of putting one step in front of the other and continuing.

We were just about done in after one try, but one of our team members Bob said, OK, let's do another!

I'm glad we did.

The second set was better--we knew what to expect.

Not necessarily better in time (my second time up was actually slower) but a better experience. I hardly double stepped the second time. I just found a nice comfortable rhythm and then walked my way up. My walking time was only 14 seconds slower than the time in which I double stepped.

The third time up was just about the same as the second, and we did an abbreviated 17 floor climb up for our fourth attempt before heading back to Tim's condo for some post practice refreshments.

Here are my times for each of the climbs:

First set of 25: 4 minutes, 5 seconds

Second set of 25: 4 minutes, 19 seconds

Third set of 25: 4 minutes, 26 seconds

Fourth set (17 flights): 2 minutes, 34 seconds

Note that it typically takes me about 6 minutes to do 25 flights of stairs in my house, because in addition to going up, I'm also going down. Extrapolating these times for the Philadelphia Fight For Air Climb, I calculated that I would finish between 8 and 9 minutes.

However, that extrapolation doesn't take into account the way each of us felt when he hit the 25th floor---like we didn't want to go any farther!

At this point, I think it's safe to say we're all a bit hesitant about our chances on March 19th.

For those of you reading my book, I heartily recommend that if you can, you find a high rise like this to practice in at least **once** before your actual climb.

It will prepare you for the real thing.

Physically, you may be ready to do the climb event, but mentally and psychologically, going straight up 25+ floors is something you need to experience.

Some organized Stair Climbs have 'practice climbs' for their contestants.

The Philadelphia Fight For Air Climb does not.

As for our team, we hope to do this at least one more time.

Notice that my overall time for the 92 floors was 15 minutes and 14 seconds.

Sunday, January 16, 2011 (Day 040---47 Flights, 658 steps, 11:12)

I did 45 flights on Friday, I was scheduled to do 46 flights yesterday, but since I was having so much fun at Tim's condo, I decided to up my count by 2 today. No problem! In fact, my pace was faster than Friday's.

Incidentally, today, while surfing the Internet, I discovered that's there's a Stair Climbing Yahoo Group. It was founded by a real Stair Climbing enthusiast David Snyder, and it has good information in it, with lots of questions asked, and a bunch of great people answering them. I don't know if you are familiar with Yahoo Groups, but they are kind of the precursor to Facebook Groups.

Two days later I would discover that David also moderates a Facebook Stair Climbing Group as well.

I've posted a link to both the Yahoo Group and the Facebook Group in Chapter 16 of this book.

Monday, January 17, 2011 (Day 041---48 Flights, 672 steps, 11:21)

In addition to a 5K run this morning I did 48 flights in the afternoon. No problem!

Tuesday, January 18, 2011 (Day 042---49 Flights, 686 steps, 11:50)

One more flight, 29 more seconds. Right on pace.

Interestingly, I discovered today that there's a Stair Climbing Facebook Group, and I've already made two new friends there.

There's a lot of activity in the group centering around upcoming Stair Climbs and a bunch of questions about training and techniques.

I've included the direct link to this Facebook group in Chapter 16 of this book.

Wednesday, January 19, 2011 (Day 043---50 Flights, 700 steps, 12:20)

In addition to a 5 mile run this morning I did 50 flights of stairs in the afternoon, 700 steps in all.

I took a moment to consider the fact that I'm halfway to 100 flights!

If I extrapolate 50 flight time for 100 flights, that would be 24 minutes and 40 seconds.

Right now, having finished 50 flights of stairs in my house, I can't imagine climbing 100 flights. I'm pretty winded by the end of my workout.

But that's the beauty of adding 1 flight of stairs a day---you can handle it.

Thursday, January 20, 2011 (Day 044---51 Flights, 714 steps, 11:27)

A Facebook Friend of mine, Lisa Kinsner Scheer suggested that I might want to vary my training by climbing 25 flights, resting, then climbing 25 flights, which is exactly what I did. In my case, I did 25 as fast as I could, rested for about 5 minutes, then did 26 as fast as I could.

The overall results, as you can see, were nearly a full minute faster than the previous day.

It's an interesting way to break up the monotony of dong what I ordinarily do which is to do all of my flights with no break.

Friday, January 21, 2011 (Day 045---52 Flights, 728 steps, 12:46)

Did the same 'split' climb as the day before, but my overall time didn't reflect it. I was a full minute <u>slower</u> than the day before.

Saturday, January 22, 2011 (Day 046---53 Flights, 742 steps, 12:53)

Back to one continuous climb. 53 flights, 1 more flight than yesterday, in just 7 extra seconds.

Sunday, January 23, 2011 (Day 047---54 Flights, 756 steps, 12:57)

1 more flight than yesterday, just 4 seconds longer. Keep it up!

Monday, January 24, 2011 (Day 048---55 Flights, 770 steps, 13:38)

Monday's can be tough for me---usually a full day of work, some traveling, and general overall fatigue.

On top of that, it's that period of time when the Winter doldrums set in, and even with an upcoming event, such as a race or climb to prepare for, it's still seems a long way off and it can make it difficult to maintain focus.

Having said that, however, once again the beauty of Stair Climbing is that you don't need to drive anywhere to do it, you don't need to go to a gym, you don't need friends to join you.

Just put on a pair of shorts and running shoes and start climbing!

That's usually enough to get you going.

Tuesday, January 25, 2011 (Day 049---56 Flights, 784 steps, 14:01)

In addition to a 5 mile run this morning, once again I hit the stairs.

1 more flight than yesterday, although 23 seconds longer.

Wednesday, January 26, 2011 (Day 050---57 Flights, 798 steps, 13:43)

57 flights of stairs in the house. 1 more flight than yesterday, but 18 seconds faster.

Thursday, January 27, 2011 (Day 051---58 Flights, 812 steps, 11:32)

I did splits for this workout, this time instead of sets of 20, I did 6 sets of 10, with a break of 1 minute between each set.

As you can see, my overall time was phenomenal, but I'm not sure how useful this technique will be in going up a 50 floor building.

I think my body reacts best to continuous effort.

Friday, January 28, 2011 (Day 052---0 Flights, 0 steps, 0:00)

We had to rush our dog Madison to the University of Pennsylvania Veterinarian Hospital for a life saving blood transfusion (she's fine now.)

Obviously, no Stair Climbing today and this is the first day I have missed since <u>December 23rd</u> (a total of 34 straight days of Stair Climbing training.)

Saturday, January 29, 2011 (Day 053---60 Flights, 840 steps, 14:29)

After a morning phone call with promising news on our Dog Madison, I did 60 flights. Another nice round number. 60% of the way there!

Sunday, January 30, 2011 (Day 054---61 Flights, 854 steps, 14:33)

I climbed 61 flights in 14 minutes and 33 seconds. I'm now approaching 15 minutes of continuous climbing on the stairs.

More exciting is the fact that in the morning we received a call that we could visit Madison, and when we got there the Vet said that we could take her home! What a nice surprise.

It was nice to see Madison in the house again as I climbed my stairs, although it would be a few days before she would once again be sitting at the front door watching me go up and down the stairs.

Monday, January 31, 2011 (Day 055---62 Flights, 868 steps, 14:40)

1 more flight, 7 more seconds. Right on pace.

I spoke with our teammate Tim today, and asked him about the possibility of a second practice session in his condo. It looks good that we will do another, but right now, the exact date is unknown.

Tuesday, February 1, 2011 (Day 056---63 Flights, 882 steps, 15:14)

I'm glad to be done with the month of January.

Winter is dark and cold (and lately, in Philadelphia, very icy and snowy.)

I started February with 63 flights of stairs, and passed the 15 minute threshold for the first time.

Wednesday, February 2, 2011 (Day 057---64 Flights, 896 steps, 15:28)

1 more flight, 14 more seconds. We're getting there!

Thursday, February 3, 2011 (Day 058---65 Flights, 910 steps, 15:47)

In addition to a 5 mile run this morning I did 65 flights of stairs in the house.

Friday, February 4 2011 (Day 059---66 Flights, 924 steps, 16:25)

66 flights in 16 minutes and 24 seconds.

Two major thresholds achieved: 66 flights is two thirds of the way to 100, and I'm now able to climb continuously for 16+ minutes.

Both of these were just a dream when I started climbing back in December!

Saturday, February 5, 2011 (Day 060---67 Flights, 938 steps, 15:46)

Now officially past two thirds of the way to my goal of 100 flights---and now under 16 minutes!

Sunday, February 6, 2011 (Day 061---68 Flights, 952 steps, 16:15)

Super Bowl Sunday! Always a fun day.

We're headed to a party later today, so I had to do my stairs a bit earlier than usual.

No problem. 68 flights, 952 steps. Closing in on 1,000 steps climbed in a single session, and shortly after that surpassing the number of steps (1,088) in the actual Bell Atlantic Tower.

Monday, February 7, 2011 (Day 062---69 Flights, 966 steps, 16:43)

It's the day after Super Bowl Sunday. It's a great day. My wife and I won a Super bowl pool, which offsets the fact that it's still a Monday ☺

69 Flights---closing in on 70, another multiple of 10, and closer to the 1000 step threshold.

Tuesday, February 8, 2011 (Day 063---70 Flights, 980 steps, 16:56)

In addition to a 5 mile run this morning I did 70 flights of stairs in the house. There are lots of significant numbers today.

70 flights means I'm 70% of the way to 100 flights.

And, today is February 8th, exactly two months since I started training.

Wednesday, February 9, 2011 (Day 064---71 Flights, 994 steps, 16:11)

Great news! Tim just confirmed our second practice session at his condo on Saturday.

This good news gives me a little extra 'pep in my step' as I head up the stairs and complete 71 flights up and down my stairs, at a good pace.

Thursday, February 10, 2011 (Day 065---72 Flights, 1,008 steps, 16:35)

72 flights---one more flight than yesterday.

What can I say? It's slow and steady for me.

Friday, February 11, 2011 (Day 066---73 Flights, 1,022 steps, 17:24)

It's the Friday before out second practice session at Tim's Condo, and I feel a bit sluggish.

One more flight climbed than yesterday, but almost a full minute longer.

Horrible---I hope I feel better tomorrow.

Saturday, February 12, 2011 (Day 067---92 Flights, 1,656 steps, 14:36)

We did another practice climb at our teammate Tim's condo.

Once again, we each did 3 sets of 25 flights, and 1 set of 17 flights (his condo is on the 17th floor), with about a 5 minute rest in between.

I felt about the same I did the last time I did his steps---but this time, I knew what was coming and was prepared for it. Also, having completed 73 flights of stairs on my own just yesterday, I'm probably in better shape than I was when I did these steps on January 15th. At least that's what my times show.

Here are my times for each of the climbs:

First Set of 25: 3 minutes, 52 seconds. (Jan 15 4 minutes, 5 seconds)

Second Set of 25: 4 minutes, 6 seconds. (Jan 15 4 minutes, 19 seconds)

Third Set of 25: 4 minutes and 7 seconds (Jan 15 4 minutes, 26 seconds_

Fourth Set (17 flights): 2 minutes, 31 seconds (Jan 15, 2 minutes, 34 seconds)

Overall, my times were 14 minutes and 36 seconds. On January 15, 15 minutes and 14 seconds, so I was nearly 1 minute faster this time.

Considering how poorly I felt the day before, this is great progress!

Sunday, February 13, 2011 (Day 068---75 Flights, 1,050 steps, 18:55)

75 flights, in nearly 19 minutes. I've reached another milestone---75% of the way to 100 flights.

Monday, February 14, 2011 (Day 069---0 Flights, 0 steps, 0:00)

What happened? No steps?

A couple of things.

First, I'm feeling great, and with the successful Condo practice on Saturday, I now know that doing OK on March 19th is probably a foregone conclusion.

Secondly, I'm beginning to treat my running in the morning as Cross Training for my stair climb, and vice versa.

I've decided that on days where I run, I won't stair climb, and on days that I climb stairs, I won't run.

Let's see how that turns out.

Tuesday, February 15, 2011 (Day 070---77 Flights, 1,078 steps, 19:28)

77 Flights of stairs in 19 minutes, and 28 seconds. I can't lie to you, today was a real effort to do this.

Today's step total, 1,078 steps, is 10 shy of the actual number in the Bell Atlantic Tower. My next climb I'll surpass it!

Wednesday, February 16, 2011 (Day 071---0 Flights, 0 steps, 0:00)

I ran 5 miles this morning, so no stair climb.

Thursday, February 17, 2011 (Day 072---79 Flights, 1,106 steps, 19:17)

79 flights, 1,106 steps!

I'm past the 1,088 steps I'll need to do about one month from today when I climb the Bell Atlantic Tower.

I guess I could just stop adding to the Stair Climbing total at this point---I've reached the step total, but 100 Flights of stairs has been my goal since I started training 72 days ago, so there's no sense stopping now!

Note the time it took me to do 79 Flights. 19 minutes and 17 seconds.

I think that would be a respectable time for the Philadelphia Fight For Air Climb, but you have to remember that two-thirds of my overall time of 19 minutes is spent coming down the steps. That should mean my Climb Day time will be faster.

Friday, February 18, 2011 (Day 073---0 Flights, 0 steps, 0:00)

I ran 5 miles this morning, so no stair climb.

Saturday, February 19, 2011 (Day 074---81 Flights, 1,134 steps, 18:48)

81 Flights of stairs---I've passed 80, another multiple of 10. And I did so in under 19 minutes. Great job!

The 2011 Philadelphia Fight For Air Climb is exactly one month from today, on March 19th!

Sunday, February 20, 2011 (Day 075---82 Flights, 1,148 steps, 19:37)

82 flights of stairs. I'm feeling good.

My workout time now consists of the climbing itself (19 minutes or so, a 5 to 10 minute cool down period and a 10 minute shower.) That's about 40 minutes to get my work out in.

This is important to know when climbing steps prior to planning to go to church or head out to a movie.

Monday, February 21, 2011 (Day 076---83 Flights, 1,162 steps, 20:31)

Wow, for the first time, I'm over 20 minutes of going up and down the stairs in my house.

I'm sure my wife Linda has noticed, but so far, she hasn't said anything about the obvious signs of wear and tear appearing on the rugs in our stairway and the top of the stairs.

She's an angel ☺

Tuesday, February 22, 2011 (Day 077---84 Flights, 1,176 steps, 20:07)

One more flight of stairs and 24 seconds less than my previous effort. Great job!

Wednesday, February 23, 2011 (Day 078---0 Flights, 0 steps, 0:00)

I ran 5 miles this morning, so no stair climb.

Thursday, February 24, 2011 (Day 079---0 Flights, 0 steps, 0:00)

I ran 5 miles this morning, so no stair climb.

Friday, February 25, 2011 (Day 080---0 Flights, 0 steps, 0:00)

No stair climb.

What was my excuse this time?

After working a full day, we had a family birthday celebration, and with my Stair Climbing workout now taking over 40 minutes, there just wasn't time.

I was concerned what missing a workout three days in a row would do to my next climbing session, but I must admit I was also a bit curious.

I hadn't gone more than 2 days without climbing since I started in December of 2010.

Tomorrow's climb will be interesting.

I'm now 3 flights "behind."

Saturday, February 26, 2011 (Day 081---88 Flights, 1,232 steps, 20:41)

Wow, I must be doing something right. Maybe that rest helped me.

I hadn't climbed any steps since Tuesday (84 flights) and I needed to do 88 today to 'catch up'.

Not only did I catch up (I seem to do pretty well on Saturday afternoons), but my time, for 3 additional flights, was only 34 seconds more.

Great job!

Sunday, February 27, 2011 (Day 082---89 Flights, 1,246 steps, 21:22)

Sunday afternoons are probably my favorite time to climb.

It usually shows in my performance.

89 flights, just 11 flights to go until 100!

Monday, February 28, 2011 (Day 083---90 Flights, 1,260 steps, 21:47)

90 Flights of stairs climbed, another multiple of 10.

And here's an interesting statistic.

Since I started training on December 8th, I have now climbed a total of 3,534 Flights of stairs, a total of 50,212 steps!

Tuesday, March 1, 2011 (Day 084---0 Flights, 0 steps, 0:00)

I ran 5 miles this morning, so no stair climb.

148

We did get good news from our team mate Tim. We'll be able to travel to his Condo and practice on his 25 floor fire escape one more time before the actual climb on March 19th.

We're all anxious to see how we will do.

Wednesday, March 2, 2011 (Day 085---92 Flights, 1,288 steps, 22:47)

92 flights of stairs—wow, it's hard to believe that I'm about a week away from 100. Still in the 22 minute range.

Thursday, March 3, 2011 (Day 086---0 Flights, 0 steps, 0:00)

I ran 5 miles this morning, so no stair climb.

Friday, March 4, 2011 (Day 087---94 Flights, 1,316 steps, 22:52)

94 flights in 22 minutes and 52 seconds. Looking forward to training at Tim's Condo tomorrow.

Saturday, March 5, 2011 (Day 088---92 Flights, 1,656 steps, 14:31)

Tim's Condo.

This was our 3rd practice session at Tim's condo, and while we trained in the basic same way as the other 2 practice sessions, we did mix things up a bit by sprinting to the elevator after our first climb, getting to the first floor as quickly as possible, and then immediately climbing to the top of his building a second time.

In other words, we eliminated as much as possible the rest period we were giving ourselves between climbs.

We figured that this would more accurately simulate the actual climb we'll be doing in exactly two weeks!

Once again, we each did 3 sets of 25 flights, and 1 set of 17 flights (his condo is on the 17th floor).

Overall, I had a 5 second improvement in my times. (14 minutes and 31 seconds.)

My first set was 11 seconds faster than my previous first set.

Here are my times for each of the climbs:

First Set of 25: 3 minutes, 41 seconds.

Second Set of 25: 4 minutes, 11 seconds.

Third Set of 25: 4 minutes and 7 seconds

Fourth Set (17 flights): 2 minutes, 31 seconds

My teammates Bob and Tim both beat me to the top each time.

Each of us is beginning to anticipate what we'll do on actual Climb Day.

I'm hoping to go under 11 minutes.

Bob, Tim and Sophorn are hoping to go under 10 minutes.

My daughter Melissa has no idea.

Sunday, March 6, 2011 (Day 089---96 Flights, 1,344 steps, 23:13)

It's my birthday, and naturally, I'm climbing stairs! 96 flights in a little over 23 minuts. 4 more flights until I hit 100.

96 flights is more than the number of flights in the Hustle Up The Hancock Tower in Chicago. which has 94 flights, but less than the number of steps. The Hustle Up The Hancock has 1632 steps.

Monday, March 7, 2011 (Day 090---0 Flights, 0 steps, 0:00)

I ran 5 miles this morning, so no stair climb.

Tuesday, March 8, 2011 (Day 091---98 Flights, 1,372 steps, 24:22)

98 flights in 24 minutes. 2 flights from 100! It's also been 3 months since I started training back in December.

Wednesday, March 9, 2011 (Day 092---0 Flights, 0 steps, 0:00)

I ran 5 miles this morning, so no stair climb.

Thursday, March 10, 2011 (Day 093---100 Flights, 1,400 steps, 24:20)

100 Flights. I've done it! And I really wanted to do 100 flights in under 25 minutes.

Friday, March 11, 2011 (Day 094---0 Flights, 0 steps, 0:00)

I ran 5 miles this morning, so no stair climb.

Saturday, March 12, 2011 (Day 095---102 Flights, 1,428 steps, 24:42)

What to do if you've reached your goal of 100 fllghts?

Do 102 of course. I don't know when I'll stop.

Exactly 1 week until the actual climb.

Sunday, March 13, 2011 (Day 096---103 Flights, 1,442 steps, 25:00)

For the first time, I've reached the 25 minute barrier.

I had predicted that it would take me about 25 minutes to do 100 Flights, but in actuality, I did it in less, 24 minutes and 20 seconds.

Today I did 103 Flights in 25 minutes. I'm happy!

Monday, March 14, 2011 (Day 097---0 Flights, 0 steps, 0:00)

I ran 5 miles this morning, so no run.

Tuesday, March 15, 2011 (Day 098---105 Flights, 1,372 steps, 25:52)

Yes, it's the IDES of March, but nothing to beware of on the stairs.

I did 105 flights in under 26 minutes.

Only 5 days until Climb Day.

Wednesday, March 16, 2011 (Day 099---106 Flights, 1,484 steps, 26:25)

Climbing two days in a row—106 flights today.

This would be the most flights I would climb, and the longest duration, before Climb Day.

Hopefully you have checked out Chapter 1, where I tell you how much longer I continued to add flights of stairs to my previous day's total.

Eventually, I would work up to 131 flights of stairs, 1834 Steps, in 32 minutes and 53 seconds.

Thursday, March 17, 2011 (Day 100---0 Flights, 0 steps, 0:00)

I ran 5 miles, so no Stair Climbing for me.

Friday, March 18, 2011 (Day 101---0 Flights, 0 steps, 0:00)

I ran 5 miles, so no Stair Climbing for me.

Saturday, March 19, 2011 (Day 102---50 Flights, 1,088 steps, 10:37)

Climb Day! What an experience!

Final results:

Tim Gradoville	31 M	9:09.86
Bob Gauss	48 M	9:24.99
Melissa Smiley	14 F	10:36.15 (2nd place in her age group)
John Smiley	56 M	10:37.82 (9th place in his age group)
Sophorn Smiley	31 F	11:10.97
Nora McCloskey	25 F	22:44.55
Danielle Turner	22 F	22:50.88

Both Nora and Danielle stopped for a bathroom break somewhere between the 20th and 25th floor.

CHAPTER FIVE

Suggested Training Plan Template

I've mentioned several times in the book that I started with 7 flights of stair in my house, then added 1 flight of stairs per day until I was daily doing more than the number of steps in the Philadelphia Fight For Air Climb.

Day	Date	Flights	Steps	Time
1	_____	_____	_____	_____
2	_____	_____	_____	_____
3	_____	_____	_____	_____
4	_____	_____	_____	_____
5	_____	_____	_____	_____
6	_____	_____	_____	_____
7	_____	_____	_____	_____
8	_____	_____	_____	_____
9	_____	_____	_____	_____
10	_____	_____	_____	_____
11	_____	_____	_____	_____
12	_____	_____	_____	_____
13	_____	_____	_____	_____

Day	Date	Flights	Steps	Time
14	_____	_____	_____	_____
15	_____	_____	_____	_____
16	_____	_____	_____	_____
17	_____	_____	_____	_____
18	_____	_____	_____	_____
19	_____	_____	_____	_____
20	_____	_____	_____	_____
21	_____	_____	_____	_____
22	_____	_____	_____	_____
23	_____	_____	_____	_____
24	_____	_____	_____	_____
25	_____	_____	_____	_____
26	_____	_____	_____	_____
27	_____	_____	_____	_____
28	_____	_____	_____	_____
29	_____	_____	_____	_____
30	_____	_____	_____	_____
31	_____	_____	_____	_____
32	_____	_____	_____	_____
33	_____	_____	_____	_____
34	_____	_____	_____	_____
35	_____	_____	_____	_____
36	_____	_____	_____	_____
37	_____	_____	_____	_____
38	_____	_____	_____	_____
39	_____	_____	_____	_____
40	_____	_____	_____	_____
41	_____	_____	_____	_____
42	_____	_____	_____	_____
43	_____	_____	_____	_____
44	_____	_____	_____	_____

Day	Date	Flights	Steps	Time
45				
46				
47				
48				
49				
50				
51				
52				
53				
54				
55				
56				
57				
58				
59				
60				
61				
62				
63				
64				
65				
66				
67				
68				
69				
70				
71				
72				
73				
74				
75				

Day	Date	Flights	Steps	Time
76	_____	_____	_____	_____
77	_____	_____	_____	_____
78	_____	_____	_____	_____
79	_____	_____	_____	_____
80	_____	_____	_____	_____
81	_____	_____	_____	_____
82	_____	_____	_____	_____
83	_____	_____	_____	_____
84	_____	_____	_____	_____
85	_____	_____	_____	_____
86	_____	_____	_____	_____
87	_____	_____	_____	_____
88	_____	_____	_____	_____
89	_____	_____	_____	_____
90	_____	_____	_____	_____
91	_____	_____	_____	_____
92	_____	_____	_____	_____
93	_____	_____	_____	_____
94	_____	_____	_____	_____
95	_____	_____	_____	_____
96	_____	_____	_____	_____
97	_____	_____	_____	_____
98	_____	_____	_____	_____
99	_____	_____	_____	_____
100	_____	_____	_____	_____

CHAPTER SIX
TEAM SMILEY ROSTER

How could I write a book and fail to mention the teammates that inspired me?

Bob Gauss

Age: 48

Residence: Flourtown, PA

What makes him special: An original climbing member of Team Smiley, Bob did his first Stair Climb, the 2011 Philadelphia Fight For Air Climb, 50 floors, 1088 steps, in 9:24, placing him 2nd in the Team Smiley competition behind Tim Gradoville. In addition to Stair Climbing, Bob has also run the Philadelphia Broad Street Run 11 times, and completed 2 Marathons, most recently the inaugural Bucks County Marathon in 3:53. Bob hopes to break the 9 minute mark in his next attempt, hopefully the 2012 Philadelphia Fight For Air Climb.

Bio: In addition to his athletic pursuits, Bob is an accomplished guitarist, playing in his own band.

Quotes:

"I was born on a Friday because I didn't want to miss the weekend.."

Jamie Gradoville

Age:

Residence: Royersford, PA

Why she's special: Jamie was pregnant during the 2011 Philadelphia Fight For Air Climb and was unable to climb, but she did attend the climb and take a bunch of pictures. Additionally, she and her husband Tim graciously offered Team Smiley the use of their 25 floor condo for practice purposes. No word yet on whether Jamie will join us in the 2012 Philadelphia Fight For Air Climb.

Bio:

Jamie is a former High School athlete. Jamie married her husband Tim in January, 2009 and they have a 7 month old son Johnathan Robert born in June of 2011.

Team Smiley anticipates Johnathan's first climb will be in the year 2018.

Tim Gradoville

Age: 31

Residence: Royersford, PA

Why he's special: An original climbing member of Team Smiley, Tim did his first Stair Climb, the 2011 Philadelphia Fight For Air Climb, 50 floors, 1088 steps, in 9:09, placing him first in the Team Smiley competition. Tim started Stair Climbing because it was challenging and different. He had never been much of a runner so Stair Climbing allowed him to compete in a race that wasn't a traditional 5K or 10K. Tim is a former professional baseball player and coach. He looks forward to breaking the 8 minute mark in the 2012 Philadelphia Fight For Air Climb.

Bio: Tim was born in Mechanicsburg, PA and grew up near Denver, CO. He graduated from Creighton University in 2002 with a degree in Management Information Systems. He was drafted by the Philadelphia Phillies in 2002, and played 6 years in the Phillies system earning a big league call-up in September of 2006. He finished his playing career with the Texas Rangers after being traded to them in 2008.

Tim was a big league bullpen catcher and minor league coach for the Philadelphia Phillies in 2009.

Tim is a Board member of a Sports Ministry called Lasting Crown

http://www.lastingcrown.com

Tim married his wife Jamie in January, 2009 and they have a 7 month old son Johnathan Robert born in June of 2011.

Team Smiley anticipates Johnathan's first climb will be in the year 2018.

Training:

Tim trains in the gym all year round, concentrating on the Nautilus StairMaster SM916. as Climb Day approaches.

Links:

http://www.lastingcrown.com

Twitter:

@lastingcrown

Nora McCloskey

Age: 25

Residence: New Jersey

What makes her special: An original climbing member of Team Smiley, Nora did her first Stair Climb, the 2011 Philadelphia Fight For Air Climb, 50 floors, 1088 steps, in 22:44, a time that included a 10 minute restroom break :)

Bio: Nora is a former High School and College Athlete, and now works in a Philadelphia Skyscraper, something that should really help her 2012 Stair Climbs. She is looking forward to competing in the 2012 Philadelphia Fight For Air Climb and has already recruited several new members for Team Smiley.

Jim Smiley

Age: 32

Residence: Philadelphia, PA

What makes him special: He didn't climb in 2011, but he did take a bunch of pictures and lend a lot of moral support, both in Condo practices and on the actual Climb Day. Jim is already signed up for the 2012 Philadelphia Fight For Air Climb. He has run the Philadelphia Broad Street Run 3 times, and completed the Philadelphia Marathon in 2010.

Bio: In his own words...

I was born on April 1st, 1978. I have a 2003 undergraduate degree from Drexel University in Computer Science.

In 2007, my father Bob and I started the Frankford Gazette, a citizen driven hyperlocal blog in Philadelphia.

http://frankfordgazette.com

In June 2008, I married my wife Sophorn. Coincidentally, at the same time I quit smoking after 13 years. I started running while training for the 2009 Philadelphia Broad Street Run (10 mile race) after being inspired by my uncle John.

I've run the 2010 Philadelphia Marathon and am training for future distance runs.

I'm active in Philadelphia's creative technology community and open data movement. I've worked on Knight Foundation projects for North East Philly and currently am at work for one with Technically Philly.

Links:

His Websites:

http://www.frankfordgazette.com

His Blogs:

http://ifatblog.com/
http://teamsmileytraining.com

Twitter:

@jimrsmiley

John Smiley

Age: 56

Residence: Cinnaminson, NJ

What makes him special: The founding member of Team Smiley, John did his first Stair Climb, the 2011 Philadelphia Fight For Air Climb, 50 floors, 1088 steps, in 10:37. In addition to Stair Climbing, he has also run the Philadelphia Broad Street Run 3 times, and in 2010 completed the Philadelphia Half Marathon.

Bio: In his own words...

John is a computer programmer by trade, and has been programming and teaching Computer Science for more than 25 years. He has written over 15 books on Computer Programming.

John is also an Adjunct Professor of Computer Science at Penn State University, Philadelphia University, and Holy Family University, and also teaches in a variety of Internet venues.

In his spare time, he runs, plays basketball, and of course climbs stairs!

He credits his wonderful wife and great family for his inspiration and energy.

Quotes:

"I'd rather sprint up 50 floors in a high-rise than run anything longer than a 5K."

"Many are called, few are chosen, and fewer heed my call to climb the stairs."

Links:

His Websites:

http://www.johnsmiley.com
http://www.johnsmiley.com/main/stairs.htm

Twitter:

@johndsmiley
@jdspublishes
@jdsteaches

Linda Smiley

Age:

Residence: Cinnaminson, NJ

Why she's special: She's John's inspiration, and without her patience, there's no doubt that Team Smiley would not exist. Few wives would tolerate the wear and tear on their carpets that she has. Linda is registered for the 2012 Philadelphia Fight For Air Climb.

Bio: Linda is as beautiful as the day her husband John first saw her in standing next to a filing cabinet at work in November of 1979.

She is a wife and mother to 3 children.

A former athlete, she hits the gym three times a week, and is currently training for the 2012 Philadelphia Fight For Air Climb.

Melissa Smiley

Age: 15

Residence: Cinnaminson, NJ

Why she's special: An original climbing member of Team Smiley, Melissa did her first Stair Climb, the 2011 Philadelphia Fight For Air Climb, 50 floors, 1088 steps, in 10:36, beating her father, John Smiley, by 1 second, good for a 3rd place finish in the Team Smiley competition, and 2nd overall for her age group in the climb. She is registered for the 2012 Philadelphia Fight For Air Climb, and if she climbs in the Elite Category this year, should easily break 10 minutes.

Bio: Melissa is a High School Athlete, currently participating in Soccer, Winter and Spring Track (the 200 and 400 Meter races are her specialty.) She is also a straight-A student, and Recording Secretary for the Sophomore Class.

Training: Melissa gets all the training she needs by participating in High School Soccer and Winter and Spring Track. In addition, she runs 3 to 5 miles several times a week, and does Yoga and stretching.

Sophorn Smiley

Age: 31

Residence: Philadelphia, PA

What makes her special: An original climbing member of Team Smiley, Sophorn did her first Stair Climb, the 2011 Philadelphia Fight For Air Climb, 50 floors, 1088 steps, in 11:10. In addition to Stair Climbing, she has run the Philadelphia Broad Street Run twice, completed 2 Marathons (2010 Philadelphia Marathon, 4:25:29, 2011 Chicago Marathon, 4:10:51,) and one Ultra Marathon, the Hagerstown Maryland JFK 50 finishing in 10 hours, 38 minutes and 16 seconds.

Bio: In her own words...

My name is Sophorn (the "h" is silent; pronounced *Suh-porn*). During the day, I work full time. My life outside my job is a runner and fitness enthusiast. I'm deeply motivated by physical fitness and a running lifestyle. I believe running provides many positive benefits to my life. I started running consistently in February 2009 with my husband Jim (married almost 3 yrs now). I've done many races within the last 2 years since moving to Philadelphia from a small town in Central PA.

I've come to enjoy competitive running.

I love the sense of accomplishment and satisfaction after finishing a race, especially a long distance race such as the Marathon. It's truly a great feeling!

The importance of achieving ultimate life goals and being physically healthy adds flavor to daily living. Thus, I have a passion to maintain a healthy mind, body, and soul. I strongly believe a healthy body requires a healthy mind.

Links:

A Distance Runner From a family that's traveled far

http://www.philly.com/philly/columnists/art_carey/20111205_Well_Being
__A_distance_runner_from_a_family_that_s_traveled_far.html

Her Blogs:

http://la-vida-smiley.blogspot.com/
http://teamsmileytraining.com

Twitter:

@PhornSmiley

Danielle Turner

Age: 23

Residence: New York

What makes her special: An original climbing member of Team Smiley, Danielle did her first Stair Climb, the 2011 Philadelphia Fight For Air Climb, 50 floors, 1088 steps, in 22:50, a time that included a 10 minute restroom break :)

Bio: Danielle is a former High School Athlete, now a school teacher in New York state. She is looking forward to competing in the 2012 Philadelphia Fight For Air Climb and improving upon her time!

CHAPTER SEVEN

Spotlights

I wanted to highlight some people mentioned in the book via these 'Spotlights'. I hope you find them interesting and inspiring. I know I did.

Over the course of the 6 months that it's taken me to write this book, I've encountered a number of really generous, interesting and noteworthy people. Most (but not all) of them have been Stair Climbers, of one kind or other, and I just wanted to take some time to highlight their accomplishments here.

Some people, like **Jennifer Lynn Thanem**, never took a climb in the stairs, but its for people like her, and the hope of saving them, that so many of us climb and raise money for great causes. Climbs are expensive propositions to put on (serving on the 2012 Philadelphia Fight For Air Climb committee has enlightened me in that aspect.) and I couldn't complete this book without putting a young face to a name to a cause. I came upon Jennifer when I was researching a West Coast climb and discovered that, 12 years after her death in 1999 at the age of 13, the Seattle Cystic Fibrosis Foundation Climb is still dedicated to her. Her family and friends didn't forget her, and neither will I.

Chris Solarz, who set the Guinness Book of World Records Record for most flights of stairs climbed in a 12 hour period

Thomas Dold, who captured the 2011 Men's World Cup Title, and in addition, can run a 10K backward faster than most people can run it forward. His backward 1-kilometer (0.6-mile) time of 3 minutes 36.07 seconds is in Guinness World Records.

Cindy Harris, considered by TowerRunning to be the greatest stair climber of all time, is still going strong at age 42. She came in 2nd in the 2011 Women's World Cup Competition. In addition to Cindy, the woman who beat her is highlighted in this section.

I encountered some very competitive older climbers in my research.

Ginette Bedard, a 73 year old Stair Climber from Howard Beach, NY, who took up Marathon Running and Stair Climbing in her 60's!

Shirley Lansing, an 82 year old, who annually climbs the Seattle Tower

But Shirley's not the oldest stair climber I found.

That would be **Chico Scimone**, who died in 2005 at the age of 93, and will never be forgotten for the zest he displayed in completing 16 Empire State Building Run Ups.

And what can you say about a 94 year old Stair Climber **Peng Hung-nian** who says he'll climb until he's 101? Incredible

I also came upon a Stair Climber, **Dwayne Fernandes**, who climbs with prosthetic legs.

My research on Stair Climbing was really helped by some very helpful advocates in the Stair Climbing World.

PJ Glassey, noted Personal Trainer and Stair Climber, who has inspired and trained a bunch of people in the Seattle area. He owns X-Gym and founded the X-Gym Stair Climbing team. It's funny how so many of the best stair climbers in the United States come out of that area, and I think he may be a big reason why. Right now, two of the best Stair Climbers in the world, Kevin Crossman and Kourtney Dexter, are members of his X-Gym team.

Sebastian Wurster and Michael Reichetzeder, who put together the TowerRunning website and The TowerRunning World Cup, both invaluable resources on Stair Climbing.

David Snyder who created both the Yahoo Stair Climbing Group and the Facebook Stair Climbing Group. Both are great resources for Stair Climbers everywhere.

Mark Trahanovsky founded the West Coast Labels Stair Climbing team. Like the X-Gym team noted above, it's another power house of United States Stair Climbers. He gets special mention for his unbridled enthusiasm for the sport of Stair Climbing.

Read on for more detail about them, and others, in this Spotlight section.

Spotlight on Erika Aklufi

Age: 34

Residence: Santa Monica, California

Why she's special: She holds the Los Angeles U.S. Bank Tower Women's record of 10 minutes, 35 seconds, set in 2011. She came in 3rd in her first Empire State Building Run Up in 2011.

Bio: Erika Aklufi is a busy person. In addition to being a phenomenal athlete, she is also an attorney and a Santa Monica police officer. She has a knack of finding new sports to try and producing phenomenal results her first time out.

Links: Here are a couple of great stories about Erika

Hometown Hero Erika Aklufi

http://susancloke.blogspot.com/2010/07/hometown-hero-erika-aklufi.html

Erika Aklufi

http://www.triathloninformer.com/undercovered/erika_aklufi.html

Spotlight on Syd Arak

Age: 66

Residence: Indianapolis

Why he's special: Ranked #7 **All Time** Stair Climber according to TowerRunning.com. He holds the 60-69 Age group record for the Sears (Willis) Tower Climb in 17:54, which he set in 2006.

Bio: A "senior citizen", he's still a force to be reckoned with. He completed the 2010 Indianapolis American Lung Association Climb in 5:04, at the age of 65, and the 2011 Indianapolis Bop To The Top in 5:24 at the age of 66. For good measure, Syd completed the Hustle Up The Hancock (94 floors) in 13:36 at the age of 65. Needless to say, he won his age group, and did so by an amazing 4 minutes. He came in 46th overall

Links: See Syd on the famous Culver City Stairs in this You Tube video

Syd on the Culver City Stairs

http://www.youtube.com/watch?v=mMCVNvtLGBU

Spotlight on Ginette Bedard

Age: 77

Residence: Howard Beach, New York

Why she's special: Ranked #37 **All Time** Stair Climber according to TowerRunning.com. Has competed in 5 consecutive Empire State Building Run Up's, and has won her age group each time. In 2011, she was the oldest participant (male or female), and once again came in 1st in her age group in 22:16. In addition to Stair Climbing, she is the world's faster Marathoner in her age group, and runs a 48 minute 10k.

Bio: Ginette gets up at **4am every day** to run on the beach. She didn't start running until she was 68. She has won 99 of the 101 New York Road Runners events she has entered.

Quotes: "When you retire, life is not just waiting to die. That's why I got involved with the New York Road Runners and the Marathon. There's more to life than getting old."

"Nothing lasts forever, but as long as my body holds up, I'm going to run. It keeps me going. I love the feeling I get from it."

Speaking of the Empire State Building Run Up, she said:

"That was a beautiful experience. It was so easy. I didn't know how to pace myself and so I started too slow. I know I could have gone under 20 minutes if I had known how to pace myself."

"When I got up there, it was like I was on my wedding day. Oh, it was beautiful."

Links:

Marathon Runner Gets Better With Age

http://articles.nydailynews.com/2008-11-01/sports/17910915_1_paula-radcliffe-year-s-marathon-paul-tergat

Interview with Ginette Bedard (includes an audio link)

http://www.maridavis.com/stories_Detail.php?id=8

Spotlight on Omar Bekkali

Age: 32

Residence: Liege, Belgium

Why he's special: Ranked #5 man in the 2011 World Cup Standings according to TowerRunning.com.

Bio: Came in 2nd in the 2011 Empire State Building Run Up Men's Division with a time of 11:25, a minute behind the winner, Thomas Dold.

Spotlight on Valentina Belotti

Age: 39

Residence: Italy

Why she's special: Ranked #7 woman in the 2011 World Cup Standings according to TowerRunning.com.

Bio: Wish I had more...

Spotlight on Jesse Berg

Age: 39

Residence: Chicago

Why he's special: Ranked #11 **All Time** Stair Climber, and #2 man in the 2011 World Cup Standings according to TowerRunning.com. In 2011, he won the Chicago American Lung Association Climb, won the Chicago Step Up for Kids Climb, won the Stair Climb for Los Angeles, came in 2nd in the Willis (Sears) Tower Climb, came in 3rd in the Hustle Up The Hancock Climb, and came in 5th in the Empire State Building Run Up. Not a bad season of Stair Climbing, was it?

Bio: Works as a fitness instructor in Chicago

Links:

Getting Schooled On The Stairs By Jesse Berg
http://www.youtube.com/watch?v=bz1Z1lrh4yI

Spotlight on Cristina Bonacina

Age: 35

Residence: Pontida, Italy

Why she's special: Ranked #1 woman in the 2011 World Cup Standings according to TowerRunning.com. The 2008 Taipei 101 was her first International Climb. She came in 2nd in the 2011 Empire State Building Run Up.

Bio: Ran the 2011 Taipei 101 with her husband Dario.

Spotlight on Hal Carlson

Age: 59

Residence: Aurora, IL

Why he's special: Ranked #9 **All Time** Stair Climber according to TowerRunning.com.

Bio: A "senior citizen", he's still a force to be reckoned with. In 2011, he started off the year by completing the 2011 Indianapolis Bop To The Top Stair Climb in 5:17 at the age of 59, coming in first in his age group and 42nd overall. He came in 2nd in the Hustle Up The Hancock (94 floors) in 12:59. He finished 1st in his age group at the Chicago Fight For Air Climb and ended his year by completing the Skyrise Chicago Climb in 16:43, winning his age group by an amazing 2 minutes. He came in 16th overall.

He's also the Fire Chief of Aurora, IL. He competes with his wife Bridget in Stair Climbs, and she's quite a Stair Climber in her own right.

Links:

Hal Carlson, Fire Chief of Aurora

http://www.aurora-il.org/detail_news.php?newsDateID=519

Spotlight on Sandra Nunez Castillo

Age: 38

Residence: Mexico City, Mexico

Why she's special: Ranked #9 woman in the 2011 World Cup Standings according to TowerRunning.com. Came in 3rd in the U.S. Bank Tower Climb in Los Angeles.

Bio: Wish I had more...

Spotlight on Tomas Celko

Age: 26

Residence: Žilina, Slovakia

Why he's special: Ranked #3 man in the 2011 World Cup Standings according to TowerRunning.com. Came in 7th in the 2011 Empire State Building Run Up.

Bio: Wish I had more...

Spotlight on Paul Crake

Age: 35

Home: Australia

Why he's special: Ranked as the #6 **All Time** Stair Climber by Tower Runing Com. Also holds the Empire State Building Run Up men's record of 9:33, set in 2003, and the Taipei 101 men's record of 10:29, set in 006. Paul won the Empire State Building Run Up 5 times in a row.

Bio: Paul turned from Stair Climbing to Professional Cycling and was tragically paralyzed in a freak biking accident in 2006. Paul believes that one day he will walk again, and I do too. He currently lives in Australia with his wife Daniella.

Quotes:

"Stair running is incredibly psychological. I don't care how strong you are in the stairs, there comes a point when it's a battle to keep running. It becomes almost impossible."

Links:

Crake Excelling In His Biggest Challenge

http://www.canberratimes.com.au/news/local/news/general/crake-excelling-in-his-biggest-challenge/2371590.aspx

Paul Crake Conquered An Empire Then Was Told He'd Never Walk Again

http://www.smh.com.au/news/sport/paul-crake-conquered-an-empire-then-was-told-hed-never-walk-again/2007/01/06/1167777323353.html

Spotlight on Kevin Crossman

Age: 27

Residence: Seattle, Washington

Why he's special: He's the #10 ranked man in the 2011 World Cup Standings according to the TowerRunning. He came in 1st in the Las Vegas Stratosphere Climb, 1st in the Seattle American Lung Association Climb, 2nd in the Chicago Step Up For Kids Climb and 2nd in the U.S. Bank Tower Climb in Los Angeles.

Bio: (In Kevin's own words)

By day I am Investment Analyst working in the real estate industry.

When I am not working or sleeping much of my focus is on the sport of Tower Running.

I finished 10th in the TowerRunning.com World Cup in 2010 and achieved top 5 results in all of all of the tower races I entered from 2010 though June 2011 (with the notable exception of the Empire State Building Run Up).

Some of my other interests include mountain running, inline skating, cooking, nutrition, sustainable agriculture and dancing like MC Hammer.

I was born in Everett, Washington in 1983 (along with my twin brother Brian) and graduated from the University of Washington in 2006 with a BS in Economics and was named a 2006 Outstanding Economics Scholar.

I also minored in Scandinavian Studies and was named That Guy Who Uses Spanish Words In Swedish Class.

Quotes;

"I don't get why people do marathons. They take forever. I don't want to run for three hours."

"I'm just not as passionate about road races as I am about tower races. There's more satisfaction there for me."

"I know I've done a good job of racing if I'm sitting by a garbage can dry-heaving for the next 15 minutes."

"What does it take to be a good stair-runner? Mental toughness. All the best stair-racers are people who can suffer," he says.

You'll generally see the regular folks out of breath, walking at the end of stair race, but "the fastest people, the best people are falling across the finish line."

Links:

His Website:

http://www.kevinclimbs.com/

His Blog:

http://www.kevinclimbs.com/blog.html

Barefoot Ted Interviews Stair Climbing Master Kevin Crossman

http://youtu.be/NlfHvdNeFI8

Forget the elevator, Snohomish's Kevin Crossman Climbs The Stairs Of Iconic Skyscrapers For Sport

http://www.heraldnet.com/article/20110426/SPORTS/704269971

Spotlight on Piero Dettin

Age: 72

Residence: Italy

Why he's special: Ranked #3 **All Time** Stair Climber according to TowerRunning.com. He finished 47th in the 2005 Empire State Building Run Up, and climbed it once again in 2011 at the age of 73. He was the oldest male participant, and came in 2nd in his age group in 18:55.

Bio: Wish I had more...

Spotlight on Kourtney Dexter

Age: 31

Residence: Washington State

Why she's special: She finished first in six United States climbs that I covered for 2011. The Cystic Fibrosis Foundation Climb in Los Angeles, Cystic Fibrosis Foundation Climb in Seattle, the American Lung Association Climb in Bennington, VT, the American Lung Association Climb in Los Angeles, the American Lung Association Climb in Seattle, and the Leukemia Society Climb in Seattle. She finished 2nd in the American Lung Association Climb at the Las Vegas Stratosphere Climb, 2nd in the U.S. Bank Tower Climb in Los Angeles, and 3rd at the Willis (Sears) Tower Climb in Chicago. What a year! She's ranked as the #4 woman in the World Cup Standings for 2011 according to the Tower Running World Cup, and the #49th ranked Stair Climber of **All Time**. That undoubtedly will change as she gets more climbs under her belt.

Bio: She's a graduate of the University of Nevada-Reno and was a personal trainer at the legendary X-Gym for sevrral years.

Links:

2010 San Francisco Bank Of America Climb

http://www.youtube.com/watch?v=WHYNXptSoDk

2011 Bennington Vermont Stair Climb

http://www.youtube.com/watch?v=0a_HoBokFIg

She Came, She Conquered, She Coughed

http://www.seattlepi.com/lifestyle/health/article/1-300-stairs-She-came-she-conquered-she-coughed-1267937.php

Big Climb Seattle 2010

http://www.youtube.com/watch?v=xTG3c4ByKmE

Spotlight on Thomas Dold

Age: 27

Residence: Germany

Why he's special: He's ranked as the #2 **All Time** Stair Climber (behind Cindy Harris) and the #1 man in the World Cup Standings for 2011 according to the Tower Running World Cup. He has won the Empire State Building Run Up a record 6 straight times, including 2011 when he finished in 10:10. He also holds the World Record for running a 10K and 1K **backward**!

Bio: In his own words...

Thomas Dold (born September 10, 1984 in Wolfach, Baden-Württemberg) is a German track and field and extreme athlete and a tower runner, stair runner, world-record holding champion backwards runner.

Dold has competed a number of times in the most prestigious tower run of the world, the Empire State Building Run Up in New York. He first participated in 2005 and finished second. The next year he won the competition, the youngest competitor ever to do so. When he participated the third time on February, 6th 2007 he was able to defend his title. In February 2008 he finished the run with his personal record time of 10 minutes, 8 seconds and won for the third time in a row. He followed it up with another win in 2009 in a time of 10 minutes and 6 seconds.

On June, 15th 2008 Thomas Dold won the tower run up 2,046 steps to the 91st level of Taipei 101, which was the highest skyscraper of the world at that time. It took him 10 minutes, 53 seconds.

Thomas Dold is also part of the world elite in backwards running, the so-called Retro-Running. His greatest success was winning two World Championship titles at any one time in 2006 in Rotkreuz/Switzerland and in 2008 in Pietrasanta/Italy.

Currently he holds 5 world records in backwards running between 400 meters and a mile.

He travels three hours to Frankfurt twice a week to run up the 56-story Main Tower.

Quotes:

"If you take one step, I guarantee you won't win, because there will be another guy who takes two."

Links:

Wikipedia Entry

http://en.wikipedia.org/wiki/Thomas_Dold

His Website

http://www.thomasdold.com/en/

Twitter (it's in German)

@thomadold

Thomas Dold Wins The Empire State Building Run Up For A Record 6th Straight Time

http://www.huffingtonpost.com/2011/02/01/thomas-dold-wins-empire-s_0_n_816958.html

Thomas Dold Interview

http://www.youtube.com/watch?v=EjQ3UWmLZcY

Spotlight on Dwayne Fernandes

Age: 26

Residence: Sydney, Australia

Why he's special: Double Amputee Climber. He did his first Stair Climb in 2008, doing 1504 steps in the Sydney Tower, setting the world record for amputees in 23:49. He since has bettered that record to 20:14. He took part in the Empire State Building Run Up in 2009, finishing with a great time of 26:12.

Bio: In his own words. He is 26 years old (10 May 1985) and is an Indian born Australian who in 2008 ran up his first building being 1,504 stairs of the Sydney Tower, setting his first world record for amputees in 23 minutes and 49 seconds. He has been part of that event in 2009 and 2010, where his new record for double amputees stands at 20mins and 14 seconds. He has partaken in a variety of tower climbs around the world as follows:

Sydney Centerpoint Tower (1,501 Stairs), Sydney
2008 23:45
2009 23.12
2010 20.14

Empire State Building (1,576 Stairs), New York
2009 26.12

Central Plaza Building (1,688 Stairs), Hong Kong
2010 28.05
2011 24.59

Eureka Tower (1,642 Stairs), Melbourne
2010 22.54
2011 24.55

Swissotel Vertical Marathon (1,336 Stairs), Singapore
2010 18.21
2011 19.34

Baiyoke Run Up (2,060 Stairs), Bangkok
2011: 30.11

Vietnam Vertical Run Bitexco Financial Tower (1,002 Stairs)
Ho Chi Minh City
2011: 14.3

His aim to travel to all the major cities and climb all the tall towers and experience the cultures of the world

Dwayne Fernandes does not consider himself to be the fastest of the runners or the fittest for that matter, however believes "life is for living" and "you got to do what you can with what you've got." That is why you will always see him participating in events, from marathons to fun nights out with friends.

He uses his blog to talk about traveling, normal life, extreme sports, amputee issues, dreams, stories, dancing; sponsors, organizers, motivation, work life balance and other sporting related stories.

www.dwaynefernandes.com.au

When Dwayne is not running up buildings you can find him public speaking about at life and motivation. He has completed a university degree in Bachelor of Business (Accounting) and has had a varied career from a Junior Field Reporter for a Television program call "What now?" in New Zealand to being on Board of Directors of the University of Western Sydney Student Association and also a fund raiser for UNICEF and Mission Australia. Some of his pastimes are travelling, rock climbing, golf, riding scooters, photography, indoor soccer, being magician assistant and most of all dancing, lots and lots of dancing.

Dwayne would like to point out that he is available for Public Speaking Engagements. Contact him via his website below.

Quotes:

"1 guy 2 false feet and a lot of towers"

"Life is for living"

"You got to do what you can with what you've got."

Links:

His Website

http://www.dwaynefernandes.com.au/

How To Take On A Tower And Win

http://www.smh.com.au/executive-style/fitness/how-to-take-on-a-tower-and-win-20110329-1cdy4.html

Amputee Takes On Empire State Building

http://blacktown-advocate.whereilive.com.au/news/story/amputee-takes-on-empire-state-building/

Men's Health Interview With Dwayne Fernandes

http://www.menshealth.com.sg/guy-wisdom/mh-interview-dwayne-fernandes

Dwayne Gets Interviewed Prior To Vietnam Vertical Run Climb

http://www.youtube.com/watch?v=5mHBaFvuzhs

Spotlight on Trevor Folgering

Age: 32

Residence: Regina, Saskatchewan

Why he's special: He's founder of StairClimbCanada.com, a valuable resource for Stair Climbers in Canada. Currently ranked #31 in the world. He completed the 2011 Empire State Building Run Up in 13:15, good for 30th place, and was the first Canadian.

Bio: In Trevor's own words

Trevor Folgering, a professional stair climber and fitness trainer based in Regina, Saskatchewan has been climbing stairs and towers professionally since 2006.

He is currently ranked 31st in the world for Stair Climbs, and he is the founder of the Canadian Stair Climb Association.

Trevor's most recent Stair Climbs include the 2011 Empire State Building Run-up, in which he completed the course of 86 stories (1576 steps) in 13 minutes and 15 seconds. Additionally, he has climbed the CN Tower in Toronto eight times, with his fastest time being 11 minutes and 19 seconds up the 144 flights of stairs in the tallest building in North America

Trevor continues to train for the love of fitness and to reach his ultimate goal of completing the CN Tower under the current world record of 7 minutes and 51 seconds and break the World Vertical Stair Climbing Record – Climbing 61,000 feet in under 24 hours.

Trevor trains 6 days a week using a very holistic approach to fitness, one that includes core strength and endurance, cardiovascular training, strength and muscular conditioning as well as postural balancing and flexibility training.

Quotes: "Stair Climbing is a new way to run.

Links:

His Websites

http://www.trevorfolgering.com
http://www.stairclimbcanada.com
http://www.stairclimbmeetups.com

His Blogs

http://optimumlifestylecenter.blogspot.com/
http://stairclimbcanada.blogspot.com/

Spotlight on Kristin Frey

Age: 28

Residence: Schaumberg, IL

Why she's special: She finished first in three United States climbs that I covered for 2011. The American Lung Association Climbs in Milwaukee, Oakbrook Terrace, and Springfield IL. She finished 2nd in the Willis (Sears) Tower Climb, 2nd in the AON Center Chicago Climb, 3rd in the Hustle Up The Hancock, and 7th in the Empire State Building Run Up. She was ranked as the #3 woman in the World Cup Standings for 2011 according to TowerRunning.com.

Bio: Graduated in 2006 from the University of Illinois. Currently, an Environmental Scientist.

Quotes:

"For a lot of us elite climbers, it's under the theory that if you're not collapsing when you get to the top then you didn't push yourself hard enough."

Links:

Her Blog (and it's tremendously good and interesting :)

http://kristinfrey.blogspot.com/

World Record Stair Runner Kristin Frey On 1035 KISS FM

http://www.youtube.com/watch?v=JnW8M19Cfks

CF Climb For Life Chicago 2011

http://www.youtube.com/watch?v=0fkXNKiyh-A

Spotlight on PJ Glassey

Age: 44

Residence: Seattle, WA

Why he's special: Ranked in the top 25 men in the United States according to TowerRunning.com. Founder of XGym.

Bio: Graduated from Seattle Pacific University. Founder and owner of XGym in Seattle. Has trained and worked out with several World ranked Stair Climbers.

Quotes: "Stairclimbing is lower impact than even walking"

"Even people with knee replacement surgery can do Stair Climbing--it's that safe and gentle on the joints---however, it's also one of the hardest events you can do on the muscles, which is good because you get stronger"

"Going up stairs will never make you sore--coming down will."

Links:

His Websites:

http://www.xygm.com
http://www.fightclubseattle.com
http://xgym.com/xtras/stair_training/

Racing To The Top

http://renton.patch.com/articles/racing-to-the-top-8

Seattle Personal Trainer Extraordinare

http://www.dennis-yu.com/seattle-personal-trainer-extraordinare-pj-glassey

His own You Tube Channel

http://www.youtube.com/user/xgym/featured

His Stair Training Guide:

http://www.lungusa.org/pledge-events/wa/seattle-climb-fy12/local/doc/fight-for-air-climb-training-manual.pdf

His Book, Cracking Your Calorie Code

http://www.amazon.com/exec/obidos/ASIN/1436345073/ref=nosim/professorsmileys

2010 Washington Results

http://www.youtube.com/watch?v=U2Kws-gQDtc

Top 7 Techniques For Stair Climbers

http://www.youtube.com/watch?v=oay_hI-4et4

Is Exercise Better Than Prozac?

http://www.westseattleherald.com/2010/11/25/features/exercise-better-prozac

The Science Of Stair Climbing

http://www.docstoc.com/docs/66962119/Stair-Climbing

Columbia Tower Stairs

http://vimeo.com/9950093

AON Staircase Los Angeles

http://www.youtube.com/watch?v=DOCqCB0-rkw

Twitter:

@xygmstairs

Spotlight On Cindy Harris

Age: 42

Residence: Indianapolis, IN

Why she's special: Ranked as the #1 Stair Climber of **All Time** according to TowerRunning.com, and the #2 Women's Stair Climber for the 2011 World Cup Standing according to TowerRunning.com. She holds the Willis (Sears) Tower record for woman, 14:57, set in 2011. She is a 5 time winner of the Empire State Building Run Up, and the American record holder of 12:45 in 2001. She is a 9 time winner of the Willis (Sears) Tower Climb, setting the Women's Record of 14:57 in 2011. She is a 12 time winner of the Hustle Up The Hancock in Chicago, setting the Women's Record of 10:51 in 2008. She is a 17 time winner of the Bop To The Top in Indianapolis, with a Women's record time of 4:26 in 2001.

Bio: Also goes by the name Cindy Moll-Harris. At the encouragement of her father and brother, Harris did her first stair race 23 years ago—the Bop To The Top, held every February at the OneAmerica Tower in downtown Indianapolis. She has since won it 17 times. To train for Stair Climbing, Harris runs 20 to 40 miles each week and stair races several times a week, going up seven to 10 times and taking the elevator back down. She has also run a Half Marathon in the time of 1:21:29.

Quotes:

"I divide the race into three parts and pace myself accordingly. I try not to pay too much attention to where I am. The first third, I relax. The next third, I keep a steady pace. The last third, I see what's left."

Links:

Stair Climber Takes Flight With Top Tips

http://articles.chicagotribune.com/2005-02-27/features/0502270483_1_stair-climbing-anaerobic-workout

Spotlight on Peng Hung-nian

Age: 94

Residence: Taiwan

Why he's special: At the age of 94, on June 5th, 2011, he participated in the Taipei 101, climbing the 2011 Taipei 101 Skyscraper (2000 steps) in 53 minutes and 38 seconds. .

Bio: Vows to continue Stair Climbing until he's 101—there's no reason to doubt him!

Links:

http://www.wantchinatimes.com/news-subclass-cnt.aspx?id=20110606000017&cid=1104

Spotlight on Matthias Jahn

Age: 27

Residence: Germany

Why he's special: Ranked #6 man in the 2011 World Cup Standings according to TowerRunning.com.

Bio: College graduate with a degree in Business Marketing. Enjoys snowboarding, diving, travelling, and everything that includes adrenaline (eg. bungee jumping, skydiving, etc.)

Quotes:

"It is the contrasts, that fascinates me about stair-running : the silence while I fight against my myself in mostly dark and sticky staircases. Also the gigantic view, the fresh air, the excitement at the finish line and the perfect happiness at the end."

"You'll never know how strong you are until you've tried it."

"Always two at a time."

Links:

His website:

http://www.matthiasjahn.com/

Spotlight on Shirley Lansing

Age: 82

Residence: Seattle, WA

Why she's special: She's 82 and she's a dynamo!

Bio: Shirley, a breast cancer survivor, owned a local Seattle company, General Employment Services, from 1957 to 1995. She was Vice President of the Seattle Chamber of Commerce and the second woman admitted to the Rainier Club. She lost her son, a helicopter pilot, in 1991 in the Persian Gulf War. Shirley trains with PJ Glassey, and XGym, in Seattle.

Training: According to Shirley: The way I keep "in shape" is to be very active .. use every opportunity to walk, climb stairs, etc. Only regular routine is with PJ Glassey on Saturdays climbing stairs, then personalized workout in his Alki gym on Sundays. I am thankful I can move easily as many of my age cannot. Since I am not a "racer" I have just begun timing my Saturday climb 40+ floors to get an idea of how to plan for the Columbia Tower in March.

Quotes:

Referring to her climb: "This was a simple thing, not a complicated thing. You just put one foot ahead of the other and up you go. My life has complexities to it, so I was excited to do something simple."

Links:

Woman, 80, Makes 69-story Climb Up Columbia Center With Others For Charity

http://seattletimes.nwsource.com/html/localnews/2011406929_lansing22 m.html

Bellevue woman will be oldest female in Sunday's Big Climb
http://www.bellevuereporter.com/sports/88438627.html

80-year-old woman Is Inspired To "keep marching"

http://bellevue.komonews.com/content/80-year-old-woman-inpired-keep-marching

80 year Old Stair Climber

http://www.youtube.com/watch?v=3w-qD8fOXqU

Shirley's Big Climb 2010

http://www.youtube.com/watch?v=pZC8AliGx_Q

81 year Old Stair Climber

http://www.youtube.com/watch?v=jnyVq5HoDBU

Tackle The Tower Practice Day

http://www.youtube.com/watch?v=H_2Tb-R-nZA

Spotlight on Sproule Love

Age: 40

Residence: Indianapolis, IN

Why he's special: Ranked as the #19 Stair Climber of **All Time** according to TowerRunning.com. Holds the Willis (Sears) Tower record for men, 13:03, set in 2011.

Bio: A graduate of Columbia University, he's Director of Business Development at Bright Power, Inc . He started climbing competitively in 1999. Finished 3rd in the 2005 Empire State Building Run Up. The first year he did it he was thrown into the banister at the start.

Quotes:

"These guys are definitely masochistic," when describing fellow stair climbers "It's basically who can suffer the most."

"It's a great conversation piece. I'll tell people I cross-country ski, run in marathons, do mountain races, and the only thing they'll remember is the Stair Climbing."

Links:

Step By Step, Stair Climbs Succeed

http://articles.orlandosentinel.com/2007-03-17/news/STAIRRACING_1_stair-climbing-races-are-run-empire-state-building

Spotlight on Andrea Mayr

Age: 52

Residence: Austria

Why she's special: Ranked as the #8 **All Time** Stair Climber by Tower Runing Com. Also holds the Empire State Building Run Up women's record of 11:23, set in 2006, and the Taipei 101 women's record of 12:38, set in 2007.

Bio: Primarily a long-distance runner, she also competes in mountain running and cycling. She set her personal best (2:30:43) in the women's marathon on April 19, 2009, winning the Vienna City Marathon. She holds the Austrian records over the half marathon and marathon distances.

Spotlight on Melissa Moon

<u>Age:</u> **42**

Residence: Wellington, New Zealand

Why she's special: Ranked as the #41 Stair Climber of **All Time**, and the #8 woman in the 2011 World Cup Standings according to TowerRunning.com. Won the Empire State Building Run Up in 2010.

Bio: Melissa Moon is a long-distance runner from Wellington, New Zealand. She is a two time World Mountain Running champion and has won 21 New Zealand athletics titles over her career. In 2001 she was named New Zealand Sportswoman of the Year. In 2008 she was named as one of ten Top Young Outstanding Persons of the World Program by the Junior Chamber International. In 2010, Moon won the women's race up the 86 flights of stairs of the Empire State Building Run Up, in a time of 13 minutes and 13 seconds.

She will usually jog five minutes from her home to the Majestic Centre in Wellington, New Zealand.

Quotes:

"I've done marathons, track, mountain running, half marathons and I've got to say this is the hardest thing mentally and physically when you're racing all out."

Links:

Her Website:

http://www.melissamoon.co.nz/

Melissa Moon To Run Up World's Second-tallest Building
http://www.3news.co.nz/Melissa-Moon-to-run-up-worlds-second-tallest-building/tabid/415/articleID/157158/Default.aspx

Empire State Stair Race Draws Pros, Amateurs, And Seniors Up 86 Flights
http://blogs.villagevoice.com/runninscared/2010/02/empire_state_st.php

The Wellington Interview: Melissa Moon

http://www.stuff.co.nz/dominion-post/news/local-papers/the-wellingtonian/3429967/The-Wellingtonian-interview-Melissa-Moon

Melissa Moon Wins 2010 Empire State Building Run

http://authspot.com/thoughts/nzer-melissa-moon-wins-empire-state-building-run/

Dwayne Fernandes, Melissa Moon And Thomas Dold Press Conference For Vietnam Vertical Run

http://www.youtube.com/watch?v=5mHBaFvuzhs

Melissa Moon To Run Up World's Second Tallest Building

http://www.3news.co.nz/Melissa-Moon-to-run-up-worlds-second-tallest-building/tabid/317/articleID/157158/Default.aspx

2010 Empire State Building Run Up

http://www.dailymotion.com/video/xc5a12_empire-state-building-run-up-2010_news

Athletes Run Up Empire State Building In Annual Race

http://news.bbc.co.uk/2/hi/8495030.stm

Kiwi Woman First Up Empire State Building

http://tvnz.co.nz/othersports-news/kiwi-woman-first-up-empire-state-building-3347640

Training Tips:
http://www.melissamoon.co.nz/uploads/media/Melissa_Moon__s_Training_Notes-1.pdf

http://www.vietnamrun.com/training/download/MelissaMoon8WeekTraining.pdf

Spotlight on Terry Purcell

Age:

Residence: Springfield, IL.

Why he's special: Ranked #5 **All Time** Stair Climber by TowerRunning.com. U.S. Bank Tower in Los Angeles Men's Record holder (along with Tim Van Orden) in 9 minutes and 32 seconds. Set his record in 2009. He has won the Chicago Hustle Up The Hancock 8 times.

Bio: Described by some as the Lance Armstrong of Stair Climbing, as of March 2011, Terry had won more stair races than any other racer in the world. Like Chris Solarz, Terry doesn't do a lot of training in the stairs.

Quotes:

"Tell people you ran a marathon and they say, 'Oh, O.K..If I say I ran up the Hancock, people are gob smacked."

"Going out too fast is the biggest mistake that both fit and unfit athletes make," said Terry Purcell. "Most people underestimate how difficult Stair Climbing really is."

"Actual training in the stairs is not an enjoyable experience-it's not like a nice run in the forest. So I try to find other activities to tax the legs and lungs."

"Tower racing is a mental sport. There's this moment when you begin to suffer, and you have a decision: You can slow down, or you can push harder."

"Most guys don't study technique anymore, which is fantastic for me. They may be fitter and have more time to train, but they waste so much energy. I see people wasting it on the turns by taking too many steps. I see people not using the railings well to save your legs. Also, the building messes with your head."

As far as competitors. "The way to kick them in the gut is to surge. But who does that? A guy who's trained to do it for the last six months."

Links:

The Tortoise And The Stair

http://www.outsideonline.com/fitness/endurance-training/The-Tortoise-and-the-Stair.html

Climbing To The Top With Terry Purcell

http://www.podcast.tv/video-episodes/climbing-to-the-top-with-terry-purcell-12832699.html

Breakfast With The Stair Titans

http://www.youtube.com/watch?v=fjlsU1ffCKo

Stair Climbing Becomes Popular Urban Sport

http://www.youtube.com/watch?v=fjlsU1ffCKo

US Bank Tower 2009

http://www.youtube.com/watch?v=mhZvwvc_PVE

US Bank Tower 2009 Pre Race Prep

http://www.youtube.com/watch?v=5HaoJxTVJp4

Helping A Good Cause, One Step At A Time

http://articles.chicagotribune.com/2009-01-22/news/0901200229_1_stair-climbers-aon-center-john-hancock-center

Climbing To The Top With Terry Purcell

http://vimeo.com/9243397

Spotlight on Michael Reichetzeder

Age: 54

Residence: Vienna, Austria

What makes him special: He is the President and founder of TowerRunning.com, one of the most informative and influential web sites in the world of Stair Climbing.

Bio: (In Michael's own words.)

My first encounter with organized sports was back in 1984 when in my hometown Vienna the inaugural Vienna City Marathon was held. My two brothers and me took the challenge, trained as we thought it right and finished some minutes before the 4:15 deadline.

Since then this marathon has become a family fixture and we hope to extend our finishing streak to 29 in April ! Besides marathon in these last nearly three decades I tried and enjoyd all the various facets of running, from 100m sprints within an Everybody Decathlon to 24 hour races. Always having trained according to feeling and without plan my 11 sub3 marathon finishes are the greatest success of my "running career".

The thing I loved most were mountain runs, besides the nature feeling going up fascinated me.

Back in 1997 then fate struck when I competed in my first stair race. It was in Vienna at the Donauturm at an event held yearly since 1992. Initially this Donauturm Treppenlauf for me was just a particularly challenging race. As it was very well organized and offered many goodies I did it again and after my third participation my interest in this special kind of race awoke.

In 1999 the internet just started to spread and I tried to find other stair races on the web. I had a small personal homepage then and just for fun I published there a list of all the races I found. This very first compilation included just ten races – among them two in the US – the Empire State Building Run Up in New York and the Bop To The Top in Indianapolis !

Meanwhile I had realized that stairs are the most effictive way to make altitude and reaching for the top is somehow a basic human desire and stair races fascinated me more and more.

2001 was the year when the domain towerrunning.com came alive and in the following decade the site slowly grew and grew. In this time I have met very interesting personalities, runners and race organizers, most virtual but many of them personally too.

I think that I can say that with all the collected inputs provided from many sources the site has developed into the source of information regarding the sport of Towerrunning. Of course I still regularly compete myself and I´m most proud of finishing on 5th position in the inaugural Mount Everest Stair Marathon in Radebeul, Germany in 2005.

The last big push on the website was – together with its developer Sebastian Wurster – the introduction of the Towerrunning World Cup in 2009.

This worldwide ranking of stair racers motivates athletes to travel and spread the sport. In 2011 the World Cup united 170 races in 25 countries culminating with an official final event in Bogota, Colombia !

Links:

http://www.towerrunning.com

Spotlight on Fabio Ruga

Age: 28

Residence: Italy

Why he's special: Ranked #7 man in the 2011 World Cup according to TowerRunning.com.

Bio: Wish I had more...

Quotes:

Links:

Ruga Rules At Vertical Rush

http://www.mudsweatandtears.co.uk/2011/03/03/ruga-rules-at-vertical-rush/

Millennium Tower Run Up 2011

http://www.runinternational.eu/race-reports/2011/105-2011/587-2nd-millenium-tower-run-up-2011-vienna

UK:Vertical Running Hits London

http://www.itnsource.com/shotlist/RTV/2010/02/09/RTV449410/?v=1&a=0

Reach For The Sky

http://content.yudu.com/Library/A1rpaz/RunningFreeApril2011/resources/37.htm

Spotlight on Chico Scimone

Age: Died at the age of 93 on April 9, 2005.

Residence: Taormina, Italy

Why he's special: Ranked #4 **All Time** Stair Climber according to TowerRunning.com. At age 80, Chico became the oldest person in the world to participate in the yearly Empire State Building Run Up (he did his first one at the age of 72 in 21:13.) In 2005, at the age of 95, he completed his 16th and final Empire State Building Run Up in 49:28, and he did so despite 5 aneurysms in his leg. His 2002 time of 39:09, at the age of 90, set the 90-99 age group record. I hope to live long enough to test it.

Bio: A varied life and career, Chico was an entertainer (piano player) and owned his own farm. He took up Stair Climbing at the age of 80. He practiced by running up the 140 steps of a parking garage four times a day. Also competed regularly in the Mediterranean Super Marathon in Palermo, attributed his feats to a regular life -- up at 6am, followed by a dip in the ocean, a simple breakfast of bread and milk, a long walk, a lunch of cheese and vegetables gathered in his own garden and a beef steak and salad in the evening.

Chico appeared on the David Letterman Show in the mid 1990's. Following the show, Chico discovered he had a daughter he had never met, who just happened to be watching the show the night Chico was on. Chico's friends include Tony Bennett, Jerry Lewis, Benny Goodman, Gay Talese and many others.

A few months before his death, Chico ran up 3 skyscrapers, after which he returned to work playing piano. Chico died on April 9, 2005 in Taormina, Sicily.

At his death the Empire State Building was illuminated for three nights with the Italian colors, in memory of Chico.

Quotes:

He said he had only one medical check-up a year -- the race up the Empire State Building. "If I get to the top, I'm OK," he said.

"Age doesn't matter. The only thing that counts is your spirit. Who you are. How you are. How you move...there aren't any more old people in this world. I don't feel old. The only people who are old are those who consider themselves old."

Links:

No Building Too Tall For These StairMasters

http://articles.nydailynews.com/2005-02-01/sports/18286927_1_empire-state-building-run-up-flights-stairs

The Race To The Top (Empire State Building 2007)

http://www.speakuponline.it/articolo/the-race-to-the-top

Chico And The Run: Empire State Building Hosts Annual Run Up

http://sports.espn.go.com/espn/page2/story?page=darcy/050211&num=0

A Race To The top

http://web.jrn.columbia.edu/studentwork/deadline/2004/empire-parekh.asp

Staying With It

http://www.goswim.tv/entries/903/staying-with-it.html

Racer Wins Empire State Building Crown (1994)

http://articles.latimes.com/1994-02-18/news/mn-24469_1_empire-state-building

94 year old Runner Heads For The Heights

http://mg.co.za/article/2005-01-26-94yearold-runner-heads-for-the-heights

Chico's Tribute Page

http://www.myspace.com/chicoscimone/blog

Spotlight on David Snyder

Age: 49

Residence: Las Vegas, NV

Why he's special: David is ranked in the top 25 US Stair Climbers of **All Time** according to TowerRunning.com. In addition to his athletic endeavors, David wins special mention for advancing the sport of Stair Climbing. About 10 years ago, David created the Yahoo Stair Climbing Group, which has provided help for many years to Stair Climbers, experienced and novices alike. I found it invaluable when I first started out. In addition, he also created and administers the Facebook Stair Climbing Group, which is equally valuable. Finally, he also created **StairClimbingSport.com**, a website with many valuable resources.

Bio: In David's own words..

David Snyder was born on a U.S. Army base in Germany to Jewish American parents, stationed there with the U.S. Army. He is part of a large segment of non-Asian convert Buddhists commonly known as JuBu (pronounced Jew-boos), meaning Buddhists of Jewish heritage.

After earning a Ph.D. from The University of Texas at Arlington in 1989, he taught sociology at Tarrant County College. Later he worked for the U.S. Department of Justice, Federal Bureau of Prisons.

Before working for the Federal Bureau of Prisons, he had to attend the Federal Law Enforcement Training Center (police academy for federal law enforcement positions). He graduated with honors in marksmanship and martial arts.

He left government service to pursue real estate investments and management which he also used to open Buddhist centers in Colorado and Nevada. A former correspondence chess champion he has invented a chess variant known as D-Chess.

Dr. Snyder is a stair climber. He runs one of the two major Stair Climbing websites around the world, promoting the sport of Stair Climbing.

A businessman and Buddhist, his political philosophy includes fiscal conservatism, not wasting money on unnecessary wars, and a mixed economy -- middle-way scope and use of government. The website Peace Through Wealth (www.peachthroughwealth.com) describes his complete political manifesto.

The Ven. Madawela Punnaji, M.D., wrote the Foreword to his bestselling book, *The Complete Book of Buddha's Lists -- Explained.*

David has lived in apartment condo mid-rises and hi-rises most of his life and he loves them. David got into the habit of taking stairs instead of the elevaotr and found it to be the most efficient exercise/sport.

David and his family currently live in a 29 story hi-rise in Las Vegas. David tries to take the 416 steps to the top floor at least three times per day. No wonder he's in such great shape!

Quotes:

"Where else can you get such a strenuous workout in such a short amount of time?"

"It started in high school when I lived on the fifth floor of a five-story building with no elevator," he said. "I had no choice and had to carry books and a bicycle up all the stairs at least twice per day."

Links:

His Website:

http//www.StairClimbingSport.com

Step By Step Stair Climbs Succeed

http://articles.orlandosentinel.com/2007-03-17/news/STAIRRACING_1_stair-climbing-races-are-run-empire-state-building

The Zen Of Stair Climbing

http://www.dhammawiki.com/index.php?title=Zen_of_stairclimbing

The Ecstasy Of The Agony

http://mg.co.za/article/2008-07-03-the-ecstasy-of-agony

Spotlight on Chris Solarz

Age: 32

Residence: New York

Why he's special: Chris is ranked in the top 25 US Men Stair Climbers of **All Time** according to TowerRunning.com. The holder of several Guinness Book Of World Records, on June 25, 2011, Chris Solarz climbed Philadelphia's Bell Atlantic Building (now known as Three Logan Square) 55 times in 11 hours, a total of 33,000 feet to break the Guinness World Record for the "Greatest Vertical Height Climbed in 12 Hours."

Bio: Chris is a 32 year old native of New York. On March 26, 2011, he climbed the stairs from the 2nd floor to the 50th floor a total of 55 times in Three Logan Square (formerly known as the Bell Atlantic Tower), taking the elevator down each time. From 7am – 7pm, Chris covered a total of 2,640 floors or 58,080 steps.

Chris's record attempt was dubbed the "Urban Everest Challenge" because his plan was to surpass 29,029 feet, the height of Mount Everest's peak above sea level.

The previous record was set in 1994 by Russell Gill, who scaled the Rhodes State Office Tower in Columbus, Ohio, 53 times for a cumulative vertical height of 26,712ft.

Chris has considerable experience in both endurance events and stairclimbing races.

He has run nearly 200 marathons and ultra marathons in 30 countries around the world.

He has also run dozens of stair races around the world, and has won 6 Stair Climbs hosted in Philadelphia's Mellon Bank Center and Three Logan Square.

Links:

Chris Solarz Sets Another World Record

http://citycoach.typepad.com/weblog/2011/06/chris-solarz-sets-another-world-record.html

Chris Solarz World Record Stair Climb

http://www.youtube.com/watch?v=b-DeG_N5Twk

Meet the Hedge Fund Manager Who Holds 5 World Records, Including 1 For Beer Drinking

http://articles.businessinsider.com/2011-09-06/wall_street/30128479_1_marathons-wedding-anniversary-subway-challenge

Marathoner To Attempt Stair Climbing Record
https://thephilanews.com/marathoner-to-attempt-stair-climbing-world-record-18055.htm

A Typical Weekend For Chris--2 Days, 3 Events, 2 Victories

http://citycoach.typepad.com/weblog/2010/03/chris-solarz-pictured-here-with-emily-kindlon-after-they-each-won-run-the-rock-in-2008-had-a-busy-couple-of-days-last-week.html

His Record Setting Subway Ride :)

http://www.youtube.com/watch?v=EiLEziw8ItE

Spotlight on Justin Stewart

Age: 24

Residence: Springfield, IL:

Why he's special: Ranked as the #9 Men's Stair Climber in the 2011 World Cup Standings according to Towerrunning. He finished 1st in 6 Stair Climbs that I covered for 2011: The Milwaukee Cystic Fibrosis Foundation Climb, the Seattle Cystic Fibrosis Foundation Climb, the Bennington Vermont American Lung Association Climb, the Los Angeles American Lung Association Climb, the Springfield IL American Lung Association Climb, and the St. Louis American Lung Association Climb. He came in 10th in the Willis (Sears) Tower Climb in Chicago.

Bio: Studied at Eastern Illinois, University. Is currently a High School Cross Country Coach.

Links:

2011 Milwaukee Stair Climb US Bank Building

http://www.youtube.com/watch?v=MFVHhyw1M-U

Justin Stewart Howe Street Stairs Record

http://www.youtube.com/watch?v=oFDV0U97dTE

Hilton Stair Workout With Justin Stewart

http://www.youtube.com/watch?v=3Gy4OEWoI6E

His own You Tube Channel

http://www.youtube.com/user/JTStew8001/feed

Jacobs Ladder Training With Justin Stewart

http://www.youtube.com/watch?v=lLrVSMODZOU

Tabata Bike Workout With Justin Stewart

http://www.youtube.com/watch?v=_1o9XNxi4Us

2011 Bennington Vermont Stair Climbing Results

http://www.youtu.be/watch?v=0a_HoBokFIg

2011 Washington Mutual Stair Climb-Seattle

http://www.youtube.com/watch?v=OQbO6eNo1q4

Springfield, IL American Lung Association Stair Climb 2012

http://www.youtube.com/watch?v=tHQbV70ZUYY

Stair Climbing Workout With Justin Stewart

http://www.youtube.com/watch?v=hrOj4mA1c9s

Culver City Stairs 4.0

http://www.youtube.com/watch?v=d_AyXi1ew6I

Jacob's Ladder Workout-First Time On the Ladder

http://www.youtube.com/watch?v=D2Nn2fQjwZc

First Time On Jacob's Ladder

http://www.youtube.com/watch?v=NqW0EhLjSJI

43 Flights Of Stairs Challenge

http://www.youtube.com/watch?v=z5nsqXfX0-A

Spotlight on Mark Trahanovsky

Age: 52

Residence: Yorba Linda, CA

Why he's special: Ranked as the #34th Stair Climber of All Time. Ranked #27 in 2011 Tower Running World Cup Standings according to Towerrunning. 50-59 Fastest Time Age Group Record at the YMCA U.S. Bank Building in Los Angeles. Founder and Team Captain of the West Coast Labels/X-Gym/Running Raw Stair Climb Team. In 2011, Mark finished 1st in two climbs I follow: the Pittsburgh American Lung Association Climb and the San Diego American Lung Association Climb.

Bio. In his own words…

Mark has been Stair Climbing since 2007, and has done 30 Stair Climbs to date.

When Mark Trahanovsky, an avid and world ranked stair climber who has resided in California for the last 28 years did Pittsburgh's 2009 Stair Climb he considered this his hometown stair climb. You see, Mr. Trahanovsky is originally from Johnstown, PA and lived in Pittsburgh in the late '70s when he attended the Art Institute of Pittsburgh.

Back then, Mark was amazed with Pittsburgh's tall buildings and even remembers one sunny spring day when he and a fellow classmate snuck through an unlocked door and went up on the roof of a 40 story Liberty Avenue Skyscraper where they ate lunch and enjoyed the view.

Little did Mark know that over 30 years later he would be enjoying many other rooftop views from skyscrapers all over the country.

Interestingly, Mark did not do his first Stair Climb until the fall of 2007. He'd had an unexpected knee surgery caused by years of running and was forced to find a non-impact form of exercising. A running friend of Mark's told him of an upcoming 75 floor Los Angeles stair climb, and with trepidation and intimidation Mark competed in that event and managed to get a 3rd place age group finish. That day he was hooked!

Since then he has done 25 Stair Climbs across the USA including Chicago's 103 floor Willis (Sears) Tower, formally known as the Sears Tower, Denver's challenging high altitude building race and recently New York City's prestigious 86 floor Empire State Building Run Up.

As a busy husband (married to Valerie), a father of 2 younger children (Amanda, age 9 and Torrey, a boy age 12), a printing sales rep for West Coast Labels in Orange County, CA and a volunteer advisor in the sport of Stair Climbing, Mark is an example that we all can still find time to exercise.

Trahanovsky believes this sport only requires 20 to 30 minutes max per day, 4-5 days a week to become very fit and well conditioned.

He always encourages cross training workouts such as spinner bike, regular bike, elliptical machines, raised treadmill, jump rope and stepper machines. This cross training brings variety to an exercise plan and prevents physical and mental burnout.

Over the past couple of years he has seen many others become physically fit and lose weight via Stair Climbing and its training.

Mark's older sister Jane is proof of that.

Since getting into this sport about two years ago, she has lost over 80 lbs.

Quotes:

"Use the rails, train hard , eat right and sleep to rebuild."

"The best thing about the sport is it fits a busy lifestyle," said the fulltime salesman and father of two. "This sport (takes) 30 minutes a day for incredible fitness. I am the same weight that I was in high school."

"There is no impact (in Stair Climbing) on your knees," Trahanovsky said. "The body is meant to climb."

Links:

7 Climbing Tips From Mark Trahanovsky

http://pittclimb.blogspot.com/2011/02/7-climbing-tips-from-mark-trahanovsky.html

West Coast Labels

http://www.youtube.com/watch?v=0FFb1F19Gsw

He Never Takes The Elevator Up

http://www.ocregister.com/articles/trahanovsky-236309-stair-climb.html

Willis (Sears Tower Climb

http://www.youtube.com/watch?v=Xv26mGY2SIM

Twitter

@labelsone

Spotlight on Tim Van Orden

Age: 43

Residence: Bennington, Vermont

Why he's special: Ranked #10 **All Time** Stair Climber according to TowerRunning.com. U.S. Bank Tower in Los Angeles Men's Record holder (along with Terry Purcell) in 9 minutes and 32 seconds. Set his record in 2009. Came in 4th in the 2011 Empire State Building Run Up. He is also was named, for the second year in a row, the Masters Mountain Runner Of The Year, and the USA Masters Trail Runner Of The Year.

Bio: Known as "Tivo" to his friends, Tim is an accomplished runner and climber. In 2005, he started the Running Raw Project, a grand experiment in diet and athletic performance. He sought to answer a simple question: Can one be an athlete while eating a 100% raw vegan diet? Tim's answer: a resounding YES!

Links:

TiVo's 2nd Run Up The Bennington Monument Stairs 2011

http://www.youtube.com/watch?v=H3rb3WSZc2c

Vegan Athlete Tim Van Orden

http://www.organicathlete.org/vegan-athlete-tim-vanorden

After 30 years, Bennington Battle Monument Opens 'iron steps'

http://www.vpr.net/news_detail/85105/after-30-years-bennington-battle-monument-opens-ir/

The Only Way Is Up

http://www.guardian.co.uk/lifeandstyle/2008/jun/03/healthandwellbeing.features

Big Climb Start And Finish

http://www.youtube.com/watch?v=sd3ZVlIawYM

Culver City Stairs

http://www.youtube.com/watch?v=SLxfTgWFbVU

Tim Van Order's You Tube Channel

http://www.youtube.com/user/runningraw

Bisbee 1000 - The Course 10/17/08

http://www.youtube.com/watch?v=MvA5JTAc5ew

2010 AON Climb Results

http://www.youtube.com/watch?v=oGCWP8Tsln0

2011 Bennington Monument Stair Race Results

http://www.youtube.com/watch?v=0a_HoBokFIg

Tim Van Orden's Website

http://www.runningraw.com/

Tim Van Orden's Blog

http://www.runingraw.com/blog

Spotlight on Sebastian Wurster

<u>Age:</u> 24

Residence: Germany

Why he's special: He's the Developer and Manager of the TowerRunning World Cup Ranking System.

Bio: Sebastian is currently studying for a degree in Medicine, Sebastian also works with Michael Reichetzeder as the Sports Director of TowerRunning Office Vienna. He is the Developer and manager of the Towerunning World Cup Ranking System.

Read more about Michael Reichetzeder and Sebastian Wurster, the TowerRunning administrators, in Chapter 7.

Links:

http://www.Towerrunning.com

CHAPTER EIGHT

Frequently Asked Questions

I had a bunch of questions before my first climb, and here I've catalogued nearly everything I can think of in 100 Frequently Asked Questions and answers.

General Questions about Stair Climbs

#1. Is the Climb a race?

Only if you want it to be.

While there are individuals who run up the stairs as fast as they can, most Stair Climbs are charitable events and welcome individuals of all athletic abilities.

You can either race as an <u>Elite Climber</u> (climbing for a time) or run or walk up the stair and go at your own pace.

#2. Why do the Climb Organizers call it a climb when we actually walk or run up?

The popular term, when it comes to going up stairs, is to say you climbed them.

Makes sense to me.

#3. Where can I find a list of buildings to climb?

<u>TowerRunning.com</u> maintains a calendar of Stair Climbing events here in the United States and also world wide.

You can also find a list of 95 U.S. Stair Climbs here in the book in Chapter 11.

#4. How difficult is this Stair Climb going to be?

If you are properly trained, it could be a walk in the park. If you're not properly trained, it could be tough.

If you were telling me you were going to run a Marathon, I would say it was going to be the hardest thing you've ever done.

However, for a Stair Climb, it's most likely going to be a 10 to 20 minute climb to the top.

It will be strenuous, but it's not 26 miles, and it's not going to last 2 hours.

#5. Will my legs hurt?

They shouldn't hurt, but your legs will burn a bit, along with your lungs.

Stair Climbs are a wonderful way to <u>temporarily</u> appreciate the pain that a sufferer of lung disease feels every day/hour of their lives.

Your discomfort will be over in 10 to 20 minutes.

#6. Has anyone ever died doing a stair climb?

To my knowledge, no one has died participating in an organized stair climb, but let's face it, it could happen.

Sadly, sometimes people die pursuing things they enjoy (love).

#7. Do you have a list of tall buildings in which I can train?

I wish I did, I've been trying to find one myself.

Finding a tall building to train in can be very tricky.

If you live in a tall building, you're in great shape. Just head out the door of your condo or apartment and start walking or running up the stairs.

If you work in a tall building, most likely you'll be able to practice in the fire escape either at lunch or after work. Scout out the fire escape and see if you can practice there.

Using a building in which you neither live or work will be a problem.

Most building managers will not permit strangers to enter their building and climb up and down the stairways.

Even if you a registered climber in an event, the managers of the event will most likely not be able to get you permission to train in the Climb Day Building. That's the case with the Philadelphia Fight For Air Climb.

But you can get creative.

Tall hotels and hospitals have stair ways that you may be able to use.

If you can't find a 50 floor building to practice in, you may be able to find a 5 floor building that is more accessible---just be careful when training alone.

As you probably know by now, I do most of my training in my house, but going up 5 floors at once can be very beneficial.

#8. What kind of training should I do?

For a stair climb, I think it's important to climb steps, and most of the best Stair Climbers in the world agree with me. To prepare for an organized Stair Climb, nothing does it like actually going up and down real stairs.

If not high stairs, then stairs in your house.

If you can't do that, then machines like the StairMaster or Jacob's Ladder.

I do my training in my house, with an occasional climb in a 25 story condo—which is really helpful.

However, Chris Solarz, the Guinness Book of World Records record holder for stairs climbed in a 12 hour period doesn't climb a lot of stairs. Most of his training is in the form of running.

For more on Chris's training advice, Check out Chapter 9.

Questions About Registration

#9. Do I need a Credit Card to register?

Not necessarily.

Even in today's world of the Internet, it's still possible to register for a Stair Climb by printing out a registration form and mailing in a check.

However, some Stair Climbs are no longer displaying a print application on their Web Site, so you may need to call them and have them either email or mail a print application to you.

But be warned.

For the most part, it's an Internet world and Credit Card registration via the Internet is the way the world is going.

#10. Can I get a refund if I am unable to attend the climb?

Most Stair Climbs consider their climb to be a fund raising event, and take a hard line on issuing refunds.

The bottom line: Be sure you can participate before you register and pay a registration fee.

#11. Can I walk up and register on Climb Day?

If the climb isn't one where the maximum number of participants has already been reached, then the answer is yes, in most cases you can.

However, if you are permitted to register on Climb Day, you will need to pay not only the Registration fee, but you will need to pay any minimum fund raising requirement on the spot as well.

#12. What is a Pledge Minimum?

A Pledge Minimum is an amount of money that the Stair Climb participant agrees to raise, in donations, over and beyond the Registration Fee.

For many Stair Climb events (particularly those sponsored by the American Lung Association,) the Registration Fee is $25 and the additional pledge minimum is $100.

The organization doesn't care if the Stair Climber pays the Pledge Minimum themselves or if they ask friends and family for it, but you won't be able to climb unless you have raised it by Climb Day.

Why so strict about the Pledge Minimum?

Most Stair Climbs are organized by Charitable Organizations, and for just about all of them, the Stair Climb is their biggest fund raiser of the year. A Pledge Minimum is their way of raising money for their cause.

Since the Charitable Organization is the one sponsoring the climb, finding a building to host it, obtaining volunteers to run it, arranging for an event timer, and providing post event food, awards and prizes, it makes sense for them to impost some sort of minimum pledge amount.

Some Stair Climbs have no minimum Pledge donation beyond the Registration Fee, but the Registration fee is higher. It's generally a tradeoff.

Many of my Stair Climbing friends don't like to ask friends and family for donations to go toward the Pledge minimum, and just pay it themselves.

My feeling is that I only ask friends and family to support one charitable venture a year. As for me, I donate to worthy causes all year long, so I'm not shy about asking friends and family to donate on my behalf, but again, I do this just once a year.

By the way, just to be sure you saw it, I'll repeat.

Most climbs won't permit you to participate in the climb unless you raise the minimum donation by the morning of the Climb.

Some, that may permit you to participate in the climb, may ban you the following year.

If you paid your Registration Fee with a Credit Card (and most of us do,) you may have 'agreed' to have your Credit Card billed for the difference between the Pledge Minimum and the amount you have raised by the morning of the climb.

#13. Where can I hand in donations?

For charitable climb events, there are ample opportunities for you to mail or make donations by credit card prior to the climb.

Of course, you can always bring donations with you on the day of the climb, and just about every climb will gladly accept donations for several weeks <u>after</u> the climb is completed.

#14. Can I get a receipt for my donors?

All donations are tax deductible, and all donors will receive a thank you acknowledgement to be used for tax purposes. Additional donor receipts can be downloaded from the event website.

Questions About Training

#15. Is two months enough time to train for my first Stair Climb?

That's really hard to say, since it depends on your current fitness level.

I've seen some Stair Climbers say that if you can currently walk a 5K (which is 3.1 miles), you can do a 30 story climb.

If that describes you, that is you can walk about 3 miles now, then with 2 months of additional training, you should be able to handle 50 floors.

Using my Training Plan, presented in Chapter 4 and 5, I believe that most people can go from couch to 100 flights of stairs in their house in 100 days.

60 days takes you to 60 flights, probably about 700 steps or so, which may be enough to prepare you for a 30 story climb.

#16. Should I try to do a Stair Climb if I haven't trained?

Unless you're a world class athlete and currently at the top of your game, I wouldn't. Even if you run regularly, do a lot of hill work, and consider yourself to be in great shape, running up stairs is something you don't want to do without at least a little practice---even if it's just a matter of running up 5 flights or so without stopping to gauge your pace for Climb Day.

If you're anything other than the type of athlete I just described in the previous paragraph, trying to do a Stair Climb without properly training for it is foolish.

If you're young, you may be able to suffer through it, but what's the point in that.

Take the time to prepare properly and enjoy yourself on Climb Day.

#17. I am concerned about injury, especially my knees.

You probably need not be too concerned.

Climbing up stairs is considered a low impact activity, just a bit more strenuous on the knees than walking..

You only need to lift your foot up to the next step (or 2nd step if you are climbing every other step).

So there is not the jarring of your legs and knees as you may experience with regular running.

#18. I'd love to climb, but my knees are 'bone on bone'.

A lot of people with sore knees self diagnose arthritic conditions. Get your knees checked out by an Orthopedist to get a true diagnosis. According to the Arthritis Foundation, only an X-Ray can confirm a diagnosis of Osteoarthritis of the knees..

If your knees truly are 'bone on bone', you need to consider a knee replacement so that you can join us next year :)

#19. Is it "OK" to just go into a tall building and begin a training session? Is it customary to ask permission from the facilities manager or other?

In these days of tight security, it can be difficult to find a place to train.

If you find a tall building that looks promising, most likely there will be Security Desk with a guard. If you ask permission to climb in the stair well, I can almost guarantee you that the answer will be no.

If you enter the building, and there is no Security Desk, and you see a stair well, give it a try.

The worse that can happen is that you will be asked to leave.

Remember, though, that many of the people who enter and successfully complete Stair Climbs do not practice on stairs in a tall building.

If you follow my advice, just going up and down the stairs in your house will be enough for you.

If you can add a training session or two in a high rise to build your confidence, and to give you an idea as to how you'll feel on Climb Day, all the better.

#20. Do you recommend a StairMaster as a good way of training?

Again, nothing is as good as training on actual stairs, in a high rise, followed by training on stairs in your house.

If you can't use actual stairs, then the stair machines in this order are best: Jacob's Ladder, StepMill, StairMaster. My team mate Tim swears by the Nautilus StairMaster SM916.

I really don't think stepper machines are a good simulation of climbing stairs, but it does get your heart pumping, and works your legs which is a good thing.

#21. What's your opinion of Machines versus Real Steps?

I like real stairs. High rise stairs, and if that's not possible, then stairs in your house.

I just don't think that stepper machines are a good simulator for actual steps.

PJ Glassey, a premier Stair Climber and owner of the X-Gym in Seattle, says the best stepper machine is an incline trainer, with a 40% incline.

Something called a Jacob's ladder intrigues me---I saw it featured on the Biggest Loser, and I have several video links to it in Chapter 16.

#22. How long will it take to get ready for a 50 floor Stair Climb?

According to my training plan, about 100 days :)

#23. What do you think about while you are climbing stairs?

While training, primarily, I think about when I will be finished :)

I also calculate my percentage rate of completion. For instance, if I'm doing 100 flights, when I finish 20 flights, I know I'm 20 percent done. I tend to note the 20, 25, 33, 50, 66, 75 and 80% thresholds. After 80 flights, I just try to hold on and finish.

On Climb Day, there's a lot more adrenaline flowing and I tend to think only of the finish. One thing I don't do on Climb Day is count flights of stairs.

I may say hello to the volunteers that I pass by.

I may wonder about the person I hear ahead of me or the person grunting behind me, but that's pretty much it.

If I remember to do so, I hit the Lap button on my iPhone Stop Watch app every 10 floors.

#24. I know what's considered an average, a good and a fabulous time for running a 5K. What are the equivalent times for a Stair Climb?

Good point. Runners tend to know what an average, good and fabulous 5K time is when they see it.

Because the 'distance' climbed in a Stair Climb is variable, based on the number of floors, there is no single standard 'fabulous' time for a Stair Climb, but again, experienced Stair Climbers will know it when they see it.

Famous climbs, such as the Empire State Building Run Up or the Willis (Sears) Tower Climbs have established, well publicized record times for getting to the top that experienced climbers have committed to memory.

For instance, the record for the Empire State Building Run Up is 9:33 for men, set by Paul Crake in 2003 and 11:23 for women, set by Andrea Mayr in 2006. For more records, check Chapter 14.

In general, top Stair Climbers will get to the top of a 50 story building in 5 to 6. The men's winner of the 2011 Philadelphia Fight For Air Climb, David Tromp, got to the top in 5:45. He was climbing 10 floors in just a little over a minute, or one floor every 7 seconds or so. That's quite a pace.

In comparison, my time up the Bell Atlantic Tower was 10:37, almost twice his time and his pace. My per floor average was about 14 seconds. Still, my time was good for 9th overall in my age group and within the range of what the Climb organizers consider an Elite Climber.

I hope to better that this year with a better technique on the handrails :)

#25. Has anyone ever trained for a Stair Climb by walking up the down escalator?

Interesting question.

No one I know has done this, but it does sound like a fabulous idea.

The big problem, I guess, where can you find a down escalator that doesn't have people coming down it?

Maybe if you're a Security guard in a building or a mall somewhere?

#26. Have you tried training with weights while running up stairs? Like 2 or 3 pound dumbbells?

I have mixed feelings about this.

If the extra weight was solely giving you extra cardio conditioning, I would jump at this. However, the extra weight may also be placing extra strain on your knees and ankles as you climb the stairs.

Remember, I've proclaimed Stair Climbing to be less impactful than running---but that's when you're carrying just your body weight up the stairs. Adding extra weight to me seems risky---although I know plenty of people do it. Most of those using extra weight are carrying a weight vest.

One day, just to experiment, I carried two 20 pounds dumbbells with me for a trip up the stairs---wow, did I feel that in my knees, and that's the key there. In the knees.

Granted, it wasn't a 2 or 3 pound dumbbell, which I would hardly feel---but if I can hardly feel it, why bother?

#27. Is there a way to make practice climbing harder?

Well, as I said above, you can try a weighted vest.

But rather than making your practice harder by carrying extra weights try this.

Like a runner doing speed work, a Stair Climber can make their workouts more intense by running sprints up the stairs for fewer floors than normal, and repeat this several times during their workout.

Another suggestion I've seen is to 'hop', double-legged up the stairs. Among others, Olympic Speed Skater Apolo Ohno hops up stairs to get an intensive leg workout. Check out how the Olympic Speed Skaters use stairs to build their power in this YouTube video

http://www.youtube.com/watch?v=CSlthImZWIk

#28. Will there be a practice climb in the actual Climb Day building?

Unfortunately, practice climbs in the Climb Day building are extremely rare.

For liability reasons, very few organizations have practice climbs in the actual building prior to Climb Day.

Some Stair Climbs offer practice sessions at local gyms, or with trainers, but these aren't the real thing. Nothing prepares you for climbing up the stairs of a skyscraper than actually doing it!

My survey of organized Stair Climbs shows that very few offer organized practice climbs. Here are the ones I've found.

American Lung Association Climb of Hartford, CT

American Lung Association Climb of New Haven, CT

American Lung Association Climb of Providence, RI

American Lung Association Climb of Stamford, CT

American Lung Association Climb in Tampa, FL

The AON Climb in Los Angeles

Some organizations that offer practice climbs require a donation to the charity to participate. Some require that you have already achieved some level of fundraising.

Questions about the Climb Itself

#29 How does the Climb work?

Basically, you stand in line, wait for your turn to go, then run or walk up the stairs..

As you begin the climb, you (and your timing chip) cross over a timing mat that records your starting time. Avoid tripping over it :)

Water stations and rest stops are provided periodically through the building (roughly every 10 floors) and Medical Personnel are stationed throughout also.

The stairwells are well lit, very clean (usually cleaned and 'dusted' sometime during the week and ventilation and air conditioning will blow down the stairwell so you don't overheat.

Because of the Air Conditioning and Ventilation fans, the thing you may notice most about the stairwells will be the noise.

#30. How long will the Climb last?

Stair Climb events can last all day long.

Stair Climbs in Los Angeles and Chicago, which tend to have the most climbers, start at 8 in the morning and last until at least 3 pm.

The 2011 Philadelphia Fight For Air Climb started at 8:30 am and the last climbers were off and finished by about noon.

Individual Climb times will vary based on the number of floors you are climbing and your conditioning.

I finished the 50 floor Philadelphia Fight For Air Climb in 10 minutes and 37 seconds. Some of my teammates took 20 minutes.

The winner go to the top in 5 minutes, 45 seconds.

Some Elite Climbers got to the top in 6 minutes.

Other climbers took about 40 minutes to complete the climb.

This much you can be certain of. It will take you a lot less time to do the city's Stair Climb than it would take you to finish their Marathon :)

#31. How many floors and steps are there in a Climb?

That depends on the particular climb you are doing.

In Chapter 11 of this book, I list the 95 major U.S. Stair Climbs with the number of floors and steps in each.

Most organized climbs are at least 30 floors, and at an average of 20 steps per climb, that would be about 600 steps.

Most tall Commercial Buildings will have some steps (10 or more), then a landing, then another set of steps for each floor.

In the Philadelphia Fight For Air Climb, held in Three Logan Square (previously known as the Bell Atlantic Tower) there are 1,088 steps over the course of 50 floors. The building configuration was 10 steps, a landing, then 10 more steps per floor.

Some tall buildings have less steps as they approach the top.

The Chicago Sears (Willis) Tower is like this, and the Empire State Building (because it is an older building) varies quite a bit in its stair configuration over the course of the building.

You may have read Stan Schwartz's information about Mechanical Floors in Chapter 3. Mechanical Floors are taller than ordinary floors, and therefore have more steps in them.

The American Lung Association Climb in Las Vegas is held in the Stratosphere Tower—its staircase is open air, and the tower itself is the equivalent of a 108 floor building.

On average, expect to climb about 20 steps per floor in a modern skyscraper.

#32. How long will it take me to climb to the top of the building?

Mainly, it depends on how many floors you will be climbing.

During my 2011 Philadelphia Fight For Air Climb, I reached the top of the building in 10 minutes and 37 seconds. Put another way, I climbed 10 flights of stairs every 2 minutes, about 1 flight of stairs every 12 seconds.

Depending upon your fitness level and experience, your time per floor may be more or less, but this can give you a rough rule of thumb for you to estimate your climb time.

#33. How steep are the steps in a high rise fire escape?

My first inclination is to say 'not very'.

Building Codes dictate the steepness of stairs in a Commercial fire escape. Residential Buildings can be even steeper.

The steepness (or slope) of a stairway is dependent on the height of the steps (referred to as riser height) and the tread depth, or how deep the step is.

Commercial Building Codes in the United States dictate a riser height of between 5 and 8.5 inches. This, in combination with the tread depth, would tell you how steep the stairs are.

Building Codes also specify the variance permitted in a stairway.

Building Codes dictate that the slope of a stairway is not permitted to change within a floor. Stair climbers get 'used to' the slope of a stairway, and changing it suddenly could cause them to trip.

As you make your way to the top of a building, particularly a very tall building, expect the slope of the stairs to change as you make your way to the top.

I've heard there are great variations in the Empire State Building (I was hoping to find out myself in 2012, but I wasn't selected for the Empire State Building Run Up.)

For the 2011 Philadelphia Fight For Air Climb, we climbed 50 floors with 1,088 steps.

That's about 20 steps per floor, 10 steps, a landing, plus 10 more steps.

I didn't notice any variation in the slope during my 50 floor ascent to the top.

However, Stan Schwartz, in Chapter 3, mentions that Mechanical Floors will have an additional step or 2.

#34. Do any of the Stair Climbs offer a breakfast?

Only one Climb that I've been able to find offers breakfast.

In 2011, the Reno, NV American Lung Association Climb offered a pancake breakfast prior to the climb.

#35. What is a vertical mile?

A vertical mile consists of multiple climbs which, in height climbed, add up to 1 mile.

Some events present this option as an added challenge to the climbers (as if climbing 50 to 100 floors of a building isn't enough?)

The Cincinnati American Lung Association Climb offers a vertical mile challenge.

#36. Can teams do the Climb Relay Style?

Relay Style means that individual members of a team climb some of the floors in the building, but not all of them.

For instance, John may climb floors 1 through 10, Rita 11 through 20, Gil 21 through 30, Leona 31 through 40, with Bill finishing the climb by doing floors 41 through 50.

Climbing Relay Style is nice in that it allows people who can't complete the entire climb to be part of the experience.

However, for logistical reasons, most climbs DO NOT permit relay style climbs---it would require that members of the relay team be in place at specific stair locations prior to the first climber going up.

For timing purposes, it would also require multiple timing chips and multiple timing mats.

The only climb that I'm aware of that offers a Relay Option is the Chicago American Lung Association Climb up the Presidential Towers.

In fact, that event, has more Climbing options of any climb I've covered.

Check Chapter 11 for more information about the Chicago event, including a link to the event Web Site.

#37. What does "Full Gear" mean to the First Responder Challenge?

Climbers who complete in either an Individual or Team First Responder Challenge (some events call them Firefighter challenges,) are expected to wear official firefighter gear: helmet, mask, suit, boots, tank. Everything except for the ax. This is called "Full Gear." See the picture below.

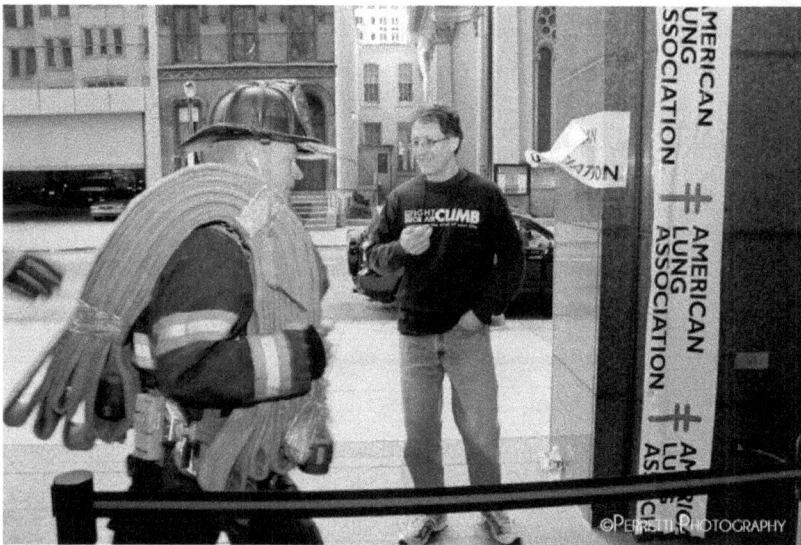

#38. What is an Elite Climber?

The definition of an Elite Climber varies by climb.

In the Philadelphia Fight For Air Climb, it's a climber who anticipates completing the 50 floor climb in 8 to 12 minutes.

Choosing to climb as an Elite Climber is nice, in that it guarantees you a staggered start, which means you'll start some seconds after the climber in front of you has started, and some seconds ahead of the climb in back of you. This means that likely you won't have to pass people or have to yield to climbers passing you.

If the climb you are interested in offer an Elite Climber category, consider choosing it if you are within their suggested finishing times.

By the way, I finished my climb in 10 minutes and 37 seconds, so my decision to climb as an Elite Climber was a good one.

#39. Should I climb with my team or as an Elite Climber?

Yes, by all means, you can climb with your team. Most organized climbs have a section of the climb set aside for Team Climbing, where team members who wish to climb together can go up together, or nearly together.

However, if some members of your team want to climb as an Elite climber, don't anticipate being able to join the rest of your team for a second climb, although there are some events that will permit this. In general, it's one climb per Registration fee.

The advantage of climbing as an Elite climber is that you are guaranteed a staggered start. The runner ahead of you will start 15 seconds before you and once you begin, the runner behind you will wait 15 seconds for you.

Team starts aren't necessarily staggered, although some are.

With a non-staggered start, you can be sure to have a bit of a crowd around you as you climb up the building.

If you are trying to get up the building fast, that's not the best way to do so.

#40. Can I climb with my friends even though we aren't on a Team together?

Most event organizers are very accommodating, and I don't see as a problem.

Last year, in the 2011 Philadelphia Fight For Air Climb, Elite Climbers went up first, and within that group, we lined up any way we wanted. Same for Individuals and Team Climbers.

Some climbs are stricter than other. Here's an excerpt from one of the Stair Climb events.

As the event gets closer and teams begin to fill up, start times will be assigned within a 5 minute window. Every person climbing, whether as an individual or a team, will be assigned within a 5 minute window. Due to safety reasons, you cannot run or walk the stairs side by side. Due to the large number of participants, specific start time requests cannot be accommodated.

The bottom line: Unless you create a team with your friends, there's no guarantee that you will be able to climb with your friends.

#41. What if I don't want to climb but I am interested in helping with an event?

All of the organizations hosting a climb will be thrilled to have you volunteer. Just email or phone the point of contact for the climb you are interested in helping out. You'll most likely even get a t-shirt.

Volunteers are always very much appreciated by the climbers---they help make things run smoothly and their enthusiasm is very encouraging as we make our way up the stairs. If you volunteer, you'll be a welcome addition to the festivities.

The volunteers at the 2011 Philadelphia Fight For Air Climb were wonderful, many of them from the Sanford-Brown School.

#42. Is water provided in the stairwells?

Small cups of water are provided at the designated water/rest stops, usually every 10 floors.

#43. How many rest stops will there be along the climb to the top

Count on one water stop/rest stop roughly every 10 floors or so.

My personal recommendation is to skip the water. You really won't get that thirsty in 10 to 15 minutes?

But use the rest stops if you need them.

By the way, don't expect to be able to use a restroom once you start your climb.

Most organized climbs don't handle 'potty' breaks during the Climb very well.

Rest Stops are manned by volunteers who can offer water and perhaps offer you a chair if you need to rest. But don't count on being able to wander the rest stop floors looking for a restroom.

If you need to visit a rest room after the climb begins, this will require an escort by a Security Officer (something one of Team Smiley's members learned last year :)

#44. What's a wave and what's a wave time?

A wave is a group of people who start up the stairs at around the same time. Waves are used to organize the climb so that everyone doesn't gather in the same place at the same time.

There may be a 9am wave, a 9:30am wave, etc.

There may also be an Elite Climber wave, a First Responder wave, a Team wave. You get the idea.

Just to warn you, your wave may begin at 10am, but if the number of climbers in your wave is large (for instance, the Team wave,) climbers towards the end of the wave may not being to climb until 11am. This is a good reason to visit the rest room before standing in your 'wave'.)

#45. Can I carry my baby in a baby pack up the stair well?

Absolutely not.

Stairwells are very narrow, some stairwells are open, with openings that would allow small objects (such as a baby) to possibly fall to the bottom.

Even a baby in a carrier isn't permitted.

It's simply too dangerous.

#46. Can I carry a small child up the stair well.?

No. For the same reason you can't carry a baby up the stairs, small children cannot be carried up the stairs.

It's just too dangerous

#47. Can my children participate?

Many events encourage family participation, including young children. Sometimes it depends if the Stair Climb is outdoors (stadium stairs) or indoors (a fire escape or stair well.)

Some Stair climbs permit children as young as 8 to climb, but only if he or she meets the minimum fundraising requirements.

Most, if not all of the climbs, seem to have settled on a minimum age of 12 to 14 to climb, some with the proviso that children need to climb with an adult or parent.

Be sure to check ahead of time when you register for the climb. You don't want to show up on Climb Day and find out that the child you brought can't participate.

By the way, if your child can't climb, young children are usually welcome to participate as volunteers.

Check with your Stair Climb event before hand.

above.

#48. Are pets allowed?

I don't know of any organized climb that will permit you to bring a pet with you to the climb.

#49. Can I climb the building multiple times?

Most Stair Climbs do not permit you to climb multiple times on Climb Day, unless you pay an additional fee for the privilege. Quite a few Stair Climbs offer the option to pay additional fees to make multiple climbs. Climbs that have a shorter building may have multiple climb options to provide a bigger challenge for the climbers.

In 2012, the Philadelphia Fight For Air Climb will offer a 'century option' in which climbers will be able to climb up the 50 floor building twice, totaling 100 floors (a century.) Climbers opting for the Century Climb option will pay twice the ordinary Registration fee.

There are 2 Climbs that appear to allow you to climb multiple times without paying an additional registration fee.

The American Lung Association Climb in Oakbrook Terrace, IL allows you to climb twice at no additional charge.

So does the Salt Lake City American Lung Association Climb. The Climb Organizers encourage you to climb multiple times without paying any additional fees. According to their Web Site: "For many of us, one climb is quite enough. However, for those of you who want to push your lungs and body a little more, consider multiple climbs."

#50. Will there be Emergency Response Technicians on hand?

Yes, there are always Emergency Personnel on hand to deal with emergencies and in addition...

Most organized climbs have a First Responders category of climbers--- Policeman, Firefighters and EMT's---who are participating as well.

This means that there are plenty of emergency personnel around (both on duty and participating in the climb) in the event that anyone gets in trouble on the stairs.

#51. Can our family and friends come and watch?

Family and friends are always welcome to come and watch you climb.

How close they can get to you may be another story.

During the 2011 Philadelphia Fight For Air Climb, family and friends were encouraged to wait at a local bar and eatery, Tír na nÓg, the location for the post-climb awards event.

The event organizers had planned on televising, on the bar's Televisions, Climbers as they reached the top of the Bell Atlantic Tower.

Friends and family were also able to watch climbers line up outside the Bell Atlantic Tower as they began their ascent in the fire escape (entry to the Bell Atlantic Tower fire escape is via an outside door.) and there were quite a few well wishers outside cheering us on.

However, friends and family were not permitted at the top of the building, and this is typical of most organized Stair Climbs.

There just isn't enough room at the top of most buildings to accommodate a large number of Climbers, plus their friends and family.

There are, however, a few select climbs that permit friends and family to wait at the top---sometimes for a price that is added to the Stair Climb event's fundraising totals.

One such event is the <u>San Francisco American Lung Association Climb</u>, whose post-event ceremony takes place at the top of the building.

Either way, feel free to invite your family and friends to come and watch your achievement, better yet, to volunteer for the event.

<u>#52. Will I get a t-shirt?</u>

Most climbs will provide you a nifty shirt to wear after the climb---some before the climb.

Some climbs only give you a shirt if you raise a minimum amount of money in donations.

Some climbs will give you an even niftier shirt if you are a high fundraiser.

Questions About Climb day

#53. What's a Climb Packet?

A packet is just your registration materials, usually consisting of your t-shirt, your bib (number), a timing chip and advertising materials that the climb organizers include in it. Sometimes your race t-shirt is included in your packet.

#54. Where is the Climb Packet Pick-up?

Most climbs give you the option of picking up your Climb Packet prior to actual Climb Day, which can be a good idea, particularly if there are a lot of materials that the climb organizers are giving you.

At the 2011 Philadelphia Fight For Air Climb, the event organizers gave us the option of picking up our Climb Packet at the Bell Atlantic Tower the day before the climb. Most likely, only those climbers who worked nearby took advantage of this opportunity. Driving into Philadelphia is no treat during a work day.

I picked up my Climb Packet on Climb Day, which meant that I needed to pin my bib on my shirt and attach my timing chip to my sneaker that morning.

The event t-shirt, sometimes included in Climb Packets, was distributed at our post climb event venue, Tír na nÓg.

#55. Can I pick up the Climb Packets for other people on my team?

Yes, as long as those team members have met the fundraising minimum.

Come Climb Organizers ask that you have your team members sign a release authorizing you to pick up their Climb Packet

#56. How will I know my start time?

Most climbs will let you know your estimated starting time a few days before the climb. The Philadelphia Fight For Air Climb sent all of the registered climbers an email a few days before the Climb with our estimated starting times.

These times will vary, usually depending upon what 'category' you are climbing in: Elite, First Responder, Individual or Team.

If you registered as a Team Climb, you'll have the thrill of climbing with your teammates :)

#57. What time should I be there?

Most climbs start between 8am and 9am, but it can take hours to get all of the climbers off and climbing.

As I said above, most climbs will inform you of a pre-assigned starting time a few days before the Climb.

You don't want to be late, neither do you want to hang around for 2 hours (as I did last year at the Philadelphia Fight For Air Climb.)

If you pick up your Climbing Packet before Climb Day, then you can show up about 30 minutes before your start time.

If you need to pick up your Climbing Pack the day of the climb, give yourself an extra 30 minutes so that you can get your timing chip, attach it to your shoes, and get a bit of a warm up in.

#58. I am volunteering, what time should I arrive and where should I go?

All volunteers will be contacted prior to the event. Plan on arriving about an hour before registration begins.

#59. What if I miss my start time?

For some events, this won't be a big deal. For others, particularly those where there are a huge number of climbers and not much 'slack room', you can get shut out. But don't despair.

If you miss your start time there is still a possibility that you can climb after the last scheduled runner at the end of your assigned wave, or if all else fails, the last scheduled climber on Climb Day. However, this cannot be guaranteed.

In particular, if you miss the last bit of the Individual Climbers wave, and the First Responders are climbing in the stair way, you may not be able to climb at all.

The bottom line: Plan to arrive at the climb at least one hour prior to your start time and be prepared to be at the start line at least 20 minutes before your assigned time.

#60. What should I eat before the climb?

I always preach caution in pre-race or pre-climb meal. Most Stair Climbs begin in the morning, so caution is the word for both the dinner (or snack) the night before the climb, and breakfast the morning of the climb.

Eat a normal dinner the night before the Stair Climb.

Remember, you aren't running a Marathon, so there's no need to carbo-load before hand. For a fifty story climb, you'll be in the stairway somewhere between 8 and 20 minutes.

Avoid anything that can dehydrate you overnight (i.e. alcohol.) For me, that means no beer with dinner the night before the climb.

Eat a normal breakfast, whatever that happens to be for you. For me, it's a bagel with some jelly, and a couple of cups of coffee.

Avoid anything that can cause you to start looking for a rest room between floors 10 and 20.

#61. Where should I park?

Most events will have plenty of available parking. Some events may have limited parking, so plan accordingly.

For the Philadelphia Fight For Air Climb, there's a parking garage underneath the Bell Atlantic Tower. It's not large, and can fill up, but if it does, on a Saturday morning, there's plenty of available parking around the building.

If you park in the Bell Atlantic Tower garage, you get reduced rate parking.

By the way, bring some cash for parking in case the Parking Garage doesn't accept a Credit Card.

#62. What should I bring with me on the day of the climb?

The charity event organizers will want you to bring, above all else, any money that you have raised for the charity, particularly if you are 'short' of the fundraising minimum required.

If you picked up your Climbing Packet before hand, be sure to bring your timing chip (attach it to your sneakers while you are still home,) your bib (number) and a few dollars for parking. Don't forget your car keys when you park.

If you want to record your climb time on the way up the top, bring a stop watch. I use my iPhone. Speaking of phones, be sure to bring one, particularly if it has a camera. You'll want to take some pictures.

Some events have water bottles for you on the ground floor of the climb. Some don't make them available until you reach the top, so you may want to bring a bottle of water to drink prior to the climb.

Again, watch the timing of your water drinking.

If you down a bottle or two of water right before the climb, you may feel nature calling on the stairs.

#63. What should I do with my personal belongings. Is there a bag check?

A bag check is a location where you can store a bag or backpack containing valuables, clothes, etc. (be sure your name is on it.) This is usually more of a big deal in events where the start and stop points are not the same, like a Marathon, for instance, and where you are less likely to carry valuables with you during the event for risk of losing them.

This really isn't an issue with Stair Climbs.

It's pretty easy to carry your car keys and cell phone up the stairs with you without dropping them in the stairway. Beyond your car keys, your cell phone and a few dollars, you really don't need to bring more than that.

However, if you need a bag check, many (but not all) events will provide a bag check area to store your belongings. Again, be sure to label your bag or pack.

All event organizers will tell you that they are not responsible for lost belongings.

The bottom line: Don't bring anything of value to the climb.

If you do, you have a choice of keeping them in your car, or using the bag check.

Your choice.

#64. What should I wear to the climb?

Climb organizers advise you to wear comfortable clothing appropriate for an intense cardio workout. Depending upon the time of year, the stairways can be hot and humid or cool and dry. However, they are extremely well ventilated and may feel a little chilly when you start.

Most of the major Stair Climbs are held in cool weather.

I've done all of my Stair Climbs in a pair of shorts and a short sleeved running shirt. I was cool at the start (particularly after standing outside for a few minutes,) but after a minute of climbing, I was plenty warm enough

#65. What kind of shoes should I wear to the Stair climb?

I wear a pair of running shoes. You need sturdy shoes, since you'll be climbing over 1,000 steps, and you also want something that will grip the steps in the fire escape.

#66. Can I dress up in funny costumes to do the climb?

You bet. Most climbs are very festive occasions.

Last year, a gentleman in the Philadelphia Fight For Air Climb wore a diaper.

This year's Philadelphia Fight For Air Climb is being held the week after St. Patrick's day, so it's possible climbers will head up the stairs dressed as leprechauns.

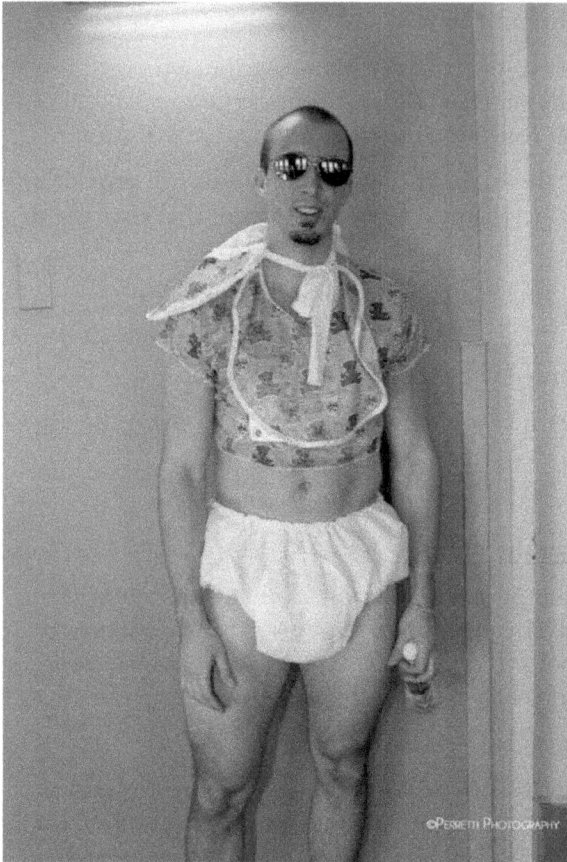
©PERRETTI PHOTOGRAPHY

#67. Where are the rest rooms?

Rest rooms, bath rooms, whatever you call them, you might need them.

You might think that in a high rise building, there would be rest rooms in the lobby. Not necessarily.

In the case of my 2011 Philadelphia Fight For Air Climb, there were no rest rooms in the lobby. Instead, to use a rest room, climbers had to take an elevator to the 5th floor. (Emphasizing the important of managing your water intake :)

Upon arriving at the Registration Desk, the first thing you ask might be the location of the restrooms.

Be aware that if you are called to line up for your turn to climb, you could be in line for 30 minutes or more, so be sure to make a nature call prior to getting in line.

One of our team members, after she began climbing, had to find a rest room somewhere between the 20th and 25th floors. Security had to be called, as there can be no unescorted climbers on floors in the building.

Questions About Getting Ready to Climb

#68. What is a bib?

A bib is a piece of paper with a climber's number on it. The bib is attached to the front of your shirt with 4 safety pins (provided at the Registration Desk.) Even though just about all events also feature timing chips that are usually attached to your shoe, you still need to wear a bib so that the climb organizers know who you are.

Typically, the reverse side of the bib has blocks for your name, your address, Emergency Contacts, etc. Fill out that information completely in case there's an emergency of some kind, and a family member or friend needs to be notified :)

By the way, bibs need to be attached to the front of your shirt. Not the back, and not to your pants or shorts.

#69. Can I trade my bib/timing device number for another one?

I'm not sure why you would want to do so, but NO, it is crucial that bibs and timing chips used during the climb correspond to those that are distributed to each participant at packet pick up. This will ensure that times and ranking are accurate for the awards ceremony.

Most organized Stair Climbs 'time' your ascent through the use of a timing chip, which records your starting and ending time as you pass over a timing mat.

Timing chips are used to measure the time it takes you to reach the top of the building. Although many climbers are climbing for charity, and don't particularly care about their official time, event organizers hire professional timers who take these things seriously.'?

Also do not bend your timing device as it will destroy the chip and you won't be credited with a climb time.

Most timing chips these days are disposable, but in some cases, timing chips must be returned after the climb---so be careful.

#70. Where do the Timing Chips go?

Some timing chips are attached to your shoes, some chips are attached to your bib.

It depends on the climb.

Be sure to use the timing chip assigned to you at registration.

If you switch chips with someone else, their time will be ascribed to you and vice versa.

Last year's Philadelphia Fight For Air climb used timing chips attached to your shoes. Here's a picture of one.

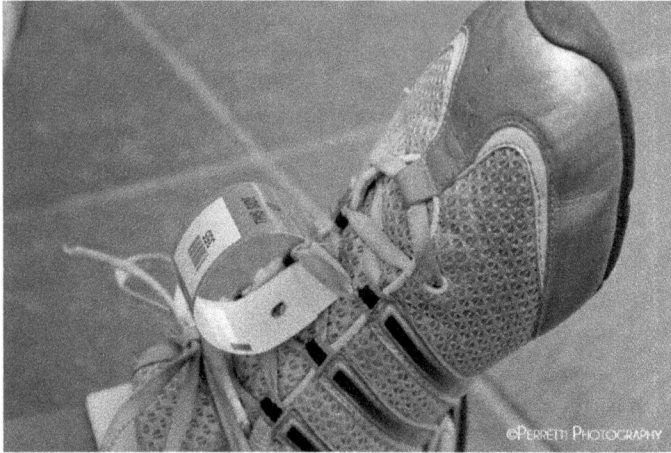

©Perretti Photography

#71. How do the Timing Chips Work?

You will receive a timing chip and a tie-wrap or ankle band to attach the timing chip at registration.

Timing chips need to be placed on your shoe or near your ankle to ensure that the chip can be read from the floor mat.

For events where climbers make multiple climbs up the building (the new Century Option for the 2012 Philadelphia Fight For Air Climb), climbers will receive a new chip every time they climb.

Firefighter and First Responder chips need to be attached as low to the floor as possible.

Staff and volunteers will be available to ensure proper timing chip placement and timing chip removal (if required.)

#72. Can we carry stuff on us while we climb?

Pets, infants and children cannot be carried with you on climb day.

In general, iPods, music devices, and heart monitors may be used, but must be worn properly. Cords must be tucked, no loose cords may dangle from your body as these could cause entanglement and injury.

If this is seen staff, volunteers or security may ask you to remove it for safety reasons.)

#73. Can we carry our things in a backpack during the climb?

Some climbs allow backpacks, some do not. I'm not sure why you would need one. Remember, it's best to leave all unnecessary personal belongings either at home, in your car, at the check bag location (if there is one,) or with a friend or family member watching the climb.

Last year, during the Philadelphia Fight For Air Climb, I didn't recall seeing any backpacks, but then in reviewing some photographs of the event, I saw a climber reaching the top of the building wearing a backpack.

I also believe I saw a climber with a Camelbak, which is a backpack that contains water for drinking.

If you think you will need to carry a backpack up the stairs, I would check with the event organizers first.

#74. Can I bring my own water bottle with me in the stair well?

For safety reasons, absolutely not.

Some stairwells have 'openings' where a dropped water bottle could fall for 50 floors. You don't want a missile like that in free fall in the stairwell.

Most people do not need to drink water on their way to the top, but if the stairwell is hot and dry, you may need to. All organized climbs will have water/rest stops, if you need them, every 10 floors or so.

Remember to properly hydrate starting 3 days prior to the climb, and drink some (not a lot) of water the morning of the climb.

#75. What about a Camelbak?

A Camelbak is a water pack that you can wear on your back. It contains a 'hands free' straw that you can drink from as you participate in your athletic event.

I'm not aware of any event that doesn't permit these, but I would check with your event organizer first.

Again, as has been my suggestion about drinking water up the stairs, because of the short length of time you'll be on the stairs, I don't see the need for one, but I may have seen one in use last year during my climb up the stairs at the Philadelphia Fight For Air Climb.

#76. Can I use an iPod or iPhone for music?

Go for it.

Most all climb events will permit you to listen to music up the stairs. And most (but not all) will permit you to wear ear buds and headphones up the stairs as well. This surprises me a bit, but right now, that's the case.

Some of my climbing friends wouldn't be able to make a trip up the stairs without their favorite playlist giving them that added incentive.

#77. Can I wear my headphones?

All but one of the climbing events I've surveyed permit you to wear headphones up the stairs. However, climb officials caution you to be conscious of other climbers and the volunteers in the stairwells.

You need to be aware that some climbers may be passing you---with ear buds and headphones, you won't hear them. You also need to be conscious that volunteers, or climb officials, may need to communicate with you during the climb, so be prepared to listen to them if need be.

One climb event that I know that specifically says 'no headphones' is the <u>Boston Climb to the Top</u> for the National Multiple Sclerosis Society

Questions About Going Up The Stairs

#78. Does everyone go up the stairs at once?

No, there are too many climbers for everyone to go up the stairs at one time.

Most organized Stair Climbs have four categories of climbers.

Elite Climbers. Individual Climbers. Team Climbers. First Responders.

Elite Climbers generally climb first, and their start times are staggered, usually 15 seconds apart. Elite climbers generally are faster climbers. In the case of the 2011 Philadelphia Fight For Air Climb, climbers designated as Elite Climbers were climbers who believed they would finish the climb in 6 to 12 minutes.

Individual Climbers are individuals, not affiliated with a team, who either have no projected finish time, or will finish at a slower pace. Individual Climbers are also generally staggered.

Team Climbers are generally what I call 'fun climbers' who may climb, in a leisurely fashion, with their team. Some event organizers also insist that Team Climbers be staggered, to reduce congestion in the stairwells. Other events permit teams to go up the stairs together.

First Responders generally go up last, and in full gear. Because of their added weight (about 40 pounds,) First Responders will almost always be the slowest to the top.

In most events, then, the only climbers who may go up all at once are the Team climbers.

The Empire State Building Run Up is an exception to rule, and generally features the best climbers in the world. It features a 'gang start'. A gang start means a rush to the stairway---watch out!

Check out Chapter 16 for a link to several videos that demonstrate how exciting (and potentially dangerous) this can be.

#79. Is it possible to get lost in the stairway?

For most people, no, but for me...

At the beginning of the Philadelphia Fight For Air Climb in the Bell Atlantic Tower, you start outside, go up 1 flight of steps and immediately encounter a long hallway. You can go left or right.

You want to go left, then connect to the main fire escape, and proceed up the rest of the stairs.

Last year, I hesitated, and this cost me about 10 seconds last year.

This year, there will be a sign in the hall way with an arrow pointing to the left :)

#80. Are the stairwells crowded?

Because most events feature staggered starts for nearly every climber, the stairwells aren't crowded. Rather than feel crowded, you may feel a bit lonely.

Last year, during the 2011 Philadelphia Fight For Air Climb, I registered as an Elite climber and after starting, I saw only 4 climbers on my 10 minute trip to the top of the building.

If you climb in the Individual category, climbers are also usually staggered but because there's a wide range of climbing capabilities in this category, you're more likely to pass another climber or be passed.

In the Team category, climbers sometimes go up the stairs as a team, so that will be your best chance to have a crowd on the stairs.

#81. Should I use the handrails to pull myself up?

The best Stair Climbers in the world use the handrails in the stairwells. Sometimes they use just one, sometimes both. My Team Smiley teammate Tim told me recently that last year, during the Philadelphia Fight For Air Climb, about half way through the climb, he started using both handrails to go up the stairs, and thought it really helped him. He's going to start that way in the 2012 climb.

If you do use the handrails, by all means practice that way. It's not something you want to try without practice.

If you do use the handrails, you may want to consider taking the advice of one of my Stair Climbing friends Lisa Kinsner Scheer---wear a pair of rubber gloves. Lisa says you will grip the handrails better, and the glover will also protect your hands from wear and tear (and germs) while gripping the handrails.

Here's a video link from premier Stair Climber, PJ Glassey. on the subject of handrails…

http://xgym.com/xtras/stair_training/

#82. When you climb, should you skip steps (double step) or do single steps?

As is the case with handrails, the best Stair Climbers in the world double step their way to the top. With the assistance of handrails, of course.

When I practice in my house, I double up the steps. This is pretty easy to do with my house stairs because as soon as I get to the top, I turn around and walk down. So I have a built-in rest period of sorts every 7 seconds or so.

Skipping or doubling up 50 floors with no break is another story altogether.

As you may have read in Chapter 1, when Team Smiley did a 25 floor practice climb at our teammate Tim's condo, I was able to double skip in his fire escape for only a few floors, and I had to do single steps the rest of the way.

In timed climbs in Tim's condo, I didn't see an appreciable difference in doubling up versus single stepping. To me, the key is to keep moving. My experience has been once I go to single steps, I can't get back to double stepping again.

On Climb Day, in the 2011 Philadelphia Fight For Air Climb, I was able to double-step for about 5 floors, then had to single step the rest of the way.

Despite that, I developed a good rhythm over the next 45 floors and finished the climb in 10 minutes and 37 seconds. Had I been able to double step all the way to the top, I'm sure I would have gone under 10 minutes, perhaps under 9. But that's the difference between me and a top Stair Climber. I just can't maintain that pace. Using the handrails may help.

This year my teammate Tim is going to try to double step all the way to the top, using handrails to assist him. Tim finished last year's climb in 9 minutes and 9 seconds. He's hoping to go under 8 minutes using this technique. I may try to do the same thing.

Ultimately, the choice whether to double step or single step may depend on whether you want to win the Stair Climb or just finish it.

#83. Can I pass someone on the Stairs?

Yes you can pass. It's perfectly fine to pass and be passed. For this reason, it's a good idea to climb single file up the stair ways to allow people to pass easily.

#84. How do I pass other climbers in the stairwells?

If you notice that you are "faster" than other climbers in front of you, about to catch up to them and wish to pass, as a courtesy shout out something like "Passing on your right" or "Passing on your left" or "Can I get by?"

It's also a common courtesy for the slower climber to move to the outside and let the fast climber pass on the inside.

#85. Can I exit the stairwell and walk in the building?

Absolutely NOT.

Stair Climbs are held in high rises that house businesses, and in the case of the Hustle Up The Hancock in Chicago, residences on the higher floors.

For this reason, under no circumstances will you be permitted to exit the stairs on your own, without a Security escort, prior to reaching the top floor of the climb.

That's not to say that you can't exit the stairs for an emergency or if you can't continue---you'll just need an escort. If you need to exit, try to get as far as a floor with a water stop and tell the volunteers there that you can't continue. If you can't get that far, let one of the other climbers behind you know that you need assistance and wait.

#86. If I can't get all the way to the top, I'll feel like a loser

Don't feel that way!.

Just about all of the Stair Climbs in the United States are held for deserving charities. As long as you raise money for a good cause, you're a winner for venturing forth into the stairway, and you should feel great about that! Some stair climb events have prizes for the person who raises the most money, and they don't even care about your time to reach the top.

If you can't go continue and need to stop after a few floors, that's OK, just try to get as far as a floor with a water stop and tell the volunteers there that you can't continue. If you can't get that far, let one of the other climbers behind you know that you need assistance and wait.

#87. Suppose I cramp up while I'm climbing up the stairs?

Cramping is usually caused by dehydration.

Be sure to properly hydrate for 3 days prior to the climb, and avoid drinking alcohol the night before the climb. If you do that, you shouldn't experience muscle cramps.

If you do happen to cramp up, slow down and if necessary stop altogether. Trying to run or climb through a muscle cramp can lead to a muscle tear. Stop climbing, and try to gently stretch your affected muscle until the muscle contraction starts to ease. You can also try to massage the cramping muscle.

Provided you can walk, try to reach a floor with a water stop on it, drink some water, and if you can, try to finish. If you continue to cramp up, think about calling it a day.

Questions About The Top Of The Building

#88. What should I expect at the finish line?

At the finish line (the top of the building,) you will be greeted with cheers and applause. You will cross the same sort of Timing Mat that you crossed when you started the climb, and if timing chips are to collected, volunteers may ask you to stop for a moment and assist you in removing it. In some cases, as with the 2011 Philadelphia Fight For Air Climb, the timing chips are disposable---you could take it home as a souvenir (which I did.)

There will be other climbers behind you reaching the top of the stairs after you, so you will want to keep moving beyond the finish line. Most likely, there will be water supplied for you, and an open area for you to rest.

If you are exhausted at the finish, try to keep moving---a sudden stop could mean muscle cramps. If you feel dizzy, you may want to find a place to sit and put your head down between your knees.

After this, you may want to hang around a bit and try to find other members of your team or find someone who can take a picture of you at the top of the building. At the 2011 Philadelphia Fight For Air Climb, there were two student photographers taking pictures throughout the climb, and Felicia Peretti was taking many pictures at the finish line.

It won't be long, though, before you will be asked to head down to the ground floor.

#89. Once we reach the top of the building, how do we get down?

This is probably the most often asked question I am asked by friends and family. Many people believe that after climbing up 50 flights of stairs, you are then asked to walk down 50 flights.

Don't worry, after climbing to the top of the building, you'll take the elevator down. You don't even have the choice of walking.

Provided that is, you aren't participating in the Bennington Tower Climb. In that case, you will need to walk down.

#90. When we reach the top of the building, will we be able to look out?

You should be able to enjoy the beautiful view for a minute or two.

However, most event organizers are in a hurry to get climbers down as fast as possible once they reach the top. Primarily, that's because space is limited up there, and there are climbers reaching the top every few seconds.

You should have an opportunity to pose for pictures with friends and team members (provided you can find them,) before you are ushered to the elevators for your ride down to the ground floor.

#91. How Much Time Will I Have at the Top to Enjoy the View?

Not much. You will have only a minute or so to enjoy the view from the top before you are asked to head down the elevator to the ground floor.

Don't forget to carry a camera or your cell phone up to the top with you so that you can get a picture of the beautiful view.

#92. Can my friends and family meet me at the top?

There are few climbs that permit family members and friends to meet you at the top. Again these are rare, and the one or two I've heard of charge a fee for the privilege of meeting you at the top.

There is one climb, the American Lung Association Climb in San Francisco that has its after event awards party at the top of the building---that's a great idea.)

Even though your friends and family can't meet you at the top, that doesn't mean they have to be shut out of the excitement of seeing you cross the finish line live.

The Philadelphia Fight For Air Climb provides a live feed of the finish line to friends and family waiting at the post climb event venue, Tír na nÓg, an Irish Bar & Grill about a block away.

Questions About After The Climb

#93. Besides being the first climber to the top, are there any other prizes awarded?

Yes. Typically, there are individual first place age group prizes awarded in addition to the first male and female climbers to the top. Just to warn you, don't expect a cash prize. Most likely, you'll receive a plaque, a medal or a medallion.

Because many climbs support charitable organizations, most of these climbs award prizes to the biggest fundraiser.

Some climbs, like the American Lung Association Palm Beach Florida climb, have prizes awarded to the team with the most members.

If I had my way, there would be prizes also awarded to the oldest male and female finishers.

#94. Where and When are the award ceremonies held?

Most times, the award ceremonies are held the same day as the climb, and sometimes in the same building as the climb.

Some climbs do hold the award ceremonies at a later date.

#95. Are there awards for the oldest climber?

None that I know of--but there should be. That's quite an effort the older climbers are making to complete the climb.

In 2011, the oldest climbers to complete a climb were 2 male climbers who were 86 years old.

James Devenney, completed the Hustle Up The Hancock (94 floors) in Chicago in 40 minutes and 14 seconds.

Anders Jacobsen, also 86 tears old, completed two Stair climbs in Seattle: The Seattle American Lung Association Climb (51 floors) in 14 minutes and 59 seconds, and the Big Climb Seattle (69 floors) in 25 minutes and 25 seconds.

The two oldest female finishers in 2011 were both 83 years old.

Marilyn Olen completed the Denver America Lung Association Climb (56 floors) in 20 minutes and 47 seconds.

Gloria Schiffler, also 83 years old, completed the 103 floor Sky Rise Chicago Climb in 1 hour and 33 seconds.

For more on older Stair Climbers, check out Chapter 15.

#96. What do participants receive?

Besides the bragging rights of doing something that most people cannot do, and for most events, raising money for a great cause, participants typically receive a commemorative t-shirt of some kind, and complementary food and beverages after the climb.

#97. What are incentive prizes?

Most climbs that raise money for a charitable cause have incentive prizes for climbers whose fundraising efforts are over and beyond the minimum necessary to climb.

It depends on the event, but as an example, raising $1,500 or more might get you a golf umbrella, $5,000 or more a gift card to a fine restaurant. You get the idea.

Incentive prizes, if they exist, vary by the event, and the event organizers would be more than happy for you to 'donate' your inventive prize back to the prize pool.

#98. How do I get my incentive prize?

After the event is complete, usually after the fund raising window has closed, you will be contacted by the event organizer and given instructions on how to get your incentive prize.

#99. When will I know my climb time?

Because all of the climbers go up at different times, there's no timing clock at the finish line.

If you remember to take a stop watch along with you to the top, you'll have a good idea of your climb time when you cross the finish line.

Last year, during the Philadelphia Fight For Air Climb, I forgot to hit the Stop button on my iPhone Stop Watch app. 5 minutes later I remembered it, but by then it was too late to get an accurate reading of my climb time. I could only estimate it.

In most cases, lists of climb times are posted somewhere at the event, since many climbs offer awards for finish times. For the Philadelphia Fight For Air Climb, they were posted on a wall in the lobby.

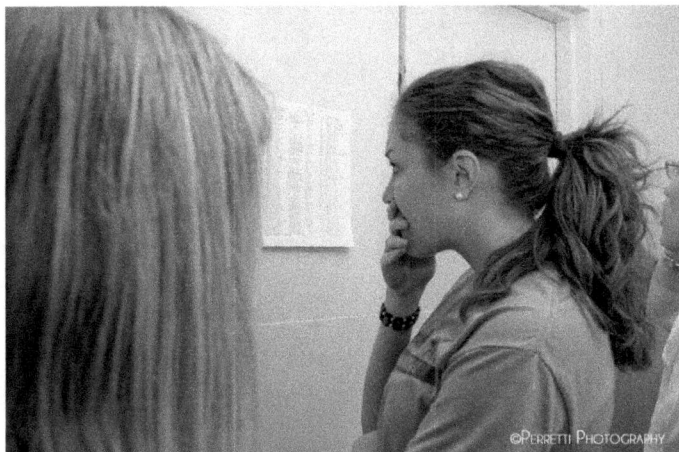
©Perretti Photography

Some time after the climb, results will be posted on the climb's web site or on the web site of the company that provides the timing for the event. Some climbs are faster than others to post results. The Philadelphia Fight For Air Climb had the results posted by 4pm on the day of the Climb.

Some climbs are very slow to post climb times. The 2011 Philadelphia Special Olympics Climb (first time it was held,) took nearly a week to post results, and even then, it took an email from me to get it from them. I'm still not sure the results are posted on their web site.

#100. Where can I see pictures from the event?

Many events post links to photos from the event on their website.

Some events have Facebook pages with photos posted there as well.

CHAPTER NINE

Tips

In this chapter I present tips from a variety of Stair Climbers, ranging from first timers, like me, to Elite, world class climbers.

Tips from John Smiley

Brief Version:

1. Climb real stairs in a high rise of the same height as your actual climb, practicing until you can climb the same amount of flights/steps.

2. If you can't find a high rise, climb stairs in your house, walking or skipping up, and walking down (never run down.) For every 10 flights in your actual climb, build up to being able to climb flights in your house for at least 5 minutes per 10 floors of your actual climb. For instance, if your actual climb is 10 floors, do 5 minutes of Stair Climbing in your house. If your climb is 20 floors, work up to 10 minutes. If your climb is 50 floors, work up to 25 minutes on your house stairs. If you're doing the Hustle Up The Hancock in Chicago, work your way up to about 50 minutes of climbing on your home stairs.

3. If you live in a one floor home or apartment, the next best thing is to either hit the gym and use a Jacob's Ladder, StairMaster, Stair Mill, or treadmill with at least a 10% incline. Work your way up to the amount of time specified in #2 above.

4. If a gym membership isn't for you, then head outside and start running. Again, as in #2 and #3, you want to concentrate on time, not distance.

More Detailed Version of Tips:

#1. The most important thing is to climb stairs.

At least I think so.

Members of my team were divided on that.

Tim, a former professional athlete, lived in the 25 floor condo building where we practiced three times, and regularly ran up the stairs for practice. Not surprisingly, his time up the Bell Atlantic Tower was the best of anyone on our team.

I climbed stairs daily, starting with 7 flights of stairs in my house on December 14th, and added one flight each day. On March 18th, the day before the actual climb, I did 123 flights in the house. In addition to the stairs I was climbing, I also did some morning runs of between 3 and 5 miles, three times a week.

My daughter Melissa is on the track team---aside from her track work, she really didn't do anything else, but she did participate in our 3 25 floor practice climbs.

Sophorn and Bob are long distance runners, and they adhered to their normal running routine. Again, like Melissa, they also participated in our three 25 floor practice climbs.

Nora and Danielle just showed up the day of the climb. Both are former High School athletes who decided to see what happened.

#2. If you can't find real stairs to train on, many climbers will tell you to train as if you are training for a 5K race.

Not bad advice. Some of the climb web sites will tell you that if you can walk 3 miles, you can climb 50 floors.

#3 Keep your training interesting

Doing the same thing every day can be boring. Last year, I varied my routine by adding 1 flight of stairs to my training each day.

This year, I'm in more of a maintenance mode, climbing 100 flights of stairs only on Sunday.

Climbing just one day a week keeps things interesting for me.

#4 Form a team and train together

Forming a team and training together for last year's ALA Philly climb really helped me. I probably could have made it to the top, but training with others was great motivation to keep going. We all pushed each other to do our best.

Although we actually only trained together 3 times, those training sessions allowed us to fine tune our individual strategies for the climb.

#5. You will have trouble forming a team.

I'd love to tell you that friends and family, once they learn of your intention to do a stair climb, will beg you to join your team. Sorry. If anything they'll avoid you.. People will come up with all sorts of excuses NOT to join your team. I just wish they would come out and say No, rather than leaving you hanging (a particular trait of young people, I must say.)

Probably your best chance of forming a team is to ask like minded inviduals to join your team.

If you belong to a gym, make up a flyer and post it on a bulletin board.

#6. Do something every day

I think it's important that you do something every day.

You don't need to climb every day---although I did last year.

If you don't climb, go out for a little jog.

Since my 2011 ALA Philly climb, on days that I don't climb, I run in the morning. When the weather is decent, I run 3 times a week (in the mornings, usually Monday-Wednesday-Friday). That means the other 4 days, I climb steps. It takes me about 23 minutes to climb 96 flights of steps, It takes me about 48 minutes to run 5 miles.

At the end of my Stair Climbing, I collapse into my easy chair, and enjoy a 5 to 7 minute Runner's high.

When I'm done my 5 mile run, I don't experience the same high. I think my body is conditioned for it

#7 Find a building and walk to the top

Stair Climbing is not stair racing. If you are lucky enough to find a high rise, walk it first. Don't be tempted to double step or skip stairs the first time up. Time yourself. See how you feel afterwards, then take the elevator down and repeat.

#8. It will be next to impossible for you to find a high rise to practice in

We were lucky that one of our team mates lived in a high rise. Other than that, unless we trespassed somewhere, it would have been very difficult. We probably would have tried a parking garage in Atlantic City.

My survey of Stair Climbs shows that very few offer organized practice climbs.

American Lung Association Climb of Hartford, CT

American Lung Association Climb of New Haven, CT

American Lung Association Climb of Providence, RI

American Lung Association Climb of Stamford, CT

Must be a New England thing.

Also, the AON climb in Los Angeles and the ALA Climb in Tampa, FL feature organized practice climbs.

#9. Look for a Support Group

If you can't form a team and train with others, there are still some great support groups out there. I recommend the Yahoo Stair Climbing Group and the Facebook Stair Climbing Page. Both of these groups are very friendly and accommodating, and will be glad to answer every question you may have. You can also use these groups to network and perhaps form a training team in your home city.

#10. Always warm up before you climb.

Team Smiley, prior to racing to the top of the Bell Atlantic Tower, ran around the tower several times before starting. Several of our team members, in particular my daughter Melissa, are staunch believers in stretching.

#11. Wear comfortable shoes

The ideal footwear to practice or climb are running shoes.

Stiff shoes, such as basketball shoes or hiking boots, are definitely not the thing to wear.

#12. Find your natural rhythm and pace

You hear the term rhythm described in athletics all the time.

When I talk to people about my climb last year, invariably I come back to finding a rhythm to climb.

You don't want to start out too fast, but I also find that the sooner I get to the point where I'm out of breath, the sooner I find that natural rhythm and pace.

In every race I do, there's a point I reach where I know I'm going to be able to finish.

#13. Avoid starting out too fast

Whether training or climbing on Climb Day, this is good advice.

Too fast will deplete your energy and your confidence.

You're unlikely to start out too fast if you have practiced in a high rise, but if all of your training has been non-stairs, more than likely you will start out too fast. It's normal to feel out of breath during the climb. In fact, most of the climb you will feel out of breath. What is NOT normal is to feel light headed. If you do, slow down, and find your pace and rhythm.

If that light headed feeling persists, seek assistance at the upcoming water stop.

#14. Oxygen Debt is normal---don't panic

Simplistically, Oxygen Debt just means that your body requires more oxygen than it can supply to meet your exercise demands. When this happens, the body starts producing energy anaerobically (without oxygen) and one effect of this is the production of lactic acid which can produce cramping. Fortunately for us, we're not running the Boston Marathon, and we're not on Heartbreak Hill when this happens. We only have a few minutes to deal with this on the stairs.

One way or other, you will feel out of breath during the climb. This is normal.

It's hard to fathom, but to your body, climbing stairs, even if you do them one step at a time at a slow pace, is as if you are sprinting on a track. Your body demands oxygen, and even if you are in the best of shape, you don't have enough to meet its demands. You will get out of breath.

#15. On Climb Day, be confident

One thing that bothers me is to have people around me, during a climb or during a race, who sound like they are going to die, or who find it necessary to tell a buddy how bad they feel, that they are about to throw up, pass out, or die.

That's the last thing I want to hear which is why last year I signed up as an elite climber for the ALA Philly climb.

Elite climbers started 15 seconds apart during the climb, and except for 2 climbers who passed me and 2 climbers I passed, there was no one to distract me at all.

#16. Visualize

It sounds corny, but I visualize myself as a steam locomotive when I'm running or climbing the stairs.

This helps me to concentrate, keep my posture and my core steady.

#17. Have fun

Most climbs will be fun experiences, with lots of friendly volunteers, music and good company. Enjoy the experience and take pleasure in knowing that you are doing something that most people cannot.

#18. I love to sweat

When I sweat, I feel alive.

#19. Skip the water stops during the climb

There are usually multiple water stops during the climb (probably one every 10 floors or so.)

Your mouth may feel very dry, but it's doubtful you'll get much relief from a cup of water at that point. At best, it will slow you down. At worst, it may make you vomit.

Resist the temptation and hold out until the top.

However, feel free to use the water stop to rest if you need to.

#20. Hydrate, Hydrate, Hydrate

Speaking of water, training gurus will tell you that an hydration is very important. How important? You probably won't realize the effects of being properly hydrated, but if you are dehydrated before starting your climb, you'll know it by the end. Drink plenty of water, starting 3 days prior to the climb.

One rule of thumb I've seen is to take your body weight, divide it by 2, and drink that amount of water (in ounces) per day.

Also, be sure to lay off alcohol 3 days prior to your actual climb.

Alcohol will dehydrate you.

#21. Avoid alcohol before the climb

Not everyone agrees with my edict to avoid alcohol the day or night before the climb, but alcohol will dehydrate you.

Some training gurus say that a dehydrated runner or climber may suffer a 10% performance degradation if dehydrated.

This means if you would have run a 24 minute 5K, a dehydrated runner may finish in 26 or 27 minutes.

For a stair climber, if you reach the top in 10 minutes, you might have done 9 minutes if you were properly hydrated.

#22. Watch what you eat

The night before you climb, have some hot chili peppers and tacos!

Sorry, just kidding, that's not for me.

It may be for you, I don't know, but as for me, I like to eat light prior to my climbs.

No big meals the night before the climb.

No alcohol.

Certainly nothing that will induce me to pop a Tums or a Maalox at 3am before the climb.

Prior to last year's ALA Philly climb, I ate a plain bagel and drank 2 cups of coffee.

I experimented with my pre-climb meal during the three 25 floor practice climbs.

The last thing you want to be worrying about when you're climbing to the top of a tall building is your stomach and what's in it.

#23. When you train on stairs, consider 'skipping' every other step, at least in the beginning of your climb.

Some Stair Climbing experts advise skipping steps on odd floors, then varying your routine by hitting every step on even floors, and so on and so forth.

My experience has been that that once I get tired, it's difficult to get back to the skipping routine.

In my practice climbs, I was able to double up (or skip) the stairs for about 10 floors. After that, it was single step all of the way to the top.

#24. One way or other, I don't feel good on my climb until my heart gets pumping.

In my training climbs, 'feeling good' sometimes took 10 seconds, sometimes a full minute. The important thing is to find that rhythm, and once you have it, hold your pace there.

#25. Don't climb alone in stairways.

Always climb with a friend. You could have a heart attack, you could trip and hurt yourself, you could be mugged.

Don't climb alone, and if you do, take a cell phone and always be sure someone knows where you are.

#26. Forget the elevator

Some scientific studies have suggested that climbing even two flights of stairs per day can lead to 6 pounds of weight loss over one year. I never take an elevator if I can avoid it.

I've seen advice that says if you have 3 floors or less to your destination, take the stairs, not the elevator.

I say why limit yourself.

My wife and I visited Chicago in June of 2011. Our room was on the 16th floor, and we took the stairs up and the stairs down.

#27. 30 minutes of running produces the same workout as 15 minutes of Stair Climbing.

I've seen those stats, and I can believe them.

I guess it depends on the individual, and the intensity of your running.

My running is more of a jog---9 minute miles.

I run 5 miles at a time 3 days per week, and I can safely say that my Sunday afternoon workout of 100 flights of stairs in my house, which takes me about 25 minutes to complete, leaves me much more drained than the 45 minutes I take to run 5 miles.

One thing I know---I can 'dog it' when I'm running 5 miles outside, but on the stairs, it's impossible. I double step my stair training, and it's either continue or stop---and I NEVER stop.

#28. Check with your doctor before embarking on a training program.

I don't want anyone reading this book to die or hurt themselves training for, or doing, a stair climb.

I recommend that everyone see their doctor at least once a year---young and old alike.

Young people die in races also, usually as a result of a hidden health problem they (or their family) didn't know they have.

The bottom line: See your doctor before you begin

#29. It hurts during the climb. I want to stop.

This is normal. I don't blame you, but please, Don't stop!

Unlike the 'no pain, no gain' mantra that drives me nuts, and is a big myth, there is a difference between pain and discomfort.

The body will feel discomfort when exercising, and when practicing for a stair climb, or actually doing it, you will experience quite a bit of discomfort.

I previously spoke of being short of, or out of breath. That's discomfort #1.

Your lungs may burn. That's discomfort #2.

Your mouth and air ways may become very dry, from your body's heavy breathing. That's discomfort #3.

Finally, your legs will ache and burn. That's discomfort #4.

Train properly, and your body will become accustomed to these discomforts and learn to deal with them for 10 minutes.

Remember, a Stair Climb lasts for only about 10 to 15 minutes.

Thanks goodness you aren't running a Marathon!

#30. There's a demon the 13th floor

The first time I practice climbed in our 25 floor condo venue, I was feeling pretty good, doubling up the stairs until about the tenth floor, then at the 13th floor, I swore that there was a demon on the 13th floor sucking the oxygen out of the stairway.

From that point forward, it was a struggle to get to the top, pretty much putting one foot in front of the other and making my way up the stairs.

The second time up the stairs, I double stepped less (stopping around the 5th floor) and single stepped my way up the rest. Guess what? The demon was still at the 13th floor.

March 19, 2011. The actual climb. 13th floor. The demon again.

It's normal. It's Oxygen Debt.

Your demon may be an earlier or later floor, but you will encounter it during the actual climb.

Better to find it during practice than during your first climb when you don't know how to handle it.

#31. Climb Day is a mental exercise

I discussed earlier the benefits of having a team and training in groups.

One of the interesting things my team and I discussed during our 25 floor training sessions was what would happen when we passed the 25th floor for the first time.

Although we had climbed nearly 100 floors during our three training sessions, we had done no more than 25 at one time---followed by an approximate 2 minute elevator ride to the first floor, and a repeat of the 25 floors.

We knew we could do 50. We had done it before.

And we knew we could do 25 floors, with 2 minutes in between, and 25 more floors.

For me, I was doing 25 floors in about 4 minutes. With the 2 minute elevator "rest" period built in, that told me at worse, even if I took a 2 minute rest at floor 25, I should be able to carry on and finish floors 26-50 in about 4 more minutes. A total of 10 minutes.

#32. Stair Climbing is easier on your joints than walking

So I've heard---it's definitely easier than running.

Think about it.

Most stairs in a fire escape are about 4 to 6 inches high.

You're climbing up all of the time---with minimal impact.

#33. Whatever you do, don't climb down stairs.

Coming down stairs is hard on your calf muscles. When you practice, take the elevator down.

#34. You will cough in the stairway.

PJ Glassey, one of the best stair climbers in the United States and a personal trainer, has coined a term called "Track Hack". He says that this cough typically starts within a few minutes of the end of an event and can last for up to 3 days, although in my experience it doesn't last that long.

He says it's caused by extreme deep and heavy breathing, combined with an elevated heart hate, and occurs because your airway becomes irritated and eroded from air passing over it with increased volume and velocity.

He says that extreme athletes (and he is one) often notice a taste of blood in their mouth after intense exertion.

Most people assume that it is due to poor air quality in the stairwell, but PJ says that is not the case.

Just about all of the major Stair Climbs will sanitize and disinfect the stairs a week or so before the climb to rid them of dust.

Be forewarned. You will cough.

Some of my Stair Climbing friends recommend sucking on a cough lozenge (don't do this during your climb.)

Others recommend those breath strips that you place on your tongue which dissolve. You can safely do this during the climb.

#35. Most Commercial Buildings have 20 steps per floor (with a landing in between.)

Just a tidbit I thought you should know.

It will help you gauge your training efforts, and what you need to do to get ready.

Our Philadelphia Fight For Air climb is 50 floors, and 1,088 steps.

20 steps per floor, and that includes a landing.

#36. Some climbs are 'turn to your left' and some climbs are 'turn to your right' as you ascend the stairs.

Bet you never thought of that one.

If you ask your Stair Climb organizer, they will tell you---not that it makes a tremendous amount of difference.

#37. Your legs will burn

I experience a burn in my legs within the first minute or so of climbing. It always passes, and then it returns sometime after the 4 minute mark. After that, it's another 6 minutes to the top.

#38. Handrails?

Handrails line the stair way. There's always one. Sometimes there are two.

Some climbers (especially the good ones) use the handrails to give themselves and extra boost to the top of the building.

The idea is that their arms do some of the work that their legs would be doing.

I don't use the handrails myself.

I didn't last year, but I do know I was passed during last year's ALA Philly climb by two climbers using the handrails. They made it look effortless as they double stepped by me.

According to PJ Glassey, Jesse Berg (#8 in the world) uses both hands on the rails at once, and pulls together.

Mark Trahanovsky (top US climber in the 50-60 age group) likes to alternate his hand grabs between both rails.

Cindy Harris and Terry Purcell (the most winning US climbers) use the inside rail only and climb it like a rope.

Javier Santiago (the Mexican national champion) and Michelle Blessing (rated top 10 in the world) use the rails only on the turns, and go hands free on the rest.

PJ Glassey uses all of these techniques and changes his method every 20 floors, so it spreads the fatigue around to as many difference muscle groups as possible.

My teammate Tim and I have pledged to try the hand rail technique this year in our practices and hopefully during our climb on March 24, 2012.

Using the rails requires some core strength, so be sure to hit the weight room also.

#39. Single step or double step?

Last year, during my actual climb, I double stepped one flight and then single stepped the remaining 49 floors.

I always double step in my house--that's not too tough since as soon as I get to the top, I need to walk down the stairs to start another cycle.

Our 25 floor practice venue was a different story, however.

Using our 25 floor practice venue, I had practiced double stepping, and was able to go as far as 10 floors or so double stepping.

In practice, I timed myself double stepping 10 floors and single stepping the remaining 15 versus single stepping 25 floors, and there was only about a 10 second difference between the two times.

I found single stepping almost from the time I started allowed me to find my pace and rhythm easier.

Having said that, there's no doubt, if I could, I would rather double step my way up to the top, and I'll be practicing double stepping in conjunction with the handrails this winter in preparation for the 2012 ALA Philly climb.

My teammate Tim also intends to double step his way to the top.

It could easily shave a minute off of our time from last year.

The great thing about double stepping in practice is that it gives you something tangible to improve upon each time out.

If you can double step 10 floors in a 25 floor condo, try for 11 or more next time.

#40. Dress light

You'll be climbing intensely, and the stair ways aren't cold to begin with.

I wear shorts and a short sleeve shirt.

#41. Wash your hands after the race

You'll be touch handrails that have been touched by hundreds of other climbers.

#42. You will be out of breath just about the entire time

Sorry, but that's the truth. Notice I didn't say you will suffocate, just that you will be out of breath. You can deal with it.

#43. If you practice in a tall building's fire escape, be prepared to get locked in

I remember a few years ago, I was taking a 'short cut' in the University of Pennsylvania's Hospital stair way, probably from the 23rd floor to the 19th.

What I didn't realize was that after entering the fire escape at the 23rd floor, there was 'no entry' again until the ground floor.

So, if you do find a stair case to practice climb in, it's possible that, once you climb to the top, you will have to climb down all the way to get out.

Some friends I know will wedge something into the doorway they use to gain entry to the stair case so they can re-enter it after their climb.

This will probably work, but you may generate a call to Security.

#44. What are the chances of getting permission to climb in a high rise?

If you're lucky, you may live in a high rise (such as our teammate Tim did last year.)

Maybe you work in a high rise.

But if you don't, what are the chances of walking into the lobby of a high rise and hitting the fire escape for practice?

With today's heightened security, it may be next to impossible. I know. I've tried.

One exception would be if you work in the building. You may be able to make arrangements with Building Management to permit you to climb at lunch time or after work before the building is secured for the evening.

Some sponsored climbs, such as the ALA and Cystic Fibrosis Foundation Climbs, have organized practice climbs, some of which are free to registered climbers, some of which charge a nominal fee that goes to the charity.

Remember, my training strategy are stairs in my house, and 3 practice climbs in a high rise. Even better would be a practice climb in the actual building you are climbing on Climb Day.

If you can't get into a high rise, there are suitable substitutions.

More likely would be a publicly accessible structure, such as a parking garage.

But be careful. You don't want to do this alone.

#45. Always take the elevator down

I think I've mentioned this already.

You don't want to take the stairs down.

It's hard on your legs (calves in particular) and it's far easier to trip down the stairs and hurt something than it is to trip up the stairs and do damage.

I know, I know, after climbing your way to the top, it seems a bit 'lazy' not to walk down, but believe me, take the elevator and get right back into the stair well and climb to the top again.

#46. Find a friend who lives in a high rise

If you can't find a high rise to practice in, ask around and see if you can find a friend who lives or works in one. You don't need much height to get a good work out (10 floors or above.)

#47. Form a team with someone who lives or works in a high rise

Form a team with someone who lives in a high rise.

#48. StairMaster? Stair Mill?

I don't care much for StairMasters or Stair mills---I just don't think they simulate the act of climbing a stair case very well.

However I've heard great things about Jacob's Ladder,

http://www.jacobsladderexercise.com/

You can buy one yourself for between $2,500 and $3.500.

Here are links to 2 You Tube videos of stair climbers using a Jacob's Ladder. It seems to simulate the action of climbing stairs much better.

http://www.youtube.com/watch?v=D2Nn2fQjwZc

http://www.youtube.com/watch?v=NqW0EhLjSJI

#49. What about Outside Public Stairs?

If you live in a city that has good outside stairs (Seattle is outstanding for this,) you are (and will be) in great shape. Use them.

Most cities don't have great outside stairs.

This website

http://www.publicstairs.com/

may help you determine if your city does.

#50. If you use a StairMaster, don't pay attention to the 'stairs climbed' read out.

Speaking of StairMasters, if you use one, don't pay attention to the 'stairs climbed' number.

It's probably not a good indicator anyway---better to pay attention to the time you are able to use the machine.

For me, it's about 10 minutes to the top of our 50 story building. 10 minutes of high intensity exercise will do it.

When I climb up AND down my stairs, I like at least 20 minutes, since half the time I'm coming down.

#51. Don't wear sweats or hats when you practice or when you climb 'for real', unless you're outside.

It drives me crazy when athletes over dress.

Of course, it may be me--I wear shorts outside to run until the temperatures drop into the teens.

As far as Stair Climbing, you're climbing inside, right?

Building are maintained at 72 degrees.

The fire escapes may be a bit cooler in the winter, warmer in the summer, but not much different.

Most organized Stair Climbs are held during the winter, spring or fall, so even if the fire escape is cool, after about 5 floors of climbing stairs, you'll be quite warmed up.

For the Philadelphia American Lung Association climb, the climb starts outside, and if the weather is cold, and you have to wait for a while to start your climb, you will get cold.

You may consider doing what I do for some of my races before they start--- wear a long sleeved "throw away" shirt that you can discard.

It may be there when you finish, it may not, but the shirts I choose are disposable in my mind.

Some races/climbs will donate discarded shirts to the homeless.

#52. To train, or not train, with weights

I can't seem to make up my mind.

I don't train with weights, yet I know other climbers who do train with a weight vest.

It's an added feature of your training.

Make up your own mind.

#53. Most organized Stair Climbs are held in fire escapes.

Another tidbit I thought you should know about.

Most organized Stair Climbs are held in high rise fire escapes.

They are well lit, well ventilated, and usually 'washed down' of excess dust a few days before the event.

Expect 20 steps per floor---10 steps, followed by a landing, and then 10 more steps.

Fire escapes will either be 'left turning' or 'right turning'.

#54. Some organized Stair Climbs are in stadiums

Some organized Stair Climbs are held, outdoors, in stadiums, and feature just about the same number of steps to climb as the indoor climbs.

#55. Prior to your actual climb, you may want to run several times around the block.

My team and I did this last year.

It served two purposes.

It got us warmed up, and it also dissipated the nervous energy we all felt waiting around to start the climb.

#56. It's possible you may want to pass someone

Most organized Stair Climbs (unless you are part of the 'fun' climb event) will have staggered starts.

That means you will start 15 seconds after the previous climber, and 15 seconds before the climber after you.

Some Stair Climbs ask you to estimate your finish time in order to arrange the climbers according to levels of abilities.

This should mean that you don't spend a lot of time either passing or being passed.

Passing requires a bit more effort on your part.

If you need to pass, hopefully the person in front of you will be close to the hand rail, not in the middle of the stairs.

Either way, say something like

"passing on your right" or "passing on your left"

to let the person in front of you know that you are passing.

#57. It's possible you will be passed

Don't worry about it.

It doesn't mean you're doing anything wrong.

If you are climbing in an open or team category, this is perfectly normal.

It's also fine if you are a climber in the Elite category and someone passes you--there's a wide variation in climbing paces and you can be passed.

Yield the right of way and he or she will be by you in no time.

Last year, in the 2011 Philadelphia Fight For Air climb, this happened to me twice, and I wound up passing one of those people later in the climb.

I'd only worry if you are the pre-climb favorite or ranked #1 in the world.

#58. There may be floor numbers on the doors at each floor you pass. Don't look at them.

No surprise there. Floor numbers must be numbered, so that emergency personnel know where they are in an emergency.

That doesn't mean you have to.

I don't know about you, but the last thing I want to see when I'm climbing to the 50th floor of a build is a sign saying I'm on the 12 floor.

Not everyone agrees.

Some of the best stair climbers pace themselves according to where they are.

That's just not for me.

Some organized Stair Climbs sell "floor sponsorships," so it's possible you won't see a floor number, but a banner advertising Mike Jones, the noted Riverton New Jersey personal trainer.

If your mind starts to wander, you can mentally check out the sponsors as you go my.

#59. Just about all organized Stair Climbs have a staggered start, not a gang start.

That's good news.

Actually, the only Stair Climb I know that features a gang start is the Empire State Building Climb, and that's limited to 25 climbers, the climbers that are going to fight it out for the first place prize.

A staggered start is one in which climbers start at a pre-determined time, 8 to 15 seconds behind the climber in front of them, 8 to 15 seconds ahead of the climber after them.

That's good news.

I really don't feel like fighting my way into a stairway, but it can make for a great You Tube video. Here's one of the Empire State Building Run Up's gang start...

http://www.youtube.com/watch?v=s1ndXZtDxlU

#60. Organized Stair Climbs are primarily fund raising events, not athletic events.

In other words, don't go crazy, and don't be an obnoxious jock.

You'll see a bunch of very fit looking people.

You'll also see some relatively unfit people who are there to raise money because a loved one has either died of a lung disease or is currently dying.

Remember how lucky you are to be able to race to the top.

Not everyone can.

#61. Carbo-loading is not necessary.

Carbohydrate loading, commonly referred to as carbo-loading or carb-loading, is a strategy used by endurance athletes, such as marathon runners, to maximize the storage of glycogen (or energy) in the muscles.

Carbo loading is generally recommended for endurance events lasting longer than 90 minutes

There's no need to Carbo Load prior to the climb. You're most likely climbing for 8 to 15 minutes. This is more of a sprint than a marathon.

#62. There's no truth in the statement, "No pain, no gain"

Along with the last chance workout, I don't think there's a single exercise mantra that repels me more.

Pain is not good.

If you are exercising, and you are in pain while you are doing it, that is not a good thing.

Stop whatever you are doing---you're either injured, or you are doing something wrong.

Pain after exercise is a different thing.

#63. If your legs are sore the day after a workout, it doesn't necessarily mean you should rest.

Not necessarily.

When I was younger, if I was sore the day after exercising, most likely it was because I wasn't exercising enough.

During your first week or two of training, you will most likely have some sore muscles. This is normal. I'd be more concerned about sore joints, ligaments and tendons which might point to poor training or overuse.

You've probably heard the expression, "listen to your body."

If you are sore, that's one thing. Grit it out and try to get a workout in. You may find that the workout actually dissipates the soreness.

If you are injured, always rest.

#64. Can't climb yourself? Consider being a Virtual Climber

A Virtual Climber isn't a volunteer---it's usually a member of a team who either physically can't climb or doesn't meet the minimum age requirement, or perhaps is stationed overseas in the military.

Virtual climbers pay the registration fee and raise the minimum in donations.

Virtual climbers are listed on the Team Roster, show up at the building on Climb Day, and attend the post climb events.

In short, they do everything a climbing team member does but they don't climb.

In some cases, they may do more, such as take a leading role in team fund raising activities, make cookies or cakes for team bake sales, you get the idea.

You have to remember the climbs are primarily fund raising activities---so it makes perfect sense to have virtual climbers.

#65. While you're waiting in line to climb on Climb Day, don't drink too much water.

Being properly hydrated is important---3 days and prior to the climb.

Drinking a bunch of water the morning of the climb is really counter productive.

If you are standing in line for an hour (the way I did last year,) you can easily finish off a quart of water due to nervous energy.

That water has to go somewhere--which could require a bathroom break prior to the climb or even worse, once your climb has started.

Take my advice, and once you stand in line, ditch your water bottle.

#66. Maintain a daily diary/log

It's been my experience that maintaining a daily diary/log is the best way to ensure that I follow through on anything.

Exercise, weight loss, book writing!

#67. Enter a Stair Climb!

The best way to ensure that you'll train and practice for a Stair Climb is to enter one!

Don't be afraid, just do it. Enter as an individual to start. If you can form a team, all the better.

#68.You may never feel ready enough

Until you do your first stair climb, you won't know for sure if you've trained enough.

If you can follow my plan, and do 100 flights of stairs without stopping, you're ready!

#69. Most likely, you will need to Fund Raise!

Last year, it cost $25 to register for the 2011 Philadelphia Fight For Air Climb, plus a commitment of another $100 in donations.

If you want, you can just put up the additional $100 yourself, or you can ask friends and family to do it.

Most people won't find the additional $100 difficult to raise.

But it's something you don't want to forget about.

Our team plans to bake some cookies and cupcakes this year and sell the cookies for 50 cents and the cupcakes for $1 to raise some team funds.

#70. When you finish, you will think it's one of the best things you've ever done

You'll feel like a million bucks after your first stair climb. Spend the next hours, days, months and even the entire year letting people know what you've done and how much you hope they join you the next year.

Tips (Anonymous, First Name Only)

Tip: Places to climb in Manhattan

Hey, I live in Manhattan, and access to stairs is a big problem here as well. I take the "don't ask, don't tell" approach. I just sneak in where I can, train, and get out of there. Smaller, less prestigious buildings are a better bet. I've tried to get into the Empire State Building, the Chrysler Building, and back in the day, the World Trade Center, but they laughed me off. Generally if you ask, you'll get shot down. I train in my office near Wall Street, which is convenient for me because it's where I work and they don't monitor the stairs. If you know someone who works or lives in a high rise, that could help. Don't carry a lot of stuff with you, maybe only keys and a cell phone in case you get locked in the stairwell or caught. Maybe Jersey City is a good option for you - there are some tall buildings near the Hudson. If you're ever downtown and want to meet up to train, let me know.

Tip: Climb Day:

I'm by no means an expert, but for me, slow and steady is recommendation. I've raced a few (this tower will be my highest climb before my Willis (Sears) Tower climb in November), but I've learned to regulate my pace, especially at first. I use the first 2-3 minutes of the climb as a "warm-up" before I begin to increase my speed. Also, I've learned to use the railing more to help me climb. Too often I've started out way too fast and then found myself winded after only a few floors. I will be keeping an eye on my stopwatch to measure how I'm doing.

Tip: Places to climb in Los Angeles

Here are some good spots for stair training in the Los Angeles area:

The 4th st. stairs in Santa Monica. Take 4th St. to the North in Santa Monica and you will see a few set of stairs of about 200 steps each. Many Santa Monica residents train there everyday.

In Hollywood area there are some more steps, see this link:

http://franklinhills.org/stairwaywalk.pdf

Tip: For those over 50

I'm a 50 plus woman who experienced the joy of Stair Climbing recently by completing a "Half Hustle" Up the Hancock in 12 minutes. (Not bad for someone who frequents the gym only to read chick lit!)

I'm now hooked and I want to do the Sears in November. My Hustle training was as follows:

5 days a week of cardio, 30 minutes each sessions alternating elliptical trainer

on the weight loss interval with 30 minutes on recumbent bike with 30 minutes of the StairMaster.

<u>5 days a week</u> of free weight training, alternating upper and lower body exercises, with a lower body focus on squats and lunges

<u>7 days a week</u> of core exercises...alternating abs and back

By the way, I'm 5 feet 8 inches, 140 lbs.

Tip: Step Master vs. StairMaster (Courtesy of Ed)

My local gym has two climbing machines: the StepMaster (which is like an escalator) and another one which has the pedals of an elliptical, but you can only move your legs up and down. You don't have the range of motion of a StairMaster.

I work in a building with 12 floors but I work out with the StairMaster.

If you can find one, the Jacob's Ladder looks like the ultimate climbing machine: you use both your arms and legs on wooden bars at a 45 degree angle. It's self-propelled.

I have yet to find a gym in my area that has it.

Tip (Courtesy of Rick)

I learned about "Go Vertical Chicago" in late '08 and thought it would be a great goal to set for myself.

I began to train for the '09 event. I live in a rural area with no tall buildings so i worked out on a stair machine. I trained hard and had gotten up to 150 floors in 20 minutes. I hated it when I found out that the event had been cancelled.

Tip (Courtesy of Louis)

The key to training is not necessarily duration, but INTENSITY.

A 12-story building is a great training venue.

However, climbing it more than 5 or 6 times per session is probably not the optimal approach.

Rather than increasing the number of climbs, increase the speed or decrease any planned rest/recovery between climbs.

Tip: Parking Garage

The best thing I have found is a parking garage its only 8 1/2
(short) floors 105 steps so you have to do a LOT if up and down and I feel that you get too much of a rest going down even if you run down as fast as you can.

The number one thing I have noticed doing actual runs (Empire State Building Run Up and Sears) is the intensity which I have not been able to recreate in training.

I have been doing real stairs at the garage 3-4 days a week and would usually head straight to the gym after doing the stairs and get on a stair climber for an additional 30-40 min just to get more cardio in.

I guess a stair climber is better than nothing but you are not actually lifting your body weight so I dont think its enough by itself to prepare you for a real climb.

Tip: Places to train outdoors near Rochester (Courtesy of Bernie)

Another great place to train outdoors is at Bloomer Park in Rochester.

There is a stair case that has 175175 steps and you can go up and down as many times as you can.

Work your self up 10 sets and you master anything!

Tip (Courtesy of Mr. Karlin)

I do a lot of different training.

I do cross training, but specifically for the stairs, I'll climb - where I live in my building,

I'll climb 450 flights and actually with a ten-pound weighted vest on. So I'll climb up from the basement to the top and take the elevator down and do 20 laps.

And that's one of my big trainings.

The other thing I might do is I may have a, also a weighted vest - maybe not 10 pounds, but a lighter vest.

And I'll just do sprints.

I'll run up 10, 15, 20 flights.

I'll sprint and then take a rest and then repeat that, and take the elevator downstairs.

I don't actually walk down the stairs.

Tip: Avoiding Injury is the Key

My main goal is not so much a best time at the next climb, but hopefully being able to last a few decades...avoiding injury is the key.

Tip: High School Bleachers

Try High School bleachers if you can't train in a high rise. If you do this, try to come down as fast as possible.

Tip: Parking Garage

Try a Parking Garage if you can't train in a high rise

Tip: If you live or work in Philadelphia

If you live or work in Philadelphia, you might be able to train on the stairs at Franklin Field on Penn's campus.

Tip from Suzannah Davidson-Alles

Background: Suzannah is one of my original Facebook Stair Climbing friends. Suzanna shares my passion for climbing house stairs---see, I'm not alone in that approach. Here she shares her tips on Stair Climbing.

I've been Stair Climbing for 20 or more years... I do 100 laps on my staircase several times a week.

My real passion is running, but when I can't get outside due to weather, this is a great alternative.

I break up the sessions into 30 laps (with a 15 minute break in between).

I am surprised at how few people consider doing this....I much prefer this and running to a gym any day!!

Tips from Trevor Folgering

Background: Trevor is the founder of StairClimbCanada.com and champion Stair Climbing. Also a Personal Trainer, Trevor is a workout maniac.

Here Trevor shares his daily diet with us.

Wake-up (4:30 am)

4:45 am - Green Tea/Almonds

5:00 am - Six Whole eggs and One Banana OR Smoothie Shake (Shake comprised of 1 Banana, 1/2 cup of mixed berries, 1 scoop of Vega Protein Powder, Almonds and water) - Will flip back and forth with these two meals depending on how my energy levels feel and my body fat levels. If I feel I am lean enough I will include smoothies more, If I feel I need to lean out I will eat the eggs. It also depends on energy levels, If I feel I need more energy then Ill have the smoothie.

Training 5:30 - 6:45 (Time Depends on Client Load, But Usually I try to book clients to start around 7 am so I can have my first meal slightly before 7am.)

7am - Meal #2 - Oatmeal/Mixed Berries and Vega Powder with almonds - This has always been a staple since I started Bodybuilding back in 1999. Its always Oatmeal and eggs or oatmeal and protein powder

10 am - Meal #3 - Super Green Smoothie Shake - Shake contains the following: Kale, Mixed Fruit Blend, almonds, Vega Powder, Water. I find this easy to have because I am usually training clients and I just sip the shake slowly throughout the hour.

It usually takes me about an hour to finish and I have learned that its way better to slowly take shakes like this in to help with digestion. Its great to actually chew your shake to help further break everything down.

Chewing produces saliva and saliva helps break food down. That's why I like adding almonds as I have to chew them more. It helps and I really believe these super shakes have helped my athletic performance.

1pm - Meal # 4 Six whole eggs and 2 grapefruits - Great meal to eat here as I am home and have no clients usually around this time. I think this is one of the perfect meals as its totally complete protein source with an amazing fruit. Grapefruit is so low in the GI index and so many positive benefits.

4pm - Meal # 5 Super Smoothie Number 2 - Same as the morning shake BUT I usually make it with spinach not Kale. Again it depends on energy levels, I might make it with Kale again as I feel Kale is superior to spinach and has higher energy levels within the body.

6:30 - 7pm. - Meal #6 - Six whole eggs and grapefruit meal. The afternoon shake can really go through me fast and I can feel really hungry by 6 -

6:30. Depending on hunger levels Ill have it when I teach stairs OR right before my 7:30 pm client.

9:00 pm - Meal #7 - Raw Oats and Vega Powder with Almonds - Last meal of the day I Usually have around 30 minutes before bed. This is a meal that I usually have that I really enjoy and its nice because its higher in carbohydrates, something my body needs after a long day of training clients and being active.

Again I used to eat no carbs after six, thinking that carbs after six isn't the smartest thing to do, however I think this meal helps me really push for my next training session and helps increase glycogen levels in the muscles. I may also have a banana as well to help level off liver glycogen levels as well. Again this is all by how I feel and how my body feels and what my training the next day is.

If its something lighter like swimming I skip out on the fruit, if its a harder training session on the stairs Ill have fruit.

Tips from Tim Gradoville

Background: Tim is a member of Team Smiley and a former professional athlete. He knows what he's talking about!

Tim was kind enough to share his Training Tips for this book.

Start training early and ease into it. Do what you can initially; too much too soon can discourage you and possibly cause injuries.

Once you have a strong training base, push yourself to go longer and quicker.

Mix in **Cross Training** like running or cardio machines to aid in your training.

If you can handle it, going two steps at a time can be beneficial.

Running with music can help keep you focused and motivate you to train longer.

Stretch after training as muscles can tense up quickly.

Lately, Tim has been training on a Nautilus StairMaster SM916.

Tips from Cindy Harris

Background: Cindy is ranked as the #1 Stair Climber of **All Time** according to TowerRunning.com, and the #2 Women's Stair Climber for the 2011 World Cup Standing according to TowerRunning.com. She holds the Willis (Sears) Tower record for woman, 14:57, set in 2011. She is a 5 time winner of the Empire State Building Run Up, and the American record holder of 12:45 in 2001. She is a 9 time winner of the Willis (Sears Tower Run up., setting the Women's Record of 14:57 in 2011. She is a 12 time winner of the Hustle Up The Hancock Tower in Chicago, setting the Women's Record of 10:51 in 2008. She is a 17 time winner of the Bop To The Top in Indianapolis, with a Women's record time of 4:26 in 2001.

Cindy was kind enough to share her Training and Racing Tips for this book.

Cindy's Training Tips

1. Practice on stairs once or twice a week.

2. Go up and take the **elevator down**, to make it easier on your knees.

3. Use the handrails.

4. Find a style of climbing that feels most comfortable for you, whether it's one step or two steps at a time, usually two steps at a time is more efficient and faster.

Cindy's racing strategy?

I divide the race into three parts and pace myself accordingly.

I try not to pay too much attention to where I am.

The first third, I relax.

The next third, I keep a steady pace.

The last third, I see what's left.

Cindy's strategy for the Empire State Building Climb

You want to be in a good position, but not necessarily first because, if you go out way too fast, you run the risk of going out too fast and just completely exhausting yourself, which isn't good.

So strategy is pretty much to be in the top five places, 'cause it's fairly easy to pass that amount of people that there are in front of you.

The strategy?

First of all you've got to train well, and be prepared and be willing to suffer 'cause it's very painful and exhausting!

Tips from John Korff

Background: John Korff is the director the NYC Triathlon. He is also the race director for the Inaugeral Ironman ® U.S. Championship coming to NYC/NJ August 11, 2012. John has been an age group champion for the Empire State Building Run Up (ESBRU.).

According to John, training is simple..

Training can include climbing a staircase, running uphill, biking uphill, using a StairMaster; and supplementing with core training, weights, and/or general fitness exercises.

The best training is climbing stairs in a tall building.

The second best training is climbing stairs in a tall building. Get it?

King Kong did it. You can too. There is no secret recipe: it's just one foot after the other.

As far as Climb Day...

You'll be fine:

It's just one foot after another until you reach the top. Below are a few tips on how to do the Run Up if you just-want-to-finish (category 1) or if you want to race (category 2). Pant, pant.

His detailed tips on training for, and doing the Empire State Building Run Up are about the best I've seen everywhere.

http://www.themmrf.org/donate-now-take-action/join-an-event/endurance-events/esbru-training-page-11-2011.pdf

His detailed tips on the Empire State Building Run Up, although specific to the Empire State Building climb, are great for every climb. Here's the link

http://www.themmrf.org/donate-now-take-action/join-an-event/endurance-events/esbru-training-race-day.pdf

Tips from Terry Purcell

Background: Ranked #5 **All Time** Stair Climber by TowerRunning.com. US Bank Tower in Los Angeles Men's Record holder (along with Tim Van Orden) in 9 minutes and 32 seconds. Set his record in 2009. He has won the Chicago Hustle Up The Hancock 8 times. He has been described by some as the Lance Armstrong of Stair Climbing, as of March 2011, Terry had won more stair races than any other racer in the world. Like Chris Solarz, Terry doesn't do a lot of training in the stairs.

Terry has publicly shared these Training Tips.

Those looking to make the leap from casual stair-climbing to a skyscraper climb should heed the advice of Terry Purcell, six-time champion of the Aon Center race: Pace yourself, or suffer the consequences.

"Those are the top three things: Start out slow, start out slow, start out slow," Purcell said.

Other tips? Suck on a mint before the race to avoid "climber's hack" the coughing or sneezing fits that often result from the combination of a stairwell's dry air and physical exertion. And use the handrails. (It's not cheating)

Tips from Lisa Kinsner Scheer

Background: Lisa is one of my original Facebook Stair Climbing friends and generously shares encouragement and advice to everyone.

I have competed in Cleveland's Tackle the Tower (37 floors).

The best training I have found is a StepMill. ot to be confused with a StairMaster.

The StepMill is similar to an escalator, with a "collapsing staircase".

Of course, real stairs are the best training, but you are in a winter climate like me. The endurance built in a spinning class or running is good too.

It is all about pace.

Don't start out too fast.

By the 8th floor, you will switch from aerobic to anaerobic activity.

You'll think you're going to die, but by the 15th or 20th floor you'll find your grove.

How about a high school stadium?

Bragging rights are worth the price!

Your friends will think you are insane. All worth it!

Here are some more great tips from Lisa

Sign up early, for a better start time. An early start means more oxygen.

Being a runner does not make you a great stair climber. The demands are different. Running helps, but does not "train you" for a climbing event.

A tall building is ideal to utilize for training.

Use the elevator to come down. Walking downstairs is hard on the knees.

No tall building?? The next best thing is to access a StepMill, which looks like a cascading staircase, NOT to be confused with a "stepper".

On the StepMill, don't use your hands. And once you are pretty good at it, carry hand weights.

Practice double stepping. Double step on event day too.

lunges, with weights are good for training too.

Don't start off too fast!!!

Use the handrails to pull yourself up.

Gloves with rubber grips or "tacky" football receiver gloves are awesome too.

It's hot and DRY in the stairwell. Dress as if it were 80 degrees outside.

Use Ayr Nasal Gel to prevent a nose bleed.

Jolly Ranchers or a cough drop are great to reduce the incredible dry mouth that you may experience.

WASH YOUR HANDS and/or remove your gloves ASAP post-race. It's germy on those handrails and in the stairwell.

HYDRATE! Beer is good post race. As is Chocolate Milk or water.

Go a second time so people think you are insane.

Once you have completed a stair climb, you are addicted to it! That is......if you are completely nuts!

It is a very humbling experience, but the bragging rights are soooo worth it!!!!!

Tips from David Snyder

Background: David is ranked in the top 25 US Stair Climbers of **All Time** according to Towerruning.com. In addition to his athletic endeavors, David wins special mention for advancing the sport of Stair Climbing. About 10 years ago, David created the Stair Climbing Yahoo Group, which has provided help for many years to Stair Climbers, experienced and novices alike. I found it invaluable when I first started out. In addition, he also created and administers the Facebook Stair Climbing Group, which is equally valuable. Finally, he also created **StairclimbingSport.com**, a website with many valuable resources.

David has generously shared his Training Tips on his website for many years.

I have made a table of the best Stair Climbing training methods (In order of preference.).

1. 60 + stories straight up the stairs

2. Shorter building, up the stairs and elevator down, repeat

3. One flight of stairs in house, repeated several times

4. Running up a steep hill

5. Cycling up a steep hill

6. Running flat or track middle distance, 2K to 5K

7. Cycling flat or track middle distance, 3K to 10K

8. Exercise stepper machines

9. Push-ups and wall-squat exercises

10. Walking down stairs

Finding the most stairs straight up with little need for repeating rounds with the elevator down is the best. You are always going up with few or no breaks. Finding a steep hill to run or cycle up are alternatives. Track or flat cycling and running are also good. I put the distance at "middle distance" in the database because middle distance running and cycling requires both sprint and endurance skills, just like Stair Climbing. Stair Climbing requires lots of explosive muscular strength as in sprints and also endurance as many famous races are 1,500 stairs or more.

You will notice that I put the exercise stepper machines way down on the list. That is because I too, have found that the steppers do not mimic the real stairs that good. Stepping machines are much easier as some of you have discovered. Real stairs do not "slide" down as you step on them, there is no "give" or "play." But in the absence of the better choices, it is still not so bad to give them a try and use the machines, especially if you already own one.

If all of the top 7 choices are still not available to you, there is always push-ups and wall-squat. Push-ups will develop your shoulder and arm muscles for pulling yourself up with the rail in a Stair Climbing race. Wall-squat is done by placing your body in a seated position (no chair) with only your back against the wall. This works the quadriceps in the legs and thighs for muscular leg strength. Try to sit for at least one minute against the wall and gradually build up to longer times.

The least preferred method (number 10 on the list) is to walk down the stairs. When you walk down, you are going with gravity and there is not much of a work-out. If you take the stairs up, don't bother to walk down, there is not much exercise there. Take the elevator down and then walk or run back to the top.

Hope this list helps you with your training. This is of course my opinion, from my experiences.

Tips from Sophorn Smiley

Background: Sophorn is a member of Team Smiley. Completed her first 50 story Stair Climb in 11:09. She would have finished faster except she cramped up around the 40th floor, something she has yet to discover the reason for.

Her weekly workout schedule consists of this routine:

Run: 3-4t times/week

Yoga: 1-2 times/week

Strength Training (Kickboxing, Cardio Circuit training, Boot camp classes, etc): 2 times/week

1 day of mandatory rest/recovery day (usually on a Friday)

Tips from Chris Solarz

Background: Chris is ranked in the top 25 US Men Stair Climbers of **All Time** according to TowerRunning.com. The holder of several Guinness Book World Records, on June 25, 2011, Chris Solarz climbed Philadelphia's Bell Atlantic Tower (now known as 3 Logan Square) 55 times in 11 hours, a total of 33,000 feet to break the Guinness World Record for the "Greatest Vertical Height Climbed in 12 Hours."

Chris generously shared his training philosophy/tips with me for this book.

I believe that general aerobic capacity is 75% of the skill set needed to be a fast stair climber.

I think that pacing and general Stair Climbing-specific knowledge is worth 15%, and I believe that specific stair training over the prior 4 months is worth 10%.

These three are not mutually exclusive.

If someone were to train each day in the stairwell and achieve the same aerobic capacity as somebody that has been running and biking outside, I believe the stair climber would have a slight (10%) advantage.

To look at it from the other side, since I cannot train in stairs, I believe that I am hardly any worse off (because I do all of my training horizontally outside) than somebody who has access to stairs.

Finally, I think the biggest mistake people make (even very experienced runners) is going out too fast and blowing up.

This is why I gave pacing a 15% weighting - you cannot win the race just on pacing, but you can certainly lose it.

When I'm training for Stair Climbing season, I usually one do only one (sometimes none at all) training session in the stairs a week. But if you are in good overall fitness and know how to pace yourself, I don't think you are generally at much of a disadvantage.

I've also found that cycling is very muscle-specific to Stair Climbing, so a healthy mixture of biking can really help, especially if you don't have access to running stairs.

Of course, my 12 hour Stair Climb was a different beast. For that, I really focused on long-term endurance.

I ran 100 miles per week + 10 hours each week of actual Stair Climbing, which didn't include time descending in elevators.

I trained 25-30 hours per week for the whole year until June, and I'm proud to say that by June 2011 I was in the best shape of my life before I attempted the record.

Tips from Mark Trahanovsky

Background: Ranked as the #34th Stair Climber of All Time. Ranked #27 in 2011 Tower Running World Cup Standings according to Towerrunning. 50-59 Fastest Time Age Group Record at the YMCA US Bank Building in Los Angeles. Founder and Team Captain of the West Coast Labels/X-Gym/Running Raw Stair Climb Team. In 2011, Mark finished 1st in two climbs I follow: the Pittsburgh American Lung Association Climb and the San Diego American Lung Association Climb.

Mark has generously shared his training tips with the public for many years.

He has 7 tips for those who are doing their first stair climb.

1. Do not start too fast. Start at a speed you believe to be a pace you can hold throughout all 37 floors. If halfway through the climb around floor 18 you are feeling energetic then pickup your pace a little. If you are going for a fast time really save any extra energy for the last 4-5 floors and finish strong.

2. If you are tall enough, participants can skip one step and take two steps at a time.

3. No matter if you are a one stepper or two stepper, you will want to pull up on the handrails as you ascend. This arm motion will save on leg energy and lactic acid buildup in the leg muscles.

4. Since our muscle fibers consists of water stay well hydrated on Climb Day, the days before the race and especially during all workouts.

5. All climbers go into the stairs at about 8-10 second intervals to make the stairwells less crowded. If you need to pass, let others know your intentions with a quick word such as "Passing" or "Coming Around" or a tap on the shoulder. If your goal is not so much a fast time but just to finish start towards the end of the line and be aware of anyone behind you on the stairs who wants to pass.

6. About 4-5 days before the climb stop exercising or taper down on any hard workouts. This will allow your muscles to be well rested.

7. MAKE IT FUN! Savor each and every moment from the time before the climb, going up the steps and especially the ecstasy of the finish and its high rise views.

Lastly, since this sport is non-impact and revolves around the everyday activity of walking up stairs it is not age limited.

Last year Mark, who is in his early 50s, encouraged his fellow 1977 Ebensburg, PA high school graduates to try this fast growing sport and some did.

This year their large numbered team cleverly named "The Pittsburgh Stairlers" not only consists of classmates, but the spouses of classmates, children of classmates and friends of these groups.

The Pittsburgh Stairlers will be wearing matching black and gold shirts and look forward to meeting all who are doing this great and healthy fundraiser!

Tips from Rick Williams Firefighter

Background: Rick Williams is a Firefighter, and these guys really rock when they climb.

Rick has shared these tips with me on the Stair Climbing Facebook Page

I've been fortunate to use our tallest building here in Portland for training, at 40 stories. They have opened the building for firefighters to train in order to prepare for the Seattle Firefighter Stair climb every March.

Anyway, I've trained there for over five years now. Coming up on 25,000 stories this month.

One training tip that I've found helpful for myself is doing various 'intervals'.

It kind of breaks up what can sometimes be monotony.

What I'll do is maybe two-step the 40 floors, next time two and one-step variation.

Or I'll do this two and one-step variation and then take a minute break half way.

After that break I'll run 5 to 10 floors and then go back to single or double steps.

The variations are endless, just using imagination in order to keep it fun.

One other tip is using shoe or <u>ankle weights</u>. I've been doing this for quite some time.

Usually when I am training for a firefighter climb I'll use ankle weights on the StairMaster until the time I start using my boots and turnouts.

But I am going to start using them on indoor and outdoor stairs as well. Not a salesman, but...I just bought a pair of '<u>SKLZ Shoe Weights</u>'.

They are a good, but simple design.

CHAPTER TEN

Surveys

The Stair Climbing Facebook Group is one of the friendliest groups I've every had the pleasure to be associated with. There's always someone on there willing to help out.

Over the course of the last few months, I've posted several survey questions to the group, and I thought I would share the results with you.

Only first names are provided in the responses...

Survey Question #1: Why did you do your first stair climb?

Lauren For the heck of it

Silvia Just for the fun and challenging .

Lisa It is a great way to keep the motivation going through a snowy Cleveland Ohio. Our local climbs typically occur in February or March. It is a also a great way to kick off the running season. Further, it was an incredible challenge that our friends said was pretty brutal. Signed up shortly after their "endorsement"! Love a challenge!!

Bob Because you dragged me there, John! Actually, I found it a nice alternative challenge to running races. Climbing 50 stories seems like a daunting task, but it's quickly over for folks who are distance runners. I found it interesting how somebody who can quickly walk 2 steps at a time can move faster than somebody like me who runs 1 step at a time.

Brenda My aunt died of lung cancer three weeks before the Lung Association Stair Climb here. I raised money and did the climb in her memory. Thanks to her I'm now hooked on Stair Climbing and have traveled to Toronto and Los Angeles just to climb stairs! It's funny how things work out.

Cass I just completed my first Stair Climb on the weekend - the Eureka Tower Climb in Melbourne Australia and it was awesome!! One of the toughest things I have done and so glad I did it! I wanted to do something really different and was up for a challenge and was also great to do something for a good cause!

David Basically, I did my first climb because I was getting fat, and I needed an activity that would force me to lose weight. :) Also, My ACL and MCL are torn. I also did stairs hoping to rehab them. Worked!

Rebecca A) I could no longer hike mountains for a period of time which I thought might be forever. I was devastated! So the tower climbing seemed like the next best thing and safe with handrails. B) I did it as a fundraiser for blood cancer and in memory of the grandpa who had just lost the fight to Myeloma a few months prior. I also did it in honor of a Team in Training friend who was going through Leukemia that same year. He passed away in 2009 so I have made a tradition of doing the climb every year in memory of him and to keep his spirit and good will alive (He was a strong supporter and participant with the Leukemia and Lymphoma Society).

Shaun My first was also the Eureka climb. 1) I thought I'd enjoy the challenge. Result YES! 2) Because I have problems with me left knee and strengthening my quads helps it. Result: My quads a LOT stronger from the training which means I can run a lot longer with less pain than before. 3) I wanted to get fit and lose some weight. Result: Nothing has achieved this as much as climbing up 250 floors a day for 2 weeks. I really loved doing the climb, I'm going to enter as many as I can, but as others have said there are limited options in Australia. I wish there were more!

Kent I did my first climb to help make myself feel better as I was going thru a very hard patch in life and I felt like I needed to accomplish something that would be a big positive. Now every time I go by or see a picture of one of the buildings I have climbed I can't help but smile and feel proud of myself for knowing what I have accomplished in that building.

Chandra 5Ks are so mundane. I was looking for something unique.

Antwanika Fitness and because I find running incredibly boring; Stair Climbing is much more fun.

Lisa The 2009 Philly Fight For Air was my first climb. After 26 years, I quit smoking while two of my co-workers were battling lung cancer. The climb gave me something to focus on while also trying to bring more awareness while fundraising and recruiting. My first year I did solo but have been creating a team (Where's the Elevator?) the past couple of years so that we can encourage each other and do this together. I am not an athlete by any means so it feels really good making it the 50 stories...and the view is a bonus.

Daniel I'm actually doing my first one in L.A. on the 3rd!! It's an art project for me. And I hope it is the first of many. I'm interested in the physical aspect and experience of the ascent of the architecture. I'm also using it as a way to better understand the tenants of the buildings. I've always been a fan of skyscrapers so now I get to have a closer look!

Kacie My first Stair Climb was the Empire State Building Run Up! I had no idea this sport even existed!! NOT the building I would recommend to anyone as their first race! Tore the lining of my lungs at floor 50 of the 86 story race!

Renard I did my first stair race to get stronger for the 400meter hurdles. I never thought I would fall in love with it though. Now I'm looking forward to placing in the top ten in the world, in addition to making the Olympic Trials.

Mary Everyone else was doing it!

Nancy Hustle Up The Hancock in Chicago. GREAT climb!

Stephen 1996 USBRU, love the competition

Marsha Needed some type of training to focus on between Marathon seasons.

Mary Jean To learn, physically, more about my lovely city (Pittsburgh).

Vern Was on vacation in Krabi, Thailand and saw the giant Buddha up on the mountain, and said... I gotta climb that.

Will Because I want to do the Gherkin (London) and thought I'd better train.

Rich .... I haven't done a competition but have run 14,200 flights so far this year ... I started doing flights as workouts nearly 15-16 years ago as it was more challenging than straight line running for miles .... next year my goal is to run 15,000 flights.

Vineet I needed some workout at my workplace. I do sets of 10 flights 6-7 a day as I have just started out. This is a way for me to stay fit.

Survey Question #2: Which is faster? Single steps or 2 at a time?

Bob I have been doing single for 5 years but just did 2 at a time for practice yesterday. I try to remember a pace using the StairMaster which is really helpful for single steps. For 2 at a time I have no idea.

Joel 2 at a time is definitely faster. It is tougher since you are pulling twice as far with your legs. I try to only climb two at a time (sometimes 3 at a time) whenever I am training.

Nancy I only climb 2 at a time. Once you get used to it, it's difficult to go back to single steps. My time got better when I switched, years ago, from single to double. You'll develop the strength in your quads fast. I even use the StepMill at my studio and take it 2 at a time when I need a break. It's mostly mental, but when I change it up, it really helps.

David 2 is better as long as your legs are strong (and I guess long enough?) Though some pretty short Elite climbers still double step. I tried doing one of my practice climbs single step a few days ago, and found maintaining the same speed as my double step climb much more tiring.

David Double step all the way! Work on doing lunges to get stronger or double step on the "rolling" style stair machines. Don't forget to use the railing to help "pull" your way up. It makes a huge difference.

Rebecca Thanks! I have been doing double steps but it is hard for me to do on the StairMaster because I have impaired balance function. So on the StairMaster I have to have it set at a lower level in order to double step without tripping. Both on the outdoor stairs and indoor I have been doing double steps lately. I use the StairMaster to learn a pace to keep at but with the double step that is hard to do Any suggestion to learn a double step pace? The largest set of outdoor steps available to me where I live is 210. So I have to do them over and over again which is still not the same. It is more like interval training because I have to go slower going down with my balance. Normally I am a long distance endurance runner and hiker, but now with those activities done, I have been doing more high intensity training and leg work with my trainer. Boy have my legs been sore! I try to run twice a week 30-35 min for maintenance.

Rebecca I have another climb coming up of 56 floors this time (the last was 51). So I will try out double stepping to see what my time will be. With a 5 floor difference it should not be TOO different so hopefully I will get a good comparison base. Whichever seems faster I will go with for my 69 floor climb in March. I am not too terribly concerned about my time in the next climb but I do want it to be the best possible for the big one.

Stephen Double stepping might be better for you

Rebecca The StairMaster is hard for me to double step but I have been doing the outdoor stairs weekly and double stepping all the way! It is interesting. Last night at the stairs a lady was sort of trying to race me! She was doing single step and I double. She ran past me but burned out before reaching the top of a 210 set of steps. I could tell she did not want me to pass her and I MUST use the handrail for my balance. So I ended up finishing the ascent right on her heels because I was behind her. I had to decrease my pace slightly. It was cool to have the experience because I saw how much more tired out she got single stepping. So I am going to double step this entire climb on December 1st to see how it goes for me. Of course the elevation gain in an actual climb is always much greater than what one practices when a large building is not available. But it will be interesting to see how I hold up double stepping 56 flights!

Sally I did the Eureka climb in Melbourne last weekend, 88 floors. My first time up, I just single stepped, because that is what I had done in training. I got to the top with extra energy (obviously didn't push myself hard enough), so I did it for a second time. The second trip up, I wanted to use it as a training exercise and try something different. I mostly double stepped and used the handrail to pull me up. I had never trained like this, but I beat my first time by 8 seconds.

David The fact that you were faster on your second climb says an awful lot. :)

Survey Question #3: Do you look at the floor numbers as you're climbing?

Chandra Nope! They're irrelevant :)

Rebecca Yes. In my mind I kind of divide them into 4ths for reminding myself not to start out to fast and for pacing. Then I try to kick it up within the last 15 floors. When I had severe anemia I started out too fast and hit the wall at about 38.

Andy Half way up for sure.

David Yes. In fact, I use an audio track that tells me when I should be on each floor.

Katy Yes, I do but probably shouldn't, but I'm at the beginning of my training.

Tom I try not to, but volunteers in the stairwell always tell you...hate it :) Would rather just go at my pace and not think about floors to go

Joel I avoid it for the most part and just focus on climbing. It is nice to know where I am and if I can't find a floor number when I expect to I am disappointed

Nancy I never look when I'm training at the building in my home town. Unfortunately, I know certain marks on the stairs and landings, so I'm usually aware of where I'm at. I prefer not to see the floor numbers. It throws me off mentally. On the stair races in Chicago, I look as I'm getting close to the top. I've been pleasantly surprised to find that I was further than I thought and completely dumbfounded when I thought I was MUCH further than I thought!! It's a mental thing with me!

Troy. Yes. I have to know when to get off on my floor.

Ryan Yes, I have to know which floor to tell the building I barfed on.

Renard I pay attention to floor count sometime, it really depends. I try to keep a good idea of where I am so I know when to pick up the pace. However I feel that consistently watching the floor numbers can be demoralizing, if you are not mentally prepared for the task at hand.

Survey Question #4: Handrails or no handrails during your climb? And, if you use handrails, how hard was it (no pun intended) to get the handle of using them.

Rebecca Handrails all the way baby! I do not have balance function, so that handrails came naturally and were a necessity. I had been using handrails on ANY stairs, for 2 and a half years prior to my first climb. In fact I was pretty scared before the first climb because I was not sure what to expect and did not know if there would be handrails. Thank God the sport was so meant for me! The conditions of tower climbing stairwells are perfect (good light, handrails on either side, great distance between the handrails/walls, and safe non-slippery steps). It was such a high and pleasantry to do my first tower climbing experience! By the way, practicing double step on the back stairs of the gym last night, I noticed that I DEFINITELY need the handrails to pull me a long. I got into a good rhythm with the ideal conditions which I can't achieve on the outdoors stairs with only one handrails and inconsistent step length. Earlier this year PJ Glassey gave us a training seminar and showed us 2 handed on one railing. I do use it that way for single stepping but find it hard to do on the outdoors stairs with two steps. You are so incredibly lucky to have a building to practice in! I have to try to make a buddy who works in a big building!

Nancy I started single steps and without the handrail. Then, I had a Stair Climbing champ watch me one day and he insisted on going double steps and using the handrail. I use it with both hands on the left side. I tried to use 2 hands on either side at the Stratosphere a couple of years ago, and I had to go back to the way I trained. It's so mental!

Sally When double stepping, Two hands on one rail, pulling myself up like pulling on a rope. One hand on the top of the rail, the other on the underside of the rail.

David Rail if you're doubling for sure. And if the hallway is narrow enough, hands on both rails;)

Lisa Handrails. Pull yourself up! Use "tacky" gloves too!

Kent I use Handrails

Chandra I always use handrails. They help.

Sarah I always have to be careful of my knees, and thought two step method would never be option for me. But recently started two steps at a time with handrails, and am amazed. The handrails take most of the pressure off knees, I am hitting new and different muscle groups, and the speed is remarkable.

Renard Handrails can be ideal when you are tired. It can serve as an extra method to propel you up the stairs.

308

Survey Question #5: Looking back, what is the biggest mistake you made either prior to your first climb or during it?

Trevor Maybe going out to hard. I did a 5 hour climb in Calgary and I should of started out slower. Regardless I did finish it and set a new course record of 28 laps completed.

Mark Not training at all for the first two I've done has been a MASSIVE mistake.

Lisa Starting off too fast. Not training enough. Thinking that being a "runner" made me a "climber". With each race I learn something new!!

Sally Not going out hard enough. Got to the 88th floor with energy left (so I did it again). So I guess it comes down to pacing

Kent Did not train for my 1st climb at all. I found out about it only about two weeks in advance. It took me a long time to finish it, but I was not going to give up. The Terminal Tower in Cleveland was my first one and I will never forget it. Since then I have only looked for taller buildings and more of a challenge.

David Like many others, going out too hard. Also, showing up to my first race deeply hung over. ;)

Chandra I started out too fast. I'd been training on only 3 flights of stairs prior to my first climb and had no concept of pacing.

Andy It helps to pace off someone, if possible, I was climbing by myself for +20 floors near end, and simply fell into a lull, only to pick it up with 7 floors to go, so lesson learned was not to get complacent if all by self.

Renard .. I honestly have to say sprinting out too fast and dying at like the 12th floor… We live and we learn.

David Pacing off someone is great. My first time up the Hancock, I was dead at ~75 and just sorta shuffling up, and a fast guy shot past me, and seeing him, I thought "all I need to do is keep up with that guy." I just tucked in behind him and stayed there until the end. Probably saved me a minute and a half...

CHAPTER ELEVEN

Organized Stair Climbs

I've surveyed 95 climbs in the United States, most of them either sponsored by the American Lung Association or the Cystic Fibrosis Foundation.

I've listed them all here, with some information about each you may find useful and interesting.

All of the information I've discovered about these climbs I have gathered by reading the Event websites. I apologize for any errors or omissions, but these are the responsibility of the event Web Sites.

Cystic Fibrosis Foundation Climbs

Cystic Fibrosis Foundation Climbs are, in general, the oldest of the organized charitable climb events in the United State.

I surveyed 17 Cystic Fibrosis Foundation Climbs that were held in 2011.

The following pages list the Climbs benefitting the Cystic Fibrosis Foundation that were held in 2011---you should be able to find one near you if you are interested.

All of the information I've discovered about these climbs I have gathered by reading the Event websites. I apologize for any errors or omissions, but these are the responsibility of the event Web Sites.

City: Albany, NY

Benefits: Cystic Fibrosis Foundation

Registration Fee: $60

Additional Fund Raising Required: $50

2011 Date: March 3, 2011

2012 Date: March 8, 2012

Location: Empire State Plaza

Floors: 42

Steps: 809

Point of Contact: Donna Clark,ne-ny@cff.org

2011 Participants: 99

Top Male Finisher: David Tromp(35),4:30:20

Top Female Finisher: Brittany Pine(24),6:48:20

Oldest Male Finisher: David Allard(63),8:26:50

Oldest Female Finisher: Lucinda Huggins(67),12:16:30

2011 Money Raised: Unknown

Website:
http://www.cff.org/Chapters/neny/index.cfm?id=18281&event=18281

Results:
http://www.albanyrunningexchange.org/results/search.php?ID=1945

Comments: 2011 was the 23rd Cystic Fibrosis Foundation Climb in held in Albany

City: Boston, MA

Benefits: Cystic Fibrosis Foundation

Registration Fee: $25

Additional Fund Raising Required: $100

2011 Date: October 23, 2011

2012 Date:

Location: 1 International Place

Floors: 46

Steps: 800

Point of Contact: Pamela Spitzer, moss-ri@cff.org

2011 Participants: 68

Top Male Finisher: David Lefcourt(30),8:03

Top Female Finisher: Melissa McManus(32),8:08

Oldest Male Finisher: Michael Feely(55),11:03

Oldest Female Finisher: Amy Powell(54),13:25

2011 Money Raised: Unknown

Website: http://www.cff.org/Chapters/mass-ri/index.cfm?id=16812&event=16812

Results:
http://www.coolrunning.com/results/11/ma/Oct23_Climbf_set4.shtml

Comments: 2011 was the 1st Cystic Fibrosis Foundation Climb in held in Boston

City: Chicago, IL

Benefits: Cystic Fibrosis Foundation

Registration Fee: $25

Additional Fund Raising Required: $200

2011 Date: December 4, 2011

2012 Date:

Location: LaSalle

Floors: 53

Steps: 1019

Point of Contact: Molly A. Rilery,illinois@cff.org

2011 Participants: Unknown

Top Male Finisher:

Top Female Finisher:

Oldest Male Finisher:

Oldest Female Finisher:

2011 Money Raised: Unknown

Website:
http://www.cff.org/Chapters/grillinois/ChapterEvents/index.cfm?ID=167
07

Results: Unknown

Comments: 2011 was the 2nd Cystic Fibrosis Foundation Climb in held in Chicago

City: Columbus, OH

Benefits: Cystic Fibrosis Foundation

Registration Fee: $50

Additional Fund Raising Required: $100

2011 Date: March 5, 2011

2012 Date: March 3, 2012

Location: Rhodes State Office Tower

Floors: 40

Steps: Unknown

Point of Contact: Susan Deutschle,central-oh@cff.org

2011 Participants: 81

Top Male Finisher: Matt Tosi(),6:06:22

Top Female Finisher: Catheine LaCourt(),6:34:54

Oldest Male Finisher: No ages provided

Oldest Female Finisher: No ages provided

2011 Money Raised: Unknown

Website:
http://www.cff.org/Chapters/centralohio/index.cfm?ID=19602&blnShow
Back=True&idContentType=1468&Event=19602

Results:
http://ohiochallengeseries.com/index.cfm?template=event&form_event_id
=2402

Comments: 2011 was the 30th Cystic Fibrosis Foundation Climb in held in Columbus

City: Dallas, TX

Benefits: Cystic Fibrosis Foundation

Registration Fee: $25

Additional Fund Raising Required: $150

2011 Date: September 24, 2011

2012 Date: September 22, 2012

Location: Bank of America Plaza

Floors: 70

Steps: 1540

Point of Contact: Tina Garcia,ne-texas@cff.org

2011 Participants: 93

Top Male Finisher: Cesar Corral(),10:45:50

Top Female Finisher: Laura Harper(),14:44:30

Oldest Male Finisher: No ages provided

Oldest Female Finisher: No ages provided

2011 Money Raised: Unknown

Website:
http://www.cff.org/Chapters/netx/index.cfm?id=20285&event=20285

Results: http://www.eteamz.com/racechiptiming/files/cfld.htm

Comments: 2011 was the 2nd Cystic Fibrosis Foundation Climb in held in Dallas

City: Fort Worth, TX

Benefits: Cystic Fibrosis Foundation

Registration Fee: $25

Additional Fund Raising Required: $100

2011 Date: September 10, 2011

2012 Date: August 25, 2012

Location: Burnett Plaza

Floors: 22

Steps: Unknown

Point of Contact: Melanie Hannah,ftworth-ne-texas@cff.org

2011 Participants: 114

Top Male Finisher: Lancy Buky(),9:45:30

Top Female Finisher: Tonya Edwards(),11:39:50

Oldest Male Finisher: No ages provided

Oldest Female Finisher: No ages provided

2011 Money Raised: Unknown

Website:
http://www.cff.org/Chapters/fortworth/index.cfm?id=20280&event=202
80

Results: http://www.eteamz.com/racechiptiming/files/climb44.htm

Comments: 2011 was the 2nd Cystic Fibrosis Foundation Climb in held in
Fort Worth

City: Los Angeles, CA

Benefits: Cystic Fibrosis Foundation

Registration Fee: $25

Additional Fund Raising Required: $100

2011 Date: December 3, 2011

2012 Date:

Location: Figueroa at Wilshire

Floors: 51

Steps: 1274

Point of Contact: Judy Ranan,so-calif-la@cff.org

2011 Participants: 180

Top Male Finisher: Eric Leninger(28),6:20

Top Female Finisher: Kourtney Dexter(31),7:16

Oldest Male Finisher: James Bromitt(65),13:10

Oldest Female Finisher: Barbara Burnett(68),22:42

2011 Money Raised: Unknown

Website: http://www.cff.org/Chapters/losangeles/index.cfm?ID=16714

Results:
http://raceresults.eternaltiming.com/index.cfm/20111203_Climb_For_Life_Los_Angeles.htm

Comments: 2011 was the 2nd Cystic Fibrosis Foundation Climb in held in Los Angeles

City: Milwaukee, WI

Benefits: Cystic Fibrosis Foundation

Registration Fee: $25

Additional Fund Raising Required: $50

2011 Date: November 17, 2011

2012 Date:

Location: US Bank Building

Floors: 47

Steps: 1034

Point of Contact:

2011 Participants: 376

Top Male Finisher: Justin Stewart(24),4:50

Top Female Finisher: Cindy Harris(42),5:55

Oldest Male Finisher: Ed Parker(73),13:21

Oldest Female Finisher: Suzanne Nason(63),15:41

2011 Money Raised: Unknown

Website:
http://www.cff.org/Chapters/wisconsin/ChapterEvents/index.cfm?ID=17
105
Results:
http://www.badgerlandstriders.org/DefaultFilePile/RaceResults/11STAIR
CLIMB_Results.txt

Comments: 2011 was the 8th Cystic Fibrosis Foundation Climb in held in
Milwaukee

City: Minneapolis

Benefits: Cystic Fibrosis Foundation

Registration Fee: $25

Additional Fund Raising Required: $50

2011 Date: February 5, 2011

2012 Date: February 4, 2012

Location: IDS Building

Floors: 50

Steps: 1280

Point of Contact:

2011 Participants: 123

Top Male Finisher: CJ Faulkner(),7:42

Top Female Finisher: Kyron Christopherson(),10:37

Oldest Male Finisher: No ages provided

Oldest Female Finisher: No ages provided

2011 Money Raised: Unknown

Website:
http://www.cff.org/Chapters/minnesota/index.cfm?ID=18969&blnShow
Back=True&idContentType=1388&Event=18969

Results:
http://www.andersonraces.com/_uls/resources/CFFFITCHALLRS2011.p
df

Comments: 2011 was the 30th Cystic Fibrosis Foundation Climb in held in
Minneapolis

City: Mobile, AL

Benefits: Cystic Fibrosis Foundation

Registration Fee: $25

Additional Fund Raising Required: $100

2011 Date: October 23, 2011

2012 Date:

Location: RSA Battlehouse Tower

Floors: 34

Steps: 650

Point of Contact: Unknown

2011 Participants: 50

Top Male Finisher: Troy Alston(),5:03

Top Female Finisher: Elaine Spruill(),7:04

Oldest Male Finisher: No ages provided

Oldest Female Finisher: No ages provided

2011 Money Raised: Unknown

Website: http://www.cff.org/Chapters/mobile/index.cfm?ID=17391

Results:
http://www.productionsbylittleredhen.com/resultsinfo_s.asp?raceid=CFST AIR11

Comments: 2011 was the 1st Cystic Fibrosis Foundation Climb in held in Mobile

City: Oklahoma City

Benefits: Cystic Fibrosis Foundation

Registration Fee: $35

Additional Fund Raising Required: $50

2011 Date: March 5, 2011

2012 Date:

Location: Oklahoma City RedHawks stadium stairs

Floors: 32

Steps: Unknown

Point of Contact: Unknown

2011 Participants: 173

Top Male Finisher: Tyler Poole(25),3:06

Top Female Finisher: Jennifer Osborne(21),4:10

Oldest Male Finisher: D.E. Brower(62),7:04

Oldest Female Finisher: Gloria Blankinship(59),9:38

2011 Money Raised: Unknown

Website: http://www.lungusa.org/pledge-events/ok/oklahoma-city-climb/local/event-information.html

Results:
http://www.productionsbylittleredhen.com/resultsinfo_s.asp?raceid=CFSTAIR11

Comments: 2011 was the 2nd Cystic Fibrosis Foundation Climb in held in Oklahoma City

City: Orlando, FL

Benefits: Cystic Fibrosis Foundation

Registration Fee: $35

Additional Fund Raising Required: $100

2011 Date: September 17, 2011

2012 Date:

Location: World Center Marriot Hotel

Floors: 28

Steps: Unknown

Point of Contact: Lisa Murphy,orlando-fl@cff.org

2011 Participants: 63

Top Male Finisher: Troy Alston(),1:44

Top Female Finisher: Yvette Amill(),3:29:00

Oldest Male Finisher: No ages provided

Oldest Female Finisher: No ages provided

2011 Money Raised: Unknown

Website: http://www.cff.org/Chapters/orlando/index.cfm?id=16747

Results: http://fleetfeetorlando.com/races/cf-climb-for-life/overall2011_male_female.html

Comments: 2011 was the 1st Cystic Fibrosis Foundation Climb in held Orlando

City: Philadelpha, PA

Benefits: Cystic Fibrosis Foundation

Registration Fee: $40

Additional Fund Raising Required: $130

2011 Date: February 27, 2011

2012 Date: February 26, 2012

Location: Mellon Bank Center

Floors: 53

Steps: 1019

Point of Contact: Eileen Miley,del-valley@cffl.og

2011 Participants: 99

Top Male Finisher: Brian Alba(16),7:02

Top Female Finisher: Kelley Peck(33),9:35

Oldest Male Finisher: John Schultz(78),16:14

Oldest Female Finisher: Maria Schaller(64),17:06

2011 Money Raised: Unknown

Website:
http://www.cff.org/Chapters/delawarevalley/index.cfm?ID=19235&blnSh
owBack=True&idContentType=1498&Event=19235

Results: http://results.active.com/pages/page.jsp?eventLinkageID=47579

Comments: 2011 was the 24th Cystic Fibrosis Foundation Climb held in
Philadelphia

City: Raleigh, NC

Benefits: Cystic Fibrosis Foundation

Registration Fee: $35

Additional Fund Raising Required: $100

2011 Date: October 29, 2011

2012 Date:

Location: Wachovia Capitol Center

Floors: 28

Steps: 1019

Point of Contact: carolinas@cff.org

2011 Participants: 99

Top Male Finisher: Troy Alston(),3:06

Top Female Finisher: Tracey Woodward(),4:27

Oldest Male Finisher: No ages provided

Oldest Female Finisher: No ages provided

2011 Money Raised: Unknown

Website: http://www.cff.org/Chapters/carolinas/index.cfm?ID=16943

Results:
http://results.active.com/pages/page.jsp?pubID=3&eventID=1974788

Comments: 2011 was the 2nd Cystic Fibrosis Foundation Climb held in Raleigh

City: San Francisco, CA

Benefits: Cystic Fibrosis Foundation

Registration Fee: $35

Additional Fund Raising Required: $100

2011 Date: November 5, 2011

2012 Date:

Location: One Sansome Street

Floors: 40

Steps: 900

Point of Contact: Cathi Conely,no-calif@cff.org

2011 Participants: 77

Top Male Finisher: Spencer Morris(),5:27

Top Female Finisher: Amanda Perez(),8:02

Oldest Male Finisher: No ages provided

Oldest Female Finisher: No ages provided

2011 Money Raised: Unknown

Website: http://www.cff.org/Chapters/nca/index.cfm?id=15938

Results: None posted

Comments: 2011 was the 2nd Cystic Fibrosis Foundation Climb held in San Francisco

City: San Antonio, TX

Benefits: Cystic Fibrosis Foundation

Registration Fee: $35

Additional Fund Raising Required: $100

2011 Date: February 26, 2011

2012 Date: February 25, 2012

Location: Tower of the Americas

Floors: 58

Steps: 952

Point of Contact: Hugh Hawthorne Farr,lone-star@cff.org

2011 Participants: 352

Top Male Finisher: Chris Aarhus(),10:37

Top Female Finisher: Virginia Herrera(),13:22

Oldest Male Finisher: Douglas Heintz(60),22:04

Oldest Female Finisher: Charlene Heintz(60),23:09

2011 Money Raised: Unknown

Website:
http://www.cff.org/Chapters/lonestar/index.cfm?ID=19567&blnShowBac
k=True&idContentType=1523&Event=19567

Results: http://rrptiming.com/2011CFFTowerClimbResults

Comments: 2011 was the 246h Cystic Fibrosis Foundation Climb held in San Antonio

City: Seattle, WA

Benefits: Cystic Fibrosis Foundation

Registration Fee: $80

Additional Fund Raising Required: None

2011 Date: December 1, 2011

2012 Date:

Location: The Tower At 1201

Floors: 56

Steps: 1120

Point of Contact: washington@cff.org

2011 Participants: 319

Top Male Finisher: Justin Stewart(24),5:29

Top Female Finisher: Kourtney Dexter(31),7:08

Oldest Male Finisher: George Burnham(69),15:26

Oldest Female Finisher: Sandy Pearson(61),14:37

2011 Money Raised: Unknown

Website:
http://stairclimb.kintera.org/faf/home/default.asp?ievent=480691

Results:
http://www.onlineraceresults.com/race/view_race.php?race_id=23092#rac
etop

Comments: 2011 was the 23rd Cystic Fibrosis Foundation Climb held in
Seattle. This climb was dedicated to the memory of Jennifer Lynn Thanem.

American Lung Association Climbs

American Lung Association Climbs are the newest of the organized charitable climb events in the United States. Many of them held in United States in 2011 were held for only their second or their year, and in some cases for the first time.

They are well organized and well run, and if you are looking for an organized Stair Climb to do, they are just in about every major Metropolitan area of the United States..

I counted 60 American Lung Association Climbs that were held in 2011.

The following pages list the Climbs benefitting the American Lung Association that were held in 2011---you should be able to find one near you if you are interested.

All of the information I've discovered about these climbs I have gathered by reading the Event websites. I apologize for any errors or omissions, but these are the responsibility of the event Web Sites.

City: Albany, NY

Benefits: American Lung Association

Registration Fee: $25

Additional Fund Raising Required: $100

2011 Date: June 12, 2011

2012 Date:

Location: 1 Commerce Plaza

Floors: Unknown

Steps: Unknown

Point of Contact: Chuck Sawyer, albanyclimb@alany.org

2011 Participants: 80

Top Male Finisher: David Tromp(35),1:33:93

Top Female Finisher: Meghan Craig(),2:08:01

Oldest Male Finisher: No ages provided

Oldest Female Finisher: No ages provided

2011 Money Raised: $30,359.00

Website: http://www.lungusa.org/pledge-events/ny/albany-climb/local/event-information.html

Results: http://www.lungusa.org/pledge-events/ny/albany-climb/local/documents/albany-climb-results.pdf

Comments: 2011 was the 4th Fight For Air Climb held in Albany

City: Albuquerque, NM

Benefits: American Lung Association

Registration Fee: $35

Additional Fund Raising Required: $100

2011 Date: February 26, 2011

2012 Date: Marvh 4, 2012

Location: Albuqueque Plaza

Floors: 19

Steps: 428

Point of Contact: None Provided

2011 Participants: 110

Top Male Finisher: Nicholas Tarasenko(),2:10:40

Top Female Finisher: Dalene Santibanez(),3:17:05

Oldest Male Finisher: No ages provided

Oldest Female Finisher: No ages provided

2011 Money Raised: $51,307.04

Website: http://www.lungusa.org/pledge-events/nm/albuquerque-climb/local/event-information.html

Results: http://www.lungusa.org/pledge-events/nm/albuquerque-climb/local/race-results.html

Comments: 2011 was the 3rd Fight For Air Climb held in Albuquerque.

City: Anchorage, AK

Benefits: American Lung Association

Registration Fee: $35

Additional Fund Raising Required: $100

2011 Date: October 15, 2011

2012 Date: October 2012

Location: Anchorage Hilton

Floors: 35

Steps: Unknown

Point of Contact: Nellie Schroder, nschroder@aklung.org

2011 Participants: 48

Top Male Finisher: Damian Schroder(),2:50

Top Female Finisher: Nina Kovac(),3:59

Oldest Male Finisher: George Burnham(69).6;56

Oldest Female Finisher: Jill Sunday(64),7:21

2011 Money Raised: $17,388.00

Website: http://www.lungusa.org/pledge-events/ak/anchorage-climb/

Results:
http://onlineraceresults.com/event/view_event.php?event_id=7628

Comments:

City: Atlanta, GA

Benefits: American Lung Association

Registration Fee: $25

Additional Fund Raising Required: $100

2011 Date: May 14, 2011

2012 Date:

Location: The Equitable Building

Floors: 32 or 64 floor option

Steps: Unknown

Point of Contact: None Provided

2011 Participants: 61 (32 floor option) 55 (64 floor option)

Top Male Finisher: Victor Serrano(33),8:19:28

Top Female Finisher: Angela Yarnish(24),11:28:03

Oldest Male Finisher: Jerry Rioux(56),8:24:83

Oldest Female Finisher: Rhonda Rhoades(55),14:09:38

2011 Money Raised: $36,684.10

Website: http://www.lungusa.org/pledge-events/ga/atlanta-climb/local/event-information.html

Results: http://www.lungusa.org/pledge-events/ga/atlanta-climb/local/2011-results.html

Comments: : 2011 was the 5th Fight For Air Climb held in Atlanta

City: Austin, TX

Benefits: American Lung Association

Registration Fee: $25

Additional Fund Raising Required: $100

2011 Date: May 14, 2011

2012 Date: May 19, 2012

Location: The Frost Bank Tower

Floors: 30

Steps: 660

Point of Contact: None Provided

2011 Participants: 355

Top Male Finisher: Christian Goy(39),3:29:86

Top Female Finisher: Megan Parsons(30),4:37:94

Oldest Male Finisher: Jim Bryce(69),8:15:46

Oldest Female Finisher: Gail Jacobs(63),8:22:50

2011 Money Raised: $123,552.00

Website: http://www.lungusa.org/pledge-events/tx/austin-climb/local/event-information.html

Results: http://www.cadencesports.com/pdf/379_overall.pdf

Comments: : 2011 was the 2nd Fight For Air Climb held in Austin

City: Bennington, VT

Benefits: American Lung Association

Registration Fee: $35

Additional Fund Raising Required: $100

2011 Date: May 21, 2011

2012 Date:

Location: The Bennington Tower

Floors: Tower

Steps: 417

Point of Contact: None Provided

2011 Participants: 107

Top Male Finisher: Justin Stewart(23),1:10

Top Female Finisher: Kourtney Dexter(30),1:27

Oldest Male Finisher: Mike Merritt(67),4:03

Oldest Female Finisher: Jane Forrest(68),4:29

2011 Money Raised: $43,830.04

Website: http://www.lungusa.org/pledge-events/vt/bennington-climb/local/event-information.html

Results:
http://www.coolrunning.com/results/11/vt/May21_Climbt_set1.shtml

Comments: 2011 was the 3rd Fight For Air Climb held in Bennington. This is not a high rise. This is the preeminent real 'tower' climb in America. It's not for the faint of heart. It's 417 circular stairs to the top. Check out the website above--you'll find a You Tube video there that will show you what you're in for if you join.

City: Birmingham, AL

Benefits: American Lung Association

Registration Fee: $25

Additional Fund Raising Required: $100

2011 Date: May 14, 2011

2012 Date:

Location: Wells Fargo Tower

Floors: 34

Steps: Unknown

Point of Contact: None Provided

2011 Participants: 75

Top Male Finisher: Charles Barr(21),3:07

Top Female Finisher: Clarissa Coe(27),5:37

Oldest Male Finisher: Phil Hammonds(60),7:30

Oldest Female Finisher: Cathy Sewell(54),17:07

2011 Money Raised: $34,750.00

Website: http://www.lungusa.org/pledge-events/al/birmingham-climb/local/event-information.html

Results:
http://www.msracetiming.com/uploads/Fight_4_Air_AL_2011_Results_List.doc

Comments: 2011 was the 1st Fight For Air Climb held in Birmingham

City: Boston, MA

Benefits: American Lung Association

Registration Fee: $25

Additional Fund Raising Required: $100

2011 Date: February 5, 2011

2012 Date: February 4, 2012

Location: One Boston Place

Floors: 41

Steps: 697

Point of Contact: None Provided

2011 Money Raised: $317,145.45

2011 Participants: 993

Top Male Finisher: Sean O'Connell(40),4:34

Top Female Finisher: Sau-Mei Leung(45),6:09

Oldest Male Finisher: John Troy(80),36:28

Oldest Female Finisher: Linda Reppucci(63),18:45

Website: http://www.lungusa.org/pledge-events/ma/boston-climb/local/event-information.html

Results:
http://www.coolrunning.com/results/11/ma/Feb5_RaceUp_set1.shtml

Comments: 2011 was the 6th Fight For Air Climb held in Boston.

City: Buffalo, NY

Benefits: American Lung Association

Registration Fee: $25

Additional Fund Raising Required: $100

2011 Date: February 12, 2011

2012 Date: March 10, 2012

Location: HSBC Center

Floors: 40

Steps: 800

Point of Contact: Lauren Maltese, buffaloclimb@alany.org

2011 Money Raised: $40,148.69

2011 Participants: 185

Top Male Finisher: Chad Krelley()3:49

Top Female Finisher: Ashley Ebert(),6:26

Oldest Male Finisher: No ages provided

Oldest Female Finisher: No ages provided

Website: http://www.lungusa.org/pledge-events/ny/buffalo-climb/local/event-information.html

Results:
http://results.active.com/pages/searchform.jsp?pubID=3&rsID=105574

Comments: 2011 was the 1st Fight For Air Climb held in Buffalo.

City: Chicago, IL

Benefits: American Lung Association

Registration Fee: $25

Additional Fund Raising Required: $100

2011 Date: March 27, 2011

2012 Date: March 11, 2012

Location: Presidential Towers

Floors: 45

Steps: 931

Point of Contact: Heidi Hoffman, Heidi.Hoffman@LungIL.org

2011 Participants: 931

Top Male Finisher: Jesse Berg(38),10:18

Top Female Finisher: Cindy Harris(42),18:26

Oldest Male Finisher: James Nasby(69),8:36

Oldest Female Finisher: Cathi Watson(77),18:24

2011 Money Raised: $263,799.32

Website: http://www.lungusa.org/pledge-events/il/chicago-climb/local/event-information.html

Results:
http://www.theracershub.com/results_view.php?id=1204&result_type=file

Comments: 2011 was the 3rd Fight For Air Climb held in Chicago. Chicago also sponsors a climb for MS, in addition to the world famous Hustle Up The Hancock. The ALA Chicago climb features a relay option. This climb has more features than any other I've seen. Be sure to check out the event information link.

City: Cincinnati, OH

Benefits: American Lung Association

Registration Fee: $25

Additional Fund Raising Required: $100

2011 Date: February 20, 2011

2012 Date: February 19, 2012

Location: The Carew Tower

Floors: 45

Steps: 804

Point of Contact: Liza Aromas-Janosik, ljanosik@ohiolung.org

2011 Participants: 407

Top Male Finisher: Bill Hoffman(),5:30

Top Female Finisher: Renee Burkhart(),6:49

Oldest Male Finisher: No ages provided

Oldest Female Finisher: No ages provided

2011 Money Raised: $136,395.11

Website: http://www.lungusa.org/pledge-events/oh/cincinnati-climb/local/event-information.html

Results: http://www.sprunning.com/2011Carew.txt

Comments: 2011 was the 6th Fight For Air Climb held in Cincinnati. Guest passes for the post-climb celebration are available for $5.

City: Cleveland, OH

Benefits: American Lung Association

Registration Fee: $25

Additional Fund Raising Required: $100

2011 Date: March 5, 2011

2012 Date: March 3, 2012

Location: The Terminal Tower

Floors: 42

Steps: 804

Point of Contact: Patty Kaplan, pkaplan@ohiolung.org

2011 Money Raised: $49,190.89

2011 Participants: 183

Top Male Finisher: Todd Suszynski(38),5:34

Top Female Finisher: Beth Darmstadter(45),6:32

Oldest Male Finisher: Richard Karberg(69),26:46

Oldest Female Finisher: Cindy Hollo(60),16:10

Website: http://www.lungusa.org/pledge-events/oh/cleveland-climb/local/event-information.html

Results: http://www.lungusa.org/pledge-events/oh/cleveland-climb/assets/images/documents/overall-results.pdf

Comments: 2011 was the 1st Fight For Air Climb held in Cleveland. Guest passes for the post-climb celebration are available for $5.

City: Columbia, SC

Benefits: American Lung Association

Registration Fee: $25

Additional Fund Raising Required: $100

2011 Date: May 21, 2011

2012 Date: June 2, 2012

Location: The Capitol Center

Floors: 40

Steps: Unknown

Point of Contact: Unknown

2011 Money Raised: $32,820.58

2011 Participants: 87

Top Male Finisher: Adam Russell(32),3:06:44

Top Female Finisher: Cindy Alyson Phillips(39),3:14:95

Oldest Male Finisher: Carl Chase(71),6:35:94

Oldest Female Finisher: Hannah Kirschenfeld(58),6:24:33

Website: http://www.lungusa.org/pledge-events/sc/columbia-climb/local/event-information.html

Results:
http://www.strictlyrunning.com/RESULTS/11ALACLIMB_C.TXT

Comments: 2011 was the 1st Fight For Air Climb held in Columbia.

City: Columbus, OH

Benefits: American Lung Association

Registration Fee: $25

Additional Fund Raising Required: $100

2011 Date: February 12, 2011

2012 Date: January 28, 2012

Location: The Rhodes Tower

Floors: 24

Steps: 453

Point of Contact: Kevin Readey, kreadey@ohiolung.org

2011 Participants: 183

Top Male Finisher: Adam Justin Milam(27),3:10

Top Female Finisher: Erica Northrup(36),4:20

Oldest Male Finisher: Mark Matson(55),5:59

Oldest Female Finisher: Sharon Roche(62),7:50

2011 Money Raised: : $23,050.74

Website: http://www.lungusa.org/pledge-events/oh/columbus-climb/local/event-information.html

Results: http://www.towerrunning.com/ergebnis/columbusffares11.txt

Comments: 2011 was the 1st Fight For Air Climb held in Columbus..

City: Dallas, TX

Benefits: American Lung Association

Registration Fee: $25

Additional Fund Raising Required: $100

2011 Date: February 26, 2011

2012 Date: February 18, 2012

Location: The Renaissance Tower

Floors: 53

Steps: Unknown

Point of Contact: Whitney Prussia, dallasevents@breathehealthy.org

2011 Participants: 506

Top Male Finisher: Zacharty Istre(28),6:06:52

Top Female Finisher: Victoria Bahr(31),8:21:23

Oldest Male Finisher: Stephen Cross(64),10:03:50

Oldest Female Finisher: Patricia Wedgeworth(64),14:35:41

2011 Money Raised: $99,000

Website: http://www.lungusa.org/pledge-events/tx/dallas-climb

Results:
http://www.runontexas.com/Results/2011/FightForAirClimb208/FightFo
rAirClimbMenu.htm

Comments: 2011 was the 1st Fight For Air Climb held in Dallas.

City: Denver, CO

Benefits: American Lung Association

Registration Fee: $25

Additional Fund Raising Required: $56

2011 Date: February 27, 2011

2012 Date: February 26, 2012

Location: The Republic Plaza

Floors: 56

Steps: 1098

Point of Contact: Unknown

2011 Participants: 1855

Top Male Finisher: Lawrence Pelo(37),6:18

Top Female Finisher: Kim Dobson(26),8:12

Oldest Male Finisher: Kenneth Ryan(78),12:41

Oldest Female Finisher: Marilyn Olen(83),20:47

2011 Money Raised: $390,309.62

Website: http://www.lungusa.org/pledge-events/co/denver-climb/local/event-information.html

Results:
http://onlineraceresults.com/race/view_race.php?race_id=17937#racetop

Comments: 2011 was the 6th Fight For Air Climb held in Denver. There will be no practice run. We recommend practicing at the Stairs at Red Rocks or at the Millennium Bridge in downtown Denver.

City: Des Moines, IA

Benefits: American Lung Association

Registration Fee: $25

Additional Fund Raising Required: $100

2011 Date: March 27, 2011

2012 Date: March 4, 2012

Location: The Des Moines Marriot

Floors: 17-35-66 floor options

Steps: 369-733-1177 options depending upon floors

Point of Contact: Unknown

2011 Participants: 486

Top Male Finisher: Luke Spencer(39),7:39

Top Female Finisher: Allison Johnson(36),8:23

Oldest Male Finisher: George Dorsey(69),20:45

Oldest Female Finisher: Cathy Crawford(60),5:42

2011 Money Raised: $147,085.21

Website: http://www.lungusa.org/pledge-events/ia/des-moines-climb/local/event-information.html

Results:
http://www.theracershub.com/results_view.php?id=1206&result_type=file

Comments: 2011 was the 7th Fight For Air Climb held in Des Moines.

City: Detroit, MI

Benefits: American Lung Association

Registration Fee: $25

Additional Fund Raising Required: $100

2011 Date: March 6, 2011

2012 Date: March 4, 2012

Location: The Renaissance Tower

Floors: 70

Steps: 1035

Point of Contact: Whitney Jessica Jimenez, jjimenez@midlandlung.org

2011 Participants: 543

Top Male Finisher: George Hudock(51),6:28

Top Female Finisher: Tricia Cockfield(32),9:17

Oldest Male Finisher: Bill Haggerty(74),17:48

Oldest Female Finisher: Bridget Morin(41),20:06

2011 Money Raised: $181,298.60

Website: http://www.lungusa.org/pledge-events/mi/detroit-climb/local/event-information.html

Results:
http://results.active.com/pages/page.jsp?eventID=1945881&pubID=3

Comments: 2011 was the 5th Fight For Air Climb held in Detroit.

City: Fort Myers, FL

Benefits: American Lung Association

Registration Fee: $35

Additional Fund Raising Required: $100

2011 Date: April 30, 2011

2012 Date: April 28, 2012

Location: High Point Place

Floors: 30

Steps: 514

Point of Contact: Kurt Goerke, KGoerke@lungfla.org

2011 Participants: 192

Top Male Finisher: Michael Peters(),2:39

Top Female Finisher: Susan Kirkham(),3:57

Oldest Male Finisher: Herm Kreiley(60),4:02

Oldest Female Finisher: Bridget Morin(41),20:06

2011 Money Raised: $41,719.33

Website: http://www.lungusa.org/pledge-events/fl/fort-myers-climb/local/event-information.html

Results:
http://www.altavistasports.com/results/2011results/alaclimbFTMYERS04302011.htm

Comments: 2011 was the 3rd Fight For Air Climb held in Fort Myers.

City: Fort Worth, TX

Benefits: American Lung Association

Registration Fee: $25

Additional Fund Raising Required: $100

2011 Date: June 11, 2011

2012 Date:

Location: Carter Burgess Tower

Floors: 40

Steps: Unknown

Point of Contact: None provided

2011 Participants: 98

Top Male Finisher: Robert Elliott(41),5:02

Top Female Finisher: Maria Quijano(40),4:14:02

Oldest Male Finisher: Robby Robertson(64),33:30:53

Oldest Female Finisher: Mili Ghose(66),10:09:61

2011 Money Raised: $35,896.67

Website: http://www.lungusa.org/pledge-events/tx/fort-worth-climb/local/faq.html

Results:
http://www.runontexas.com/Results/2011/FightForAirClimbFW260/FightForAirClimbMenu.htm

Comments: 2011 was the 2nd Fight For Air Climb held in Fort Worth.

City: Ft. Lauderdale, FL

Benefits: American Lung Association

Registration Fee: $25

Additional Fund Raising Required: $100

2011 Date: November 12, 2011

2012 Date:

Location: 110 Tower

Floors: 30

Steps: 529

Point of Contact: Paula Prendergast, ppredergast@lungfla.com

2011 Participants: 164

Top Male Finisher: Troy Alston(),3:37:00

Top Female Finisher: Alexis Evolga(),4:26:00

Oldest Male Finisher: No ages provided

Oldest Female Finisher: No ages provided

2011 Money Raised: $147,085.21

Website: http://www.lungusa.org/pledge-events/fl/fort-lauderdale-climb-fy12/local/event-information.html

Results: http://fleetfeetorlando.com/races/fight-for-air-5k-ft-lauderdale/climboverall_results.HTM

Comments: 2011 was the 3rd Fight For Air Climb held in Des Moines.

City: Greenville, SC

Benefits: American Lung Association

Registration Fee: $25

Additional Fund Raising Required: $100

2011 Date: April 9, 2011

2012 Date: April 14, 2011

Location: One & Two Liberty Square

Floors: 30

Steps: Unknown

Point of Contact: None Provided

2011 Participants: 78

Top Male Finisher: Robbie McCoy(17),3:25:25

Top Female Finisher: Mandy Howard(24),4:32:34

Oldest Male Finisher: Denis McKevitt(63),4:07:22

Oldest Female Finisher: Carole Eshenbaugh(67),13:53:32

2011 Money Raised: $24,647.55

Website: http://www.lungusa.org/pledge-events/sc/greenville-climb/local/faq.html

Results:
http://www.strictlyrunning.com/RESULTS/11ALACLIMB_G.TXT

Comments:

City: Hartford, CT

Benefits: American Lung Association

Registration Fee: $25

Additional Fund Raising Required: $100

2011 Date: March 26, 2011

2012 Date: March 30, 2012

Location: Hartford 21

Floors: 34

Steps: 688

Point of Contact: None Provided

2011 Participants: 394

Top Male Finisher: David Tromp(35),3:15

Top Female Finisher: Kendra Frederick(31),4:15

Oldest Male Finisher: John Chalupa(71),8:56

Oldest Female Finisher: Candie Martikainen(63),10:44

2011 Money Raised: $108,225.00

Website: http://www.lungusa.org/pledge-events/ct/hartford-climb/local/event-information.html

Results:
http://www.coolrunning.com/results/11/ct/Mar26_Tackle_set1.shtml

Comments: 2011 was the 4th Fight For Air Climb held in Hartford

City: Hershey, PA

Benefits: American Lung Association

Registration Fee: $25

Additional Fund Raising Required: $100

2011 Date: April 16, 2011

2012 Date: April 29, 2012

Location: Hershey Park Stadium

Floors: Stadium

Steps: Unknown

Point of Contact: Tracy Ingram, tingram@lunginfo.org

2011 Participants: 76

Top Male Finisher: Daniel O'Conor(),9:09

Top Female Finisher: Kelly Fisher(),12:20

Oldest Male Finisher: No ages provided

Oldest Female Finisher: No ages provided

2011 Money Raised: $2,997.29

Website: http://www.lungusa.org/pledge-events/pa/hershey-climb/local/event-information.html

Results: http://www.towerrunning.com/ergebnis/hershey11.xlsx

Comments: 2011 was the 2nd Fight For Air Climb held in Hershey

City: Houston, TX

Benefits: American Lung Association

Registration Fee: $25

Additional Fund Raising Required: $100

2011 Date: May 21, 2011

2012 Date: March 24, 2012

Location: First City Tower

Floors: 48

Steps: Unknown

Point of Contact: Tracy Jamie Roll, jroll@breathehealthy.org

2011 Participants: 303

Top Male Finisher: Chisholm MacDonald(44),7:21

Top Female Finisher: Deyna Aguilera(48),8:37

Oldest Male Finisher: Tony Cavender(71),26:27

Oldest Female Finisher: Otilia Sanchez(63),20:14

2011 Money Raised: $108,006.70

Website: http://www.lungusa.org/pledge-events/tx/houston-climb/local/event-information.html

Results: http://www.athleteguild.com/tower-climb/houston-tx/2011-fight-for-air-climb-in-houston/results

Comments: 2011 was the 2nd Fight For Air Climb held in Houston. No persons under the age of 10 may participate in the Stairclimb. Participants between the ages of 10 and 16 must climb with a parent or guardian. Participants between the ages of 16-18 must have a parent or guardian on site the day of the event.

City: Indianapolis, IN

Benefits: American Lung Association

Registration Fee: $25

Additional Fund Raising Required: $100

2011 Date: March 12, 2011

2012 Date: March 10, 2012

Location: One Indiana Square

Floors: 35

Steps: Unknown

Point of Contact: Liz Zuercher, liz.zuercher@lungin.org

2011 Participants: 358

Top Male Finisher: Michael Hoess(26),4:25

Top Female Finisher: Shelley Gulley(36),6:21

Oldest Male Finisher: William Blanchard(68),6:41

Oldest Female Finisher: Joanne Keaton(78),10:46

2011 Money Raised: $169,922.28

Website: http://www.lungusa.org/pledge-events/in/indianapolis-climb/local/event-information.html

Results: http://www.theracershub.com/files/474-1194.txt

Comments: 2011 was the 2nd Fight For Air Climb held in Indianapolis.

City: Jackson, MS

Benefits: American Lung Association

Registration Fee: $25

Additional Fund Raising Required: $100

2011 Date: March 12, 2011

2012 Date: February 25, 2012

Location: Trustmark Park, Braves Stadium

Floors: Stadium

Steps: Unknown

Point of Contact: Merle Eldridge, meldridge@breathehealthy.org

2011 Participants: 102

Top Male Finisher: Rob Oates(37),19:09

Top Female Finisher: Makenna Morris(14),24:17:60

Oldest Male Finisher: Larry Sykes(66),30:43:70

Oldest Female Finisher: Linda Clausel(70),40:01:80

2011 Money Raised: $59,324.46

Website: http://www.lungusa.org/pledge-events/ms/jackson-climb-fy12/local/event-information.html

Results:
http://www.msracetiming.com/uploads/Fight_for_Air_Climb_Overall_2011.doc

Comments: The climb route is a 5K route (3.1 miles) with 1 mile being in the stadium running the stairs. The mile is actually broken up into two separate 1/2 mile sections. Participants in this portion of the event will be timed by MS Race Timing Company.

City: Jacksonville, FL

Benefits: American Lung Association

Registration Fee: $25

Additional Fund Raising Required: $100

Benefits: American Lung Association

2011 Date: February 5, 2011

2012 Date: February 25, 2012

Location: Trustmark Park, Braves Stadium

Floors: 42

Steps: 838

Point of Contact: jaxevents@lungfla.org

2011 Participants: 492

Top Male Finisher: Chad Krelley(),4:55

Top Female Finisher: Giselle Carson(),6:34

Oldest Male Finisher: Bob McKenna(70),9:45

Oldest Female Finisher: Gloria Barnes(70),24:55

2011 Money Raised: $132,637.54

Website: http://www.lungusa.org/pledge-events/fl/jacksonville-climb/local/event-information.html

Results:
http://www.altavistasports.com/results/2011results/alaclimbJAX02052011.htm

Comments: 2011 was the 3rd Fight For Air Climb held in Jacksonville. Participants 17 and under are not allowed to climb the stairs more than THREE times in a practice session. Participants 15 and under must be accompanied by an adult while in the stairwells and cannot climb the stairs more than THREE times in a practice session. Firefighters and police officers may climb in full gear if they so desire. Police officers are ONLY allowed to carry their side arms. No riffles will be allowed.

City: Kansas City, MO

Benefits: American Lung Association

Registration Fee: $25

Additional Fund Raising Required: $100

Benefits: American Lung Association

2011 Date: Postponed

2012 Date: April 14, 2012

Location: Town Pavilion

Floors: 34

Steps: Unknown

Point of Contact: Lisa Gentleman, lgentleman@breathehealthy.org

2011 Participants: Climb was postponed

Top Male Finisher:

Top Female Finisher:

Oldest Male Finisher:

Oldest Female Finisher:

2011 Money Raised: Climb was postponed.

Website: http://www.lungusa.org/pledge-events/mo/kansas-city-climb/local/faq.html

Results:

Comments: The 2011 climb was postponed.

City: Las Vegas, NV

Benefits: American Lung Association

Registration Fee: $50

Additional Fund Raising Required: $250

Benefits: American Lung Association

2011 Date: March 12, 2011

2012 Date: March 3, 2012

Location: Stratosphere Hotel Tower

Floors: None--it's a Tower.

Steps: 1644

Point of Contact: None provided

2011 Participants: 271

Top Male Finisher: Kevin Crossman(),7:26

Top Female Finisher: Erica Schramm(),8:58

Oldest Male Finisher: Luis Altimiarano Shehab(60),10:34

Oldest Female Finisher: Susan Opas(61),18:36

2011 Money Raised: $100,000

Website: http://www.lungusa.org/pledge-events/nv/las-vegas-climb/

Results:
http://onlineraceresults.com/event/view_event.php?event_id=6194

Comments: 2011 was the 3rd Fight For Air Climb held in Las Vegas. This is the most complicated of all of the ALA climbs. The FAQ and Event links contain pages of information. Minimum age to climb is 18.

"Scale the Strat" is the American Lung Association in Nevada's competitive stair climb. Individuals and teams will race up the Stratosphere Observation Tower's staircase to raise money to fund lung health research, education, and advocacy in Southern Nevada. This climb is not for beginners.

Climbers will climb 1455 steps which equals 108 floors! Once the climbers are in the tower core, there is no exit point unless there is a medical emergency. The first 26 flights are configured like a typical stairwell, but the upper flights are suspended inside the middle of a hollow tower with open air on each side.

Because of the unique location of the climb, special considerations need to be taken before you should register.

Are you someone who is afraid of heights, suffers from vertigo, or claustrophobic?

You are ascending at a rate of approximately 15 ft in height every flight. If you are afraid of heights, claustrophobic, or suffer with motion sickness, this is not the climb for you.

You must be fit

If you are fit enough to run three miles (five kilometers) in 30 minutes or climb 1,000 steps on a stair machine without stopping, you should be physically able to participate in the climb.

City: Little Rock, AR

Benefits: American Lung Association

Registration Fee: $25

Additional Fund Raising Required: $100

2011 Date: May 14, 2011

2012 Date: May 5, 2012

Location: Metropolitan Tower

Floors: 39

Steps: Unknown

Point of Contact: Courtney Newell, cnewell@breathehealthy.org

2011 Participants: 174

Top Male Finisher: Kenny Bell(37),5:27

Top Female Finisher: Angela Martin(35),6:45

Oldest Male Finisher: Ed Rhodes(63),21:32

Oldest Female Finisher: Hallie Simmins(74),23:49

2011 Money Raised: $64,886.31

Website: http://www.lungusa.org/pledge-events/ar/little-rock-climb/local/event-information.html

Results:
http://www.onlineraceresults.com/event/view_event.php?event_id=6558

Comments: 2011 was the 3rd Fight For Air Climb held **in Jacksonville.**

City: Los Angeles, CA

Benefits: American Lung Association

Registration Fee: $25

Additional Fund Raising Required: $100

2011 Date: April 30, 2011

2012 Date: May 31, 2012

Location: AON Tower

Floors: 63

Steps: 1,377

Point of Contact: Vanessa Petersen, vpetersen@alac.org

2011 Participants: 549

Top Male Finisher: Justin Stewart(23),8:16

Top Female Finisher: Kourtney Dexter(30),9:44

Oldest Male Finisher: James Dohn(64),17:52

Oldest Female Finisher: Carole Lambert(68),35:36

2011 Money Raised: $139,987.39

Website: http://www.lungusa.org/pledge-events/ca/los-angeles-climb/local/event-information.html

Results:
https://www.runraceresults.com/Secure/RaceResults.cfm?ID=RCPJ2011

Comments: 2011 was the 4th Fight For Air Climb held in Los Angeles.

City: Miami, FL

Benefits: American Lung Association

Registration Fee: $25

Additional Fund Raising Required: $100

2011 Date: April 16, 2011

2012 Date: April 14, 2012

Location: Southeast Finance Center

Floors: 55

Steps: Unknown

Point of Contact: None Provided

2011 Participants: 383

Top Male Finisher: Lawrence Pelo(37),6:27

Top Female Finisher: Julienne Betsy(),9:11:00

Oldest Male Finisher: Frank Nicolosi(60),10:52

Oldest Female Finisher: Mirella Ruiz(60),13:32:00

2011 Money Raised: $124,485.13

Website: http://www.lungusa.org/pledge-events/fl/miami-climb/

Results: http://www.lungusa.org/pledge-events/fl/miami-climb/local/overall-climb-results.pdf

Comments: 2011 was the 7th Fight For Air Climb held in Miami

City: Milwaukee, WI

Benefits: American Lung Association

Registration Fee: $25

Additional Fund Raising Required: $100

2011 Date: March 27, 2011

2012 Date: March 17, 2012

Location: US Bank Center

Floors: 45

Steps: 585

Point of Contact: Stacy Schmidt, stacy.schmidt@lungwi.org

2011 Participants: 1,274

Top Male Finisher: Alex Docta(25),5:23

Top Female Finisher: Kristin Frey(27),6:35

Oldest Male Finisher: Larry Cerny(66),11:45

Oldest Female Finisher: Laura Sutherland(66),12:15

2011 Money Raised: $312,274.91

Website: http://www.lungusa.org/pledge-events/wi/milwaukee-climb/local/event-information.html

Results: http://www.theracershub.com/files/476-1203.txt

Comments: 2011 was the 3rd Fight For Air Climb held in Milwaukee.

City: Minneapolis, MN

Benefits: American Lung Association

Registration Fee: $25

Additional Fund Raising Required: $100

2011 Date: February 26, 2011

2012 Date: February 25, 2012

Location: Accenture Tower

Floors: 30

Steps: 660

Point of Contact: Maura Studer, maura.studer@lungmn.org

2011 Participants: 422

Top Male Finisher: Chad Kreiley(33),3:20

Top Female Finisher: Heather Hubert(19),5:44

Oldest Male Finisher: James Elder(67),8:04

Oldest Female Finisher: Martha Mayer(68),7:44

2011 Money Raised: $159,990.61

Website: http://www.lungusa.org/pledge-events/mn/minneapolis-climb/local/event-information.html

Results:
http://www.theracershub.com/results_view.php?id=1188&result_type=file

Comments: 2011 was the 4th Fight For Air Climb held in Minneapolis.

City: New Haven, CT

Benefits: American Lung Association

Registration Fee: $35

Additional Fund Raising Required: $100

2011 Date: March 26, 2011

2012 Date: February 11, 2012

Location: 360 State Street

Floors: 32

Steps: 413

Point of Contact: Amanda Laffin, alaffin@lungne.org

2011 Participants: 394

Top Male Finisher:

Top Female Finisher:

Oldest Male Finisher:

Oldest Female Finisher:

2011 Money Raised: Unknown

Website: http://www.lungusa.org/pledge-events/ct/new-haven-climb-fy12/local/event-information.html

Results: Unknown

Comments: You will be given two opportunities to test your run at 360 State Street prior to the climb- Saturday, December 3, 2011 and Saturday, January 21, 2012 from 10:00 AM- 12:00 PM. The building will be open for climbers and prospective participants to climb as many times as desired!

City: New York, NY

Benefits: American Lung Association

Registration Fee: $50

Additional Fund Raising Required: $250

2011 Date: None held

2012 Date: January 21, 2012

Location: One Penn Plaza

Floors: 55

Steps: Unknown

Point of Contact: nycclimb@alany.com

2011 Participants: None held

Top Male Finisher:

Top Female Finisher:

Oldest Male Finisher:

Oldest Female Finisher:

2011 Money Raised: Not held

Website: http://www.lungusa.org/pledge-events/ny/new-york-climb/local/event-information.html

Results:

Comments: 2012 will be the first year for this event

City: North Charleston, SC

Benefits: American Lung Association

Registration Fee: $25

Additional Fund Raising Required: $100

2011 Date: July 30, 2011

2012 Date: July 28, 2012

Location: North Charleston Coliseum Stadium

Floors: Stadium

Steps: 1,544

Point of Contact: charlestonevents@lungsc.org

2011 Participants: 85

Top Male Finisher: Troy Alston(24),7:39:80

Top Female Finisher: Mandy Howard(34),10:09:44

Oldest Male Finisher: David McCommon(57),12:58:63

Oldest Female Finisher: Rosalind Giddens(61),15:17:15

2011 Money Raised: $34,866.01

Website: http://www.lungusa.org/pledge-events/sc/north-charleston-climb/local/event-information.html

Results:
http://www.strictlyrunning.com/RESULTS/11CLIMB_CHAS.TXT

Comments:

City: Oakbrook Terrace, IL

Benefits: American Lung Association

Registration Fee: $25

Additional Fund Raising Required: $100

2011 Date: February 13, 2011

2012 Date: February 12. 2012

Location: Oakbrook Terrace Tower

Floors: 31

Steps: 680

Point of Contact: Erin Petschow, erin.petschow@lungil.org

2011 Participants: 572

Top Male Finisher: Jesse Berg(38),2:48

Top Female Finisher: Kristin Frey(27),3:58

Oldest Male Finisher: Charles Coleman(82),10:47

Oldest Female Finisher: Joanne Keaton(78),8:49

2011 Money Raised: $120.570.11

Website: http://www.lungusa.org/pledge-events/il/oakbrook-terrace-climb/local/event-information.html

Results: http://www.theracershub.com/files/470-1184.txt

Comments: 2011 was the 8th Fight For Air Climb held in Oakbrook Terrace.

City: Oklahoma City, OK

Benefits: American Lung Association

Registration Fee: $25

Additional Fund Raising Required: $100

2011 Date: March 5, 2011

2012 Date:

Location: First National Center

Floors:

Steps:

Point of Contact:

2011 Participants: 161

Top Male Finisher: Tyler Poole(25);3:06

Top Female Finisher: Jennifer Osborn(21),4:10

Oldest Male Finisher: D.E. Brower(62),7:04

Oldest Female Finisher: Gloria Blankinship(59),9:38

2011 Money Raised: $42,446.99

Website: http://www.lungusa.org/pledge-events/ok/oklahoma-city-climb/local/event-information.html

Results:
http://www.onlineraceresults.com/race/view_plain_text.php?race_id=1801
2

Comments: 2011 was the 2nd Fight For Air Climb held in Oklahoma City.

City: Orlando, FL

Benefits: American Lung Association

Registration Fee: $25

Additional Fund Raising Required: $100

2011 Date: November 12, 2011

2012 Date:

Location: Bank of America Tower

Floors: 25

Steps: 512

Point of Contact: Victoria Vighetto, vvighetto@lungfla.org

2011 Participants: 318

Top Male Finisher: Chad Krelley(33),2:33:00

Top Female Finisher: Shandy Plicka(),4:00:00

Oldest Male Finisher: John Garcia(60),4:29

Oldest Female Finisher: Carol Kirkland(60),5:19

2011 Money Raised: $91,343.65

Website: http://www.lungusa.org/pledge-events/fl/orlando-climb-fy12/local/event-information.html

Results: http://fleetfeetorlando.com/races/fight-for-air-orlando/climb_results2011.html

Comments: 2011 was the 5th Fight For Air Climb held in Orlando. Join us every Thursday at5:30 PM_at Florida Hospital's Ginsberg Tower (601 East Rollins Street Orlando, FL 32803) for climb training!

City: Palm Beach, FL

Benefits: American Lung Association

Registration Fee: $25

Additional Fund Raising Required: $100

2011 Date: November 19, 2011

2012 Date:

Location: Phillips Point

Floors: 20

Steps: 440

Point of Contact: eventspalmbeach@lungfla.org

2011 Participants: 98

Top Male Finisher: Thomas Scott(),1:57:00

Top Female Finisher: Pam Sharp(),2:42

Oldest Male Finisher: Dan Brown(60),2:51:00

Oldest Female Finisher: Tracy Vosburgh(60),5:38:00

2011 Money Raised: $40,647.47

Website: http://www.lungusa.org/pledge-events/fl/palm-beach-climb-fy12/local/event-information.html

Results: http://www.fleetfeetorlando.com/races/fight-for-air-palm-beach/2011/result_2011.html

Comments: 2011 was the 3rd Fight For Air Climb held in Palm Beach.

City: Philadelphia, PA

Benefits: American Lung Association

Registration Fee: $25

Additional Fund Raising Required: $100

2011 Date: March 19, 2011

2012 Date: March 24, 2012

Location: Three Logan Square

Floors: 50

Steps: 1088

Point of Contact: Sherri Fiorentino, sfiorentino@lunginfo.org

2011 Participants: 641

2011 Participants: 318

Top Male Finisher: David Tromp(35),5:45:80

Top Female Finisher: Caitlin Coleman(21),8:50.41

Oldest Male Finisher: Butch Brees(66),16:18:87

Oldest Female Finisher: Judy Cheng(73),28:41:67

2011 Money Raised: $140,361.17

Website: http://www.lungusa.org/pledge-events/pa/philadelphia-climb/local/event-information.html

Results: http://www.compuscore.com/cs2011/march/phlstair.htm

Comments: 2011 was the 5th Fight For Air Climb held in Philadelphia.

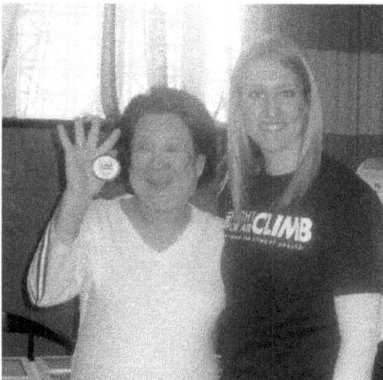

Judy Cheng, oldest Female Finisher in the 2011 Philadelphia Fight For Air Climb, along with Climb Organizer Rachael Pettigrove

City: Phoenix, AZ

Benefits: American Lung Association

Registration Fee: $25

Additional Fund Raising Required: $100

2011 Date: November 13, 2011

2012 Date:

Location: Renaissance Square

Floors: 53

Steps: 1272

Point of Contact: Janelle Tassart, jtassart@lungarizona.org

2011 Participants: 178

2011 Participants: 318

Top Male Finisher: Steve Stermer(53),7:33.46

Top Female Finisher: Danielle Kealy(27),8:21:70

Oldest Male Finisher: George Burnham(69),15:29:22

Oldest Female Finisher: Devora Krischer(64),25:07:46

2011 Money Raised: $42,310.50

Website: http://www.lungusa.org/pledge-events/az/phoenix-climb-fy12/local/event-information.html

Results:
http://results.active.com/pages/page.jsp?eventID=1982227&pubID=3

Comments: 2011 was the 3rd Fight For Air Climb held in Phoenix.

City: Pittsburgh, PA

Benefits: American Lung Association

Registration Fee: $25

Additional Fund Raising Required: $100

2011 Date: March 19, 2011

2012 Date:

Location: Gulf Tower

Floors: 38

Steps: 760

Point of Contact: Tiffany Villalba, tvillalba@lunginfo.org

2011 Participants: 238

Top Male Finisher: Mark Trahanovsky(52),4:43

Top Female Finisher: Jane Trahanovsky(54),6:54

Oldest Male Finisher: Robert Trozzo(68),1:15:15

Oldest Female Finisher: Carol Dvorchak(63),10:57

2011 Money Raised: $59,321.05

Website: http://www.lungusa.org/pledge-events/pa/pittsburgh-climb/local/event-information.html

Results: http://runhigh.com/2011RESULTS/R031911DA.html

Comments: 2011 was the 5th Fight For Air Climb held in Pittsburgh.

City: Providence, RI

Benefits: American Lung Association

Registration Fee: $25

Additional Fund Raising Required: $100

2011 Date: February 26, 2011

2012 Date: February 25, 2012

Location: One Financial Place

Floors: 28

Steps: 595

Point of Contact: Elise Kerrigan, ekerrigan@lungne.org

2011 Participants: 355

Top Male Finisher: Paul Currley(55),3:11

Top Female Finisher: Rachel Boudreau(26),3:45

Oldest Male Finisher: Mike Mollo(76),7:22

Oldest Female Finisher: Nydia Caruso(63),9:51

2011 Money Raised: $135,051.35

Website: http://www.lungusa.org/pledge-events/ri/providence-climb/local/event-information.html

Results:
http://www.coolrunning.com/results/11/ri/Feb26_Peakth_set1.shtml

Comments: 2011 was the 3rd Fight For Air Climb held in Providence.

City: Reno, NV

Benefits: American Lung Association

Registration Fee: $25

Additional Fund Raising Required: $100

2011 Date: April 17, 2011

2012 Date: April 15, 2012

Location: Silver Legacy Resort Casino

Floors: 36

Steps: 579

Point of Contact: Maryann Mcauliffe, mmcauliffe@lungnevada.org

2011 Participants: 228

Top Male Finisher: Chris Badolato(33),3:29

Top Female Finisher: Beth Kirland(27),5:03

Oldest Male Finisher: George Burnham(68),9:28

Oldest Female Finisher: Virginia Craig(69),10:20

2011 Money Raised: $54,398.64

Website: http://www.lungusa.org/pledge-events/nv/reno-climb/local/event-information.html

Results:
http://onlineraceresults.com/event/view_event.php?event_id=6357

Comments: 2011 was the 3rd Fight For Air Climb held in Providence. NEW IN 2011: A pancake feed and live band! The Climb will be held on Sunday, April 17 and it begins at 8:15 sharp! We advise being in the expo area no later than 7:30 to ensure you are ready and in line for your start time. The pancake feed will run from 7:45 - 11:00. The first wave of participants will be "elite" status participants (that means *fast*!) followed by the firefighters.

City: Sacramento, CA

Benefits: American Lung Association

Registration Fee: $25

Additional Fund Raising Required: $100

2011 Date: None held in 2011. Postponed from November 2010 to March 2012.

2012 Date: March 24, 2012

Location: Wells Fargo Center

Floors: Unknown

Steps: Unknown

Point of Contact: Julie Lautsch, jlautsch@alac.org

2011 Participants:

Top Male Finisher:

Top Female Finisher:

Oldest Male Finisher:

Oldest Female Finisher:

2011 Money Raised: Postponed

Website: http://www.lungusa.org/pledge-events/ca/sacramento-climb-fy12/local/event-information.html

Results: Postponed

Comments:

City: Salt Lake City, UT

Benefits: American Lung Association

Registration Fee: $25

Additional Fund Raising Required: $100

2011 Date: February 26, 2011

2012 Date: February 26, 2012

Location: Wells Fargo Center

Floors: 23

Steps: 598

Point of Contact: Spencer Slade, sslade@lungutah.org

2011 Participants: 370

Top Male Finisher: Bryce Astill(),3:30:30

Top Female Finisher: Natalie Garcia(),4:21:70

Oldest Male Finisher: George Sumner(65),7:51:30

Oldest Female Finisher: Dioane Teece(71),10:11:60

2011 Money Raised: $59,561.34

Website: http://www.lungusa.org/pledge-events/ut/salt-lake-city-climb/local/event-information.html

Results: http://milliseconds.com/races/detail/1402

Comments: 2011 was the 6th Fight For Air Climb held in Salt Lake City.

City: San Diego, California

Benefits: American Lung Association

Registration Fee: $25

Additional Fund Raising Required: $100

2011 Date: February 27, 2011

2012 Date: March 18, 2012

Location: Omni Hotel San Diego

Floors: 31

Steps: 561

Point of Contact: Kathlene Seymour,kseymour@alac.org

2011 Participants: 216

Top Male Finisher: Mark Trahanovsky(52),2:58

Top Female Finisher: Kacie Fischer(25),3:00

Oldest Male Finisher: David Emmanuel(71),5:51

Oldest Female Finisher: Kandy Lee(64),7:35

2011 Money Raised: $48,917.01

Website: http://www.lungusa.org/pledge-events/ca/san-diego-climb/local/event-information.html

Results:
http://raceresults.eternaltiming.com/index.cfm/20110227_Fight_For_Air_Stair_Climb_-_San_Diego.htm?Fuseaction=Results&Class=Stair%2BClimb%2BIndividual~All

Comments: 2011 was the 6th Fight For Air Climb held in San Diego.

City: San Francisco, CA

Benefits: American Lung Association

Registration Fee: $25

Additional Fund Raising Required: $100

2011 Date: March 26, 2011

2012 Date: March 31, 2012

Location: 555 California Street

Floors: 52

Steps: 1197

Point of Contact: Carrie Nash, cnash@alac.org

2011 Participants: 1192

Top Male Finisher: Sean Falconer(30),8:00

Top Female Finisher: Heather Newberry(41),9:54

Oldest Male Finisher: Tony Yacek(81),32:08

Oldest Female Finisher: Charlotte Prozan(74),29:21

2011 Money Raised: $453,600.12

Website: http://www.lungusa.org/pledge-events/ca/san-francisco-climb/local/event-information.html

Results:
http://results.active.com/pages/displayNonGru.jsp?orgID=218713&rsID=107191

Comments: 2011 was the 5th Fight For Air Climb held in San Francisco. Post climb event celebration is held at the top of the building.

City: Seattle, WA

Benefits: American Lung Association

Registration Fee: $25

Additional Fund Raising Required: $100

2011 Date: October 23, 2011

2012 Date: October 28, 2012

Location: 2 Union Square

Floors: 51

Steps: 1010

Point of Contact: Bridgett Herzog, bherzog@lungmtpacific.org

2011 Participants: 177

Top Male Finisher: Kevin Crossman(),5:09

Top Female Finisher: Kourtney Dexter(31),6:18

Oldest Male Finisher: Anders Jacobsen(86),14:59

Oldest Female Finisher: Sue Elliott(70),21:21

2011 Money Raised: $59,476.77

Website: http://www.lungusa.org/pledge-events/wa/seattle-climb-fy12/local/event-information.html

Results:
http://www.onlineraceresults.com/event/view_event.php?event_id=7688

Comments: 2011 was the 1st Fight For Air Climb held in Seattle.

City: Springfield, IL

Benefits: American Lung Association

Registration Fee: $25

Additional Fund Raising Required: $100

2011 Date: February 19, 2011

2012 Date: February 18, 2012

Location: Hilton Springfield

Floors: 30

Steps: Unknown

Point of Contact: Kelsey Dyckman,keysey.dyckman@lungil.org

2011 Participants: 416

Top Male Finisher: Justin Stewart(23),2:21

Top Female Finisher: Kristin Frey(27),3:20

Oldest Male Finisher: Dale Murray(69),12:00

Oldest Female Finisher: Loretta Durbin(65),13:37

2011 Money Raised: $120,981.41

Website: http://www.lungusa.org/pledge-events/il/springfield-climb/local/event-information.html

Results:
http://www.theracershub.com/results_view.php?id=1185&result_type=file

Comments: 2011 was the 2nd Fight For Air Climb held in Springfield.

City: Springfield, MA

Benefits: American Lung Association

Registration Fee: $25

Additional Fund Raising Required: $100

2011 Date: March 5, 2011

2012 Date: March 3, 2012

Location: One Monarch Place

Floors: 24

Steps: 528

Point of Contact: Bianca Walker,bwalker@lungne.org

2011 Participants: 186

Top Male Finisher: David Tromp(35),2:14

Top Female Finisher: Emily Curley(16),3:13

Oldest Male Finisher: Forrest Cramer(68),9:30

Oldest Female Finisher: Barbara Vanderhoff(61),6:31

2011 Money Raised: $48,424.81

Website: http://www.lungusa.org/pledge-events/ma/springfield-climb/local/event-information.html

Results:
http://www.coolrunning.com/results/11/ma/Mar5_ClimbS_set1.shtml

Comments: 2011 was the 3rd Fight For Air Climb held in Springfield.

City: St. Louis, MO

Benefits: American Lung Association

Registration Fee: $25

Additional Fund Raising Required: $100

2011 Date: March 19, 2011

2012 Date: March 10, 2012

Location: The Metropolitan Building

Floors: 42

Steps: 1000

Point of Contact: Jamie Roberts,jroberts@breathehealthy.org

2011 Participants: 1226

Top Male Finisher: Justin Stewart(23),4:17

Top Female Finisher: Cynthia Sansone(31),6:40

Oldest Male Finisher: Bill Coyne(68),9:12

Oldest Female Finisher: Rita Hellich(66),11:36

2011 Money Raised: Unknown

Website: http://www.lungusa.org/pledge-events/mo/st-louis-climb-fy12/local/event-information.html

Results:
http://www.fleetfeetstlouis.com/racetiming/results/masterthemet.htm

Comments: 2011 was the 4th Fight For Air Climb held in St. Louis

City: Stamford, CT

Benefits: American Lung Association

Registration Fee: $25

Additional Fund Raising Required: $100

2011 Date: November 19, 2011

2012 Date:

Location: Trump Parc

Floors: 34

Steps: 588

Point of Contact: Britney Martin, bmartin@lungne.org

2011 Participants: 159

Top Male Finisher: Alexander Workman(35),2:46:86

Top Female Finisher: Lauren Jacko(27),4:07:80

Oldest Male Finisher: Michael Passeero(59),14:40:59

Oldest Female Finisher: Ann Reding(61),10:05:90

2011 Money Raised: $52,287.77

Website: http://www.lungusa.org/pledge-events/ct/stamford-climb-fy12/local/event-information.html

Results: https://lungne.box.com/s/anii71tn4sku13mi8aab

Comments: 2011 was the 2nd Fight For Air Climb held in Stamford. You will be given two opportunities to test your run at Trump Parc prior to the climb.

City: Tampa, FL

Benefits: American Lung Association

Registration Fee: $25

Additional Fund Raising Required: $100

2011 Date: March 26, 2011

2012 Date: March 24, 2012

Location: Bank of America Plaza

Floors: 42

Steps: 914

Point of Contact: Danielle Cohen, dcohen@lungfla.org

2011 Participants: 915

Top Male Finisher: Tim Van Order(),4:38

Top Female Finisher: Stephanie Miles(),6:05

Oldest Male Finisher: Frank Nicolosi(70),7:40

Oldest Female Finisher: Cheri Donohoe(60),11:12

2011 Money Raised: $165,000.00

Website: http://www.lungusa.org/pledge-events/fl/tampa-climb-fy12/local/event-information.html

Results:
http://www.altavistasports.com/results/2011results/alaclimbtampa03262011.htm

Comments: 2011 was the 3rd Fight For Air Climb held in Tampa. Climb is capped at 1000 climbers.

City: Tulsa, OK

Benefits: American Lung Association

Registration Fee: $25

Additional Fund Raising Required: $100

2011 Date: April 2, 2011

2012 Date: April 7, 2012

Location: BOK Tower

Floors: 50

Steps: Unknown

Point of Contact: Kerrie Adams,kadams@breathehealthy.org

2011 Participants: 925

Top Male Finisher: Michael Peters(),6:29

Top Female Finisher: Teresa Mabarde(),7:18

Oldest Male Finisher: Jim McIntosh(72),16:02

Oldest Female Finisher: Patti Kastle(62),15:12

2011 Money Raised: $68,743.30

Website: http://www.lungusa.org/pledge-events/ok/tulsa-climb-fy12/local/event-information.html

Results:
http://www.onlineraceresults.com/race/view_race.php?race_id=18293&rel ist_record_type=result&lower_bound=0&upper_bound=190&use_previou s_sql=1&group_by=default#racetop

Comments: 2011 was the 2nd Fight For Air Climb held in Tulsa.

City: Wichita, KS

Benefits: American Lung Association

Registration Fee: $35

Additional Fund Raising Required: None

2011 Date: April 9, 2011

2012 Date: April 21, 2012

Location: Intrust Ball Arena

Floors: 34

Steps: 828

Point of Contact: Abby Brungardt,abrungardt@breathehealthy.org

2011 Participants: 200

Top Male Finisher: David Schonberg(30),11:27

Top Female Finisher: Lisa Dunn(38),13:25

Oldest Male Finisher: William Buchanan(66),17:55

Oldest Female Finisher: Jane Byrnes(66),25:14

2011 Money Raised: $46,000.00

Website: http://www.lungusa.org/pledge-events/ks/wichita-climb-fy12/local/event-information.html

Results:
http://www.mrsnv.com/uploads/evt/stp/3038/uploads/UpdatedResults.pdf

Comments: 2011 was the 2nd Fight For Air Climb held in Wichita.

City: Wilkes-Barre, PA

Benefits: American Lung Association

Registration Fee: $25

Additional Fund Raising Required: $100

2011 Date: March 19, 2011

2012 Date: March 24, 2012

Location: Mohegan Sun Arena

Floors: Stadium

Steps: 612

Point of Contact: Donna Ray-Reifler,dreilfer@lunginfo.org

2011 Participants: 94

Top Male Finisher: Ray Ricke(),6:51

Top Female Finisher: Kimberly Romoser()8:59

Oldest Male Finisher: No ages provided

Oldest Female Finisher: No ages provided

2011 Money Raised: $15,67.50

Website: http://www.lungusa.org/pledge-events/pa/wilkes-barre-climb/local/event-information.html

Results: http://www.lungusa.org/pledge-events/pa/wilkes-barre-climb/assets/images/2011-climbers-times.xls

Comments: 2011 was the 3rd Fight For Air Climb held in Wilkes Barre.

Multiple Sclerosis Climbs

There are 4 Multiple Sclerosis Society Climbs in the United States.

Like the American Lung Association Climbs, these are relatively new.

The following pages list the Multiple Sclerosis that were held in 2011.

All of the information I've discovered about these climbs I have gathered by reading the Event websites. I apologize for any errors or omissions, but these are the responsibility of the event Web Sites.

City: Boston, MA

Name: 2nd Climb to the Top

Benefits: National Multiple Sclerosis Society

Registration Fee: $35

Additional Fund Raising Required: $250

2011 Date: September 17, 2011

2012 Date: March 3, 2012

Location: John Hancock Tower

Floors: 61

Steps: 1220

Point of Contact: Unknown

2011 Participants: 101

Top Male Finisher: Alex Worman (35), 7:58

Top Female Finisher: Lisa Johnson (42), 10:25

Oldest Male Finisher: Peter Kennedy(65),13:01

Oldest Female Finisher: Mary Beth Forbes(53),22:38

2011 Money Raised: Unknown

Website: http://www.nationalmssociety.org/chapters/MAM/fundraising-events/climb/index.aspx

Results:

http://www.coolrunning.com/results/11/ma/Sep17_MSClim_set1.shtml

Comments: 2011 was the 2nd Climb to the Top in Boston. Even though you finish on the 60th floor, you will climb 61 flights of stairs, because you start on the basement level of the John Hancock Tower. Headphones and the use of cell phones are not permitted while climbing.

City: New York City, NY

Name: Climb To The Top

Benefits: Multiple Sclerosis Society

Registration Fee: $35

Additional Fund Raising Required: $250

2011 Date: February 27, 2011

2012 Date: March 4, 2012

Location: Rockefeller Center

Floors: 66

Steps: Unknown

Point of Contact: Unknown

2011 Participants: 1,027

Top Male Finisher: Paul Teti(34),8:27

Top Female Finisher: Jimena Barrera(36),11:41

Oldest Male Finisher: Herb Rozansky(80),38:12

Oldest Female Finisher: Judith Kostman(68),27:42

2011 Money Raised: Unknown

Website:

http://www.rockefellercenter.com/events/2012/03/04/ms-climb-top/

Results:

http://eventnyn.nationalmssociety.org/site/DocServer/overall_results_201
1__updated_2-28-11_.pdf?docID=51768

Comments: 2011 was the 8th Climb To The Top in New York City.
Special mention to Dwayne Richardson. Look for a Spotlight on Dwayne in
the 2013 Edition of this book.

City: Virginia Beach, VA

Name: 1st Go Vertical for MS

Benefits: Multiple Sclerosis Society

Registration Fee: $25

Additional Fund Raising Required: $100

2011 Date: September 24, 2011

2012 Date:

Location: Westin Virginia Beach Town Center

Floors: 36

Steps: Unknown

Point of Contact: Unknown

2011 Participants: 23

Top Male Finisher: Chris Sponheimer(),4:34

Top Female Finisher: Dana Weate (),5:01

Oldest Male Finisher: No ages provided

Oldest Female Finisher: No ages provided

2011 Money Raised: Unknown

Website:

http://eventvax.nationalmssociety.org/site/PageServer?pagename=GEN_ VAX_homepage

Results:

http://its-go-time.com/wp-content/uploads/2011/09/MSS-Division-results.pdf

Comments: 2011 was the 1st Go Vertical for MX in Virginia Beach

City: Winston-Salem, NC

Name: 2nd Power up the Tower

Benefits: Multiple Sclerosis Society

Registration Fee: $25

Additional Fund Raising Required: $100

2011 Date: February 5, 2011

2012 Date: February 25, 2012

Location: Winston Tower

Floors: 30

Steps: Unknown

Point of Contact: Unknown

2011 Participants: 227

Top Male Finisher: Eric Koehrsen(30),3:17

Top Female Finisher: Robyn Holland(40),4:37

Oldest Male Finisher: Paul Lanier(67),6:11

Oldest Female Finisher: Valerie Gardner(65),14:16

2011 Money Raised: Unknown

Website:

http://www.nationalmssociety.org/chapters/ncc/fundraising-events/climb-ms/index.aspx

Results:

http://www.onthemarksports.com/results/2011/2011_02_05_oa.htm

Comments: 2011 was the 2nd Power up the Tower in Winston-Salem

Other Major Climbs

These are the other major United States Climbs. Most of them are affiliated with a charity.

Some, like the Empire State Building Run Up, the Willis (Sears Tower Climb and the Hustle Up The Hancock Climb are the premier Stair Climbs in the country and the world

I've also included the Toronto Canada CN Tower Climb which the premier climb in Canada, raising over 1.2 million dollars last year for the Canadian Wildlife Fund.

All of the information I've discovered about these climbs I have gathered by reading the Event websites. I apologize for any errors or omissions, but these are the responsibility of the event Web Sites.

City: Charlotte, NC

Name: 1st Race to the Top

Benefits: Levine Children's Hospital

Registration Fee: $35

Additional Fund Raising Required: None

2011 Date: March 26, 2011

2012 Date: March 24, 2012

Location: Duke Energy Center

Floors: 49

Steps: 1194

Point of Contact: Chris Raynor,craynor@charlottesports.org

2011 Participants: 444

Top Male Finisher: Michael Creason (39), 7:29

Top Female Finisher: Stephanie Hucko (39), 8:20

Oldest Male Finisher: Bill Clayter(69),12:09

Oldest Female Finisher: Joanne Stanley(59),14:25

2011 Money Raised: Unknown

Website: http://www.charlottesports.org/racetothetop/

Results:
http://results.active.com/pages/page.jsp?eventID=1950058&pubID=3

Comments: 2011 was the first Race to the Top in Charlotte. The 2012 Race to the Top will be capped at **750** participants

City: Chicago, IL

Name: 3rd Skyrise Chicago

Benefits: Rehab Institute of Chicago

Registration Fee: $50

Additional Fund Raising Required: $100

2011 Date: November 6, 2011

2012 Date:

Location: Willis (Sears) Tower

Floors: 103

Steps: 2109

Point of Contact: Unknown

2011 Participants: 2231

Top Male Finisher: Sproule Love (40), 13:03

Top Female Finisher: Cindy Harris (42), 14:57

Oldest Male Finisher: Piero Dettin(74),23:16

Oldest Female Finisher: Gloria Schiffler(83),1:00:33

2011 Money Raised: Unknown

Website:
http://ric.convio.net/site/PageServer?pagename=event_information

Results:

http://www.theracershub.com/results_view.php?id=1503&result_type=fil

Comments: 2011 was the 3rd Skyrise Chicago Climb.

This climb features a Stair Climb option, a hand cycle option (computer simulation), and a brain power option :)

Because of limited space, spectators will not be allowed up to the Skydeck, but are invited to wait for their event participants in the lobby area.

City: Chicago, IL

Name: Hustle Up The Hancock

Benefits: Respiratory Health Association

Registration Fee: $55

Additional Fund Raising Required: $85

2011 Date: February 27, 2011

2012 Date: February 26, 2012

Location: John Hancock Center

Floors: 94

Steps: 1632

Point of Contact: Unknown

2011 Participants: 2948

Top Male Finisher: Terry Purchell (40), 10:03

Top Female Finisher: Cindy Harris (42), 11:21

Oldest Male Finisher: James Devenney(86),40:14

Oldest Female Finisher: Gail Bruffee(72),22:06

2011 Money Raised: Unknown

Website:

http://www.hustleupthehancock.org/eventinfo.htm

Results:

http://www.lungchicago.org/hustle-results11

Comments: 2011 was the 14th Hustle Up The Hancock in Chicago

City: Chicago, IL

Name: 14th Step up for Kids

Benefits: Children's Memorial Center

Registration Fee: $45

Additional Fund Raising Required: $55

2011 Date: January 30, 2011

2012 Date: January 29, 2012

Location: AON Center

Floors: 80

Steps: 1643

Point of Contact:

2011 Participants: 1949

Top Male Finisher: Jesse Berg(38), 9:56

Top Female Finisher: Bridget Carlson(), 12:40

Oldest Male Finisher: No ages provided

Oldest Female Finisher: No ages provided

2011 Money Raised: Unknown

Website:

http://www.heroesforlife.org/site/TR?sid=1190&fr_id=1240&pg=informa
tional

Results:
http://results.active.com/pages/displayNonGru.jsp?pubID=3&rsID=1051
88

Comments: 2011 was the 14th Step up for Kids in Chicago. The climb is
capped at 3,000.

City: Cleveland, OH

Name: 9th Tackle the Tower

Benefits: Ronald McDonald House of Cleveland

Registration Fee: $25

Additional Fund Raising Required: None

2011 Date: February 5, 2011

2012 Date: February 4, 2012

Location: Galleria and Tower at Erieview

Floors: 38

Steps: 646

Point of Contact: Unknown

2011 Participants: 600

Top Male Finisher: Max Haiss(17),4:17:40

Top Female Finisher: Beth Darmstadter(45),5:10:60

Oldest Male Finisher: John Popp(70),13:59:70

Oldest Female Finisher: Jean Toth(74),9:39:10

2011 Money Raised: Unknown

Website:

http://www.hermescleveland.com/roadracing/events/tower.asp

Results:

http://www.hermescleveland.com/roadracing/results/2011/TACKLE.HT
M

Comments: 2011 was the 9th Tackle the Tower in Cleveland

City: Dallas, TX

Name: 3rd Big D Climb

Benefits: Leukemia Society

Registration Fee: $25

Additional Fund Raising Required: None

2011 Date: January 29, 2011

2012 Date: January 28, 2012

Location: Fountain Place

Floors: 52

Steps: 1040

Point of Contact: Stacey Russell, Stacey.Russell@lls.org

2011 Participants: 673

Top Male Finisher: Zachary Istre(20), 6:00:90

Top Female Finisher: Shanna Moody(30), 8:26:70

Oldest Male Finisher: Ken Raggio(60),7:58

Oldest Female Finisher: Susan Istre(60),15:15

2011 Money Raised: $100,000

Website: http://www.bigdclimb.org

Results:

http://www.mychiptime.com/searchevent.php?id=5351

Comments: 2011 was the 3rd Big D Climb in Dallas

City: Indianapolis, IN

Name: 28th Bop To The Top

Benefits: Riley's Hospital for Children

Registration Fee: $22

Additional Fund Raising Required: None

2011 Date: January 22, 2011

2012 Date: January 21, 2012

Location: One America Tower

Floors: 36

Steps: 806

Point of Contact: Unknown

2011 Participants: 1211

Top Male Finisher: Marty Wilker(45), 3:55:20

Top Female Finisher: Cindy Harris(42), 4:43:70

Oldest Male Finisher: Bob Terry(83),14:36

Oldest Female Finisher: Ilonka Herber(67),10:36

2011 Money Raised: $30,000

Website:

http://www.tuxbro.com/entry-info/BoptoTopInfo.htm

Results:

http://www.tuxbro.com/results/2011/Bop11ind.html

Comments: 2011 was the 28th Bop To The Top in Indianapolis

City: Los Angeles, CA

Name: 18th Stair Climb for Los Angeles

Benefits: YMCA

Registration Fee: None. Included in Fund Raising.

Additional Fund Raising Required: $100

2011 Date: September 23, 2011

2012 Date:

Location: U.S. Bank Tower.

Floors: 75

Steps: 1500

Point of Contact: Unknown

2011 Participants: 2103

Top Male Finisher: Jesse Berg(38),9:38

Top Female Finisher: Erika Aklufi (),10:35

Oldest Male Finisher: Tom Kutrosky(76),8:19

Oldest Female Finisher: Jaon Kramer(69),23:32

2011 Money Raised: $434,000

Website:

http://www.kintera.org/faf/home/default.asp?ievent=474861

Results:

http://www.onlineraceresults.com/event/view_event.php?event_id=7402

Comments: 2011 was the 18th Stair Climb for Los Angeles

City: New York, NY

Name: 2nd Story by Story

Benefits: InMotion

Registration Fee: None. Fundraising only.

Additional Fund Raising Required: $100

2011 Date: October 6, 2011

2012 Date: Unknown

Location: 144 Broadway 39

Floors: 42

Steps: Unknown

Point of Contact: Unknown

2011 Participants: 1022

Top Male Finisher: Joe Michels(),4:37:10

Top Female Finisher: Casey Rash(),6:45:00

Oldest Male Finisher: No ages provided

Oldest Female Finisher: No ages provided

2011 Money Raised: $684,422

Website:

http://community.inmotiononline.org/Page.aspx?pid=483

Results:

http://www.inmotiononline.org/assets/pdfs/SxS-2011/SxS-2011_Timing-Chip-Results.pdf

Photos:

http://www.flickr.com/photos/66743311@N03/sets/

Comments: 2011 was the 2nd Story by Story Climb in New York

City: New York, NY

Name: 34th Empire State Building Run Up

Benefits: Unknown

Registration Fee: $100

Additional Fund Raising Required: None

2011 Date: February 1, 2011

2012 Date: February 8, 2012

Location: Empire State Building

Floors: 86

Steps: 1576

Point of Contact: Unknown

2011 Participants: 440

Top Male Finisher: Thomas Dold(26), 10:10

Top Female Finisher: Alice McNamara(24),13:03

Oldest Male Finisher: Piero Dettin(73),18:55

Oldest Female Finisher: Ginette Bedard(77),22:15

2011 Money Raised: Unknown

Website:

http://www.nyrr.org/races/2012/r0208x00.asp

Results:

http://web2.nyrrc.org/cgi-bin/start.cgi/aes-
programs/results/startup.html?result.id=b10201&result.year=2011

Comments: 2011 was the 34th Empire State Building Run Up in New
York. Limited to 600 entrants. Entry is by random drawing.

City: Norfolk, VA

Name: 2nd Step Up for the Up Center

Benefits: The Up Center

Registration Fee: $35

Additional Fund Raising Required: None

2011 Date: April 3, 2011

2012 Date: March 25, 2012

Location: Dominion Tower

Floors: 100

Steps: 2320

Point of Contact: Jessica Oulahan, jessica.oulahan@theupcenter.org

2011 Participants: 200

Top Male Finisher: Bobby Crawford(45),13:00:35

Top Female Finisher: Jackie Propst(37),16:07:70

Oldest Male Finisher: Robert Grouche(76),44:28:15

Oldest Female Finisher: Janet Dobson(51),25:58:65

2011 Money Raised: Unknown

Website:

http://www.theupcenter.org/How_to_Help/Step_Up/index.htm

Results:

http://results.active.com/pages/page.jsp?pubID=3&eventLinkageID=1289
64&year=2011

Comments: 2011 was the 2nd Step up for the Up Center in Norfolk

City: Omaha, NE

Name: 5th Trek up the Tower

Benefits: WELCOM

Registration Fee: $45

Additional Fund Raising Required: None

2011 Date: February 26, 2011

2012 Date: February 25, 2012

Location: First National Tower

Floors: 40

Steps: 870

Point of Contact: Unknown

2011 Participants: 1417

Top Male Finisher: Bobby Crawford(45),13:00:35

Top Female Finisher: Jackie Propst(37),16:07:70

Oldest Male Finisher: Hess Dyas(73),12:01

Oldest Female Finisher: Judy Hess(73),17:45

2011 Money Raised: Unknown

Website:

http://www.trekupthetower.org/

Results:

http://www.onlineraceresults.com/race/view_plain_text.php?race_id=1792
8

Comments: 2011 was the 5th Trek Up the Tower in Omaha

City: P:hiladelphia, PA

Name: 1st Special Olympics Stair Climb Philadelphia

Benefits: Special Olympics

Registration Fee: $25

Additional Fund Raising Required: $100

2011 Date: December 4, 2011

2012 Date:

Location: Mellon Bank Card Center

Floors: 53

Steps: 1019

Point of Contact: Unknown

2011 Participants: 63

Top Male Finisher: Michael Karlin(),7:15

Top Female Finisher: Wilfredro Ruiz(),9:28

Oldest Male Finisher: No ages provided

Oldest Female Finisher: No ages provided

2011 Money Raised: Unknown

Website:

http://www.climbphilly.org/

Results:
http://www.parunners.com/2011%20RESULTS/2011%20PHILLY%20ST
AIR%20CLIMB.htm

Comments: 2011 was the 1st Special Olympics Stair Climb in Philadelphia

City: Seattle, WA

Name: 25th Big Climb Seattle

Benefits: Leukemia Society

Registration Fee: $40

Additional Fund Raising Required: $50

2011 Date: March 20, 2011

2012 Date:

Location: The Columbia Center

Floors: 69

Steps: 1311

Point of Contact: Unknown

2011 Participants: 3315

Top Male Finisher: Shawn Stephens-Whale(21),7:08

Top Female Finisher: Kourtney Dexter(30),9:16

Oldest Male Finisher: Anders Jacobsen(86),25:25

Oldest Female Finisher: Shirley Lansing(81),36:49

2011 Money Raised: Unknown

Website:

http://www.llswa.org/site/PageNavigator/BC_homepage

Results:

http://racecenter.s3.amazonaws.com/res_bcfl11.htm

Comments: 2011 was the 25th Big Climb in Seattle. Event is capped at 6,000 participants.

City: Toronto, Canada

Name: 21st Annual Canada Life CN Tower Climb

Benefits: Leukemia Society

Registration Fee: Unknown

Additional Fund Raising Required: Unknown

2011 Date: April 16, 2011

2012 Date: April 21, 2012

Location: CN Tower, Toronto

Floors: 144

Steps: 1776

Point of Contact: Unknown

2011 Participants: 6200

Top Male Finisher: Unknown

Top Female Finisher: Unknown

Oldest Male Finisher: Unknown

Oldest Female Finisher: Unknown

2011 Money Raised: 1.1 Million

Website:

http://publicclimb.wwf.ca/event_details/

Results:

Comments: 2011 was the 21st Annual Canada Life Climb ion Toronto.

CHAPTER TWELVE

Major Climb Results

I thought I would present the results of the 6 highest climbs in the United States, along with my home town climb, the 2011 Philadelphia Fight For Air Climb.

The Philadelphia Fight For Air Climb

March 19, 2011

Results

1.David Tromp	Glenmont,NY	35 M	5:45.80
2.Dan Speirs	Media,PA	30 M	6:31.77
3.Stephen Marsalese	Rye Brook NY	45 M	6:48.52
4.Francisco Logo	Ocala,FL	42 M	6:53.54
5.Alexander Covington	,PA	26 M	7:12.97
6.James Mcnamara	Fanwood,NJ	55 M	7:30.39
7.Jason Pantano	Norristown,PA	32 M	7:37.68
8.Christopher Fath	Philadelphia,PA	33 M	7:41.15
9.Matthew Zacharkow	Roebling,NJ	27 M	7:43.82
10.Brian Turdo	Phillipsburg,NJ	32 M	7:46.79
11.Benjamin Jakus	Philadelphia,PA	27 M	7:54.15
12.John Wright	King Of Prussia,PA	32 M	7:54.44
13.Keith Schmitt	Doylestown,PA	22 M	7:54.92
14.Andrew L Miller	Philadelphia,PA	25 M	7:56.27
15.Eric Charles	Martinsville,NJ	26 M	7:59.78
16.Karl Neumann	,	50 M	8:00.29
17.Justin Duff	Philadelphia,PA	31 M	8:01.21
18.Daniel Mcconnell	Wilmington,DE	32 M	8:02.81
19.Nicholas Rosamilia	Philadelphia,PA	17 M	8:03.94
20.Michael O'rourke	Philadelphia,PA	30 M	8:05.10
21.Sean Mcmenamin	Cheltenham,PA	40 M	8:06.97
22.Padraig Cullen	Newtown Square,PA	23 M	8:08.92
23.Christopher Santanie	Philadelphia,PA	26 M	8:13.50
24.David Ortega	Woodbury Height,NJ	30 M	8:14.07
25.Warren Jefferis	Downingtown,PA	54 M	8:15.23
26.Hoan Thai	Philadelphia,PA	27 M	8:15.48
27.Charles Ruchalski	Philadelphia,PA	38 M	8:18.62
28.Eric Burke	Philadelphia,PA	26 M	8:18.86

29.Todd Sautter	Cherry Hill,NJ	33 M	8:20.21
30.Stefan Samulewicz	Kennett Square,PA	46 M	8:22.67
31.Will Climber	Philly Fire Pea,	99 M	8:23.62
32.Kenneth Cairns	Warrington,PA	29 M	8:24.78
33.2 Climber	Haddonfield,NJ	99 M	8:25.84
34.Gavin Kramer	Ewing,NJ	47 M	8:29.24
35.Ryan Decker	Philadelphia,PA	27 M	8:32.37
36.John Shields	Philadelphia,PA	25 M	8:36.82
37.Mark Mariski Jr.	Philadelphia,PA	26 M	8:38.77
38.Anthony Nardini	Philadelphia,PA	30 M	8:40.50
39.Charles Ruchalski	Philadelphia,PA	38 M	8:40.53
40.1 Climber	Haddonfield,NJ	99 M	8:40.63
41.Patrick Hansen	Cheyney,PA	25 M	8:42.37
42.Matthew Kelly	Aston,PA	25 M	8:42.81
43.Dick Climber	Philly Fire Pea,	99 M	8:43.29
44.Luke Stewart	Moorestown,NJ	16 M	8:43.84
45.Paul Archambault	Philadelphia,PA	29 M	8:46.21
46.Steve Duc	Philadelphia,PA	28 M	8:46.70
47.Tom Picerno	Ewing,NJ	40 M	8:47.56
48.Allen Boxer	Philadelphia,PA	25 M	8:48.21
49.Ryan Gallatig	Philadelphia,PA	32 M	8:50.07
50.Caitlin Coleman	West Chester,PA	21 F	8:50.41
51.Sheryl Leonard-schne	Wauwatosa,WI	46 F	8:50.56
52.Brian Climber	Philly Fire Pea,	99 M	8:50.80
53.Climber Second ,		99 M	8:53.03
54.Dianne San Luis	Philadelphia,PA	32 F	8:53.96
55.Alan Lloyd	Swedesboro,NJ	34 M	8:55.12
56.Dennis Cullen	Cheltenham,PA	40 M	8:59.61
57.John Shields	Philadelphia,PA	25 M	9:00.76
58.Climber Third ,		99 M	9:02.69
59.Third Climber ,		99 M	9:03.01
60.Climber Fourth ,		99 M	9:05.66

61.Gene Shaffer	Ambler,PA	42 M	9:06.28
62.Peter Camburn	Philadelphia,PA	33 M	9:06.83
63.Jonathan Gildea	Reading,PA	34 M	9:07.95
64.Sally Troy	Philadelphia,PA	27 F	9:09.76
65.Tim Gradoville	**Reading,PA**	**31 M**	**9:09.86**
66.Richard Pomager	Spring City,PA	38 M	9:10.74
67.Francis Costello	Philadelphia,PA	24 M	9:11.10
68.Christopher Witt	Milltow,NJ	36 M	9:11.62
69.Briana Wight	Downingtown,PA	18 F	9:11.96
70.Charles Smith	Philadelphia,PA	37 M	9:12.58
71.Russel Walters	Philadelphia,PA	35 M	9:12.96
72.Climber First	,	99 M	9:15.87
73.Michael Damiano	Prospect Park,PA	26 M	9:15.93
74.Thomas Remaize	West Chester,PA	33 M	9:16.06
75.Kyle Whalon	Lansdale,PA	11 M	9:16.41
76.Butch Dougherty	Oakford,PA	99 M	9:16.74
77.Brenden Dorley	Havertown,PA	39 M	9:19.34
78.Dianne San Luis	Philadelphia,PA	32 F	9:19.48
79.Garrett Fardelmann	Philadelphia,PA	31 M	9:20.08
80.Scott Chappe	Staten Island,NY	52 M	9:22.54
81.Casey Meizinger	Philadelphia,PA	24 F	9:23.42
82.Joe Ernst	Hatfield,PA	51 M	9:24.80
83.Ken Myers	Lafayette Hill,PA	42 M	9:24.92
84.Bob Gauss	Flourtown,PA	48 M	9:24.99
85.Dan Carlson	Philadelphia,PA	21 M	9:27.97
86.Robert Mcdermott	Gloucester City,NJ	27 M	9:28.24
87.Ethan Clearfield	Richboro,PA	13 M	9:28.36
88.Climber Fourth	,	99 M	9:29.52
89.Quoc Luu	Philadelphia,PA	29 M	9:30.29
90.Todd Grant	Philadelphia,PA	35 M	9:30.99
91.Joseph Lynch	Philadelphia,PA	52 M	9:32.19
92.Nicholas Watt	Baltimore,MD	30 M	9:35.40

93.Michele Jones	,	49 F	9:37.79
94.James Wise	Huntingdon Vall,PA	30 M	9:38.18
95.Michael Garozzo	Philadelphia,PA	40 M	9:38.93
96.Michael L Carr	Perkasie,PA	33 M	9:39.43
97.Brian Hamilton	Wyndmoor,PA	13 M	9:39.81
98.Mary Pawlowski	Philadelphia,PA	49 F	9:39.99
99.James Donaghue	West Chester,PA	35 M	9:41.17
100.Drew Deblasio	Ewing,NJ	47 M	9:41.74
101.Ricky Pellegrino	Norristown,PA	20 M	9:41.86
102.Christine Kasprzak	Philadelphia,PA	30 F	9:42.50
103.CalebEyster Pa	Furnace,PA	12 M	9:44.04
104.Climber Second	,	99 M	9:44.10
105.Amber Newton	Media,PA	32 F	9:44.86
106.Climber First ,		99 M	9:45.44
107.Ben Chera	West Chester,PA	21 M	9:46.46
108.Justin Santi	Sewell,NJ	23 M	9:48.69
109.Derek Graeber	Wayne,PA	38 M	9:49.81
110.Fourth Climber ,		99 M	9:51.02
111.Zachary Risler	Norristown,PA	25 M	9:53.51
112.Stephanie Wilsey	Philadelphia,PA	23 F	9:54.26
113.Devon Curry	Telford,PA	21 M	9:55.45
114.Larry Boyle	Philadelphia,PA	48 M	9:56.22
115.Bonnie Kizis	Warrington,PA	23 F	9:56.50
116.Susan Bednar	Jeffersonville,PA	33 F	9:56.67
117.Reed Costello	Audubon,NJ	40 M	9:57.34
118.Ryan Bailey	Philadelphia,PA	32 M	9:58.01
119.John Bianchi	Philadelphia,PA	47 M	9:59.67
120.Robert Boyles	Philadelphia,PA	25 M	10:00.03
121.Scott Hanson	Philadelphia,PA	25 M	10:01.37
122.Rob Janecek	West Milford,NJ	40 M	10:01.89
123.Jaclyn Russell	Philadelphia,PA	23 F	10:02.53
124.Jeffrey P Metcalf	Philadelphia,PA	33 M	10:02.75

125.Matthew Marinzoli	Philadelphia,PA	29 M	10:04.90
126.Marcia Monaco	Martinsville,NJ	56 F	10:07.15
127.Jeanine Dankoff	Philadelphia,PA	36 F	10:07.3
128.Jason Kufta	Philadelphiia,PA	30 M	10:07.44
129.Lisa Neyen	Allentown,PA	45 F	10:07.74
130.Carly Conti	Conshohocken,PA	27 F	10:08.39
131.Dennis Pomager	Chester Springs,PA	36 M	10:10.03
132.Mike Vanderslice	Newark,DE	33 M	10:11.18
133.Dan Bornstein	Newtown,PA	43 M	10:11.87
134.Jeff Carrick	Titusville,NJ	36 M	10:14.49
135.1 Climber	Haddonfield,	99 M	10:15.12
136.Eli Rivera	Pennsauken,NJ	26 M	10:16.01
137.Second Climber	,	99 M	10:18.26
138.Mitchell Cheng	Perkasie,PA	16 M	10:18.42
139.Jacqueline Christie	Philadelphia,PA	34 F	10:18.47
140.Ashley Panicker	Philadelphia,PA	23 M	10:18.68
141.Michael Warren	Moorestown,NJ	21 M	10:21.08
142.Ralph O'neill	Philadelphia,PA	59 M	10:22.69
143.Andrew Pomager	Philadelphia,PA	28 M	10:23.24
144.Monique Morgan	Drexel Hill,PA	25 F	10:23.46
145.First Climber	,	99 M	10:23.63
146.Stephanie Ruzicka	Madison,NJ	45 F	10:23.90
147.Sean Ball	Haddon Township,NJ	12 M	10:24.27
148.Tony Payton Jr	Philadelphia,PA	30 M	10:24.57
149.Craig Hubert	Ringoes,NJ	46 M	10:24.78
150.Chris Camburn	Villanova,PA	37 M	10:25.19
151.Christina Smoker	Lititz,PA	37 F	10:25.91
152.Jessica Camacho	Philadelphiia,PA	26 F	10:26.09
153.4 Climber	Haddonfield,NJ	99 M	10:28.46
154.Joseph Lynch	Philadelphia,PA	52 M	10:29.18
155.Kyle Eno	Wilmington,DE	27 M	10:29.36
156.Santo Caruso	Philadelphia,PA	26 M	10:30.01

157.Geralynne Steffenino	Collegeville,PA	44 F	10:31.24
158.Eric Miller	Philadelphia,PA	31 M	10:31.38
159.Janet Disalvo	Glenside,PA	30 F	10:33.06
160.Randy Lobasso	Philadelphia,PA	27 M	10:33.22
161.Mark Bhasin	New York,NY	36 M	10:34.79
162.**Melissa Smiley**	Cinnaminson,NJ	14 F	10:36.15
163.Matt Hess	Glenside,PA	25 M	10:36.85
164.Franco Boffice	Philadelphia,PA	45 M	10:37.22
165.**John Smiley**	Cinnaminson,NJ	56 M	10:37.82
166.Laurie Pietrini	Robbinsville,NJ	45 F	10:39.43
167.David Dimatteo	Havertown,PA	38 M	10:39.74
168.Brian Plodizyn	Haddonfield,NJ	29 M	10:42.99
169.Bob King	Audubon,NJ	20 M	10:43.73
170.Mark Bushey	Philadelphia,PA	24 M	10:46.04
171.Climber Fourth	,	99 M	10:46.69
172.Jason Carty	Mount Holly,NJ	34 M	10:48.33
173.Climber Third	,	99 M	10:48.54
174.Sean Devens	Philadelphia,PA	29 M	10:49.40
175.Keith Zimecki	Cinnaminson,NJ	37 M	10:50.26
176.Claire Riordan	Media,PA	24 F	10:50.48
177.Janelle Johnson	Philadelphia,PA	24 F	10:51.10
178.Rohan Defonseka	Ocean,NJ	40 M	10:51.95
179.Michael Ortiz	Philadelphia,PA	27 M	10:53.96
180.Denise Catini	Morristown,NJ	40 F	10:54.21
181.Larry Durland	King Of Prussia,PA	31 M	10:54.66
182.Henry Ford	Delran,NJ	46 M	10:54.90
183.Rebecca Harvey	Philadelphia,PA	28 F	10:55.32
184.Jim Corey	Warrington,PA	50 M	10:56.46
185.Felecia Wiley	Philadelphia,PA	45 F	10:57.56
186.James Cummings	Philadelphia,PA	47 M	10:57.95
187.Arielle Evans	Meadowbrook,PA	23 F	10:59.54
188.John Daskilewicz	Philadelphia,PA	26 M	11:05.11

189.Johnny Picerno	Ewing,NJ	15 M	11:05.14
190.James Rydarowski	Eastampton,NJ	29 M	11:07.10
191.Stephanie Miller	Titusville,NJ	24 F	11:07.28
192.Mark Campi	Coatesville,PA	39 M	11:08.04
193.Jennifer Pomager	Spring City,PA	35 F	11:08.31
194.Darrin Pietrini	Robbinsville,NJ	45 M	11:08.99
195.Christopher Galasso	Philadelphia,PA	21 M	11:09.31
196.**Sophorn Smiley**	Philadelphia,PA	31 F	11:10.97
197.Megan Quinlan	Philadelphia,PA	29 F	11:12.11
198.Ramsey Moorman	Silver Spring,MD	31 M	11:12.15
199.Amy Courter	Allentown,PA	40 F	11:12.24
200.Carolyn Richardson	Jeff Sta,NY	31 F	11:12.51
201.James Darr	Croydon,PA	31 M	11:12.69
202.Marco Catini	Morristown,NJ	40 M	11:13.07
203.Matthew Letourneau	Philadelphia,PA	35 M	11:16.47
204.Ngoc (jen) Nguyen	Philadelphia,PA	26 F	11:18.15
205.Nicole Oneill	Morrisville,PA	29 F	11:18.99
206.Alicia Rennie	Medford,NJ	37 F	11:19.37
207.Jeff Ham	Philadelphia,PA	28 M	11:20.74
208.Brian Gardner	Lumberton,NJ	40 M	11:20.80
209.Ellen Lyons	Aldan,PA	22 F	11:22.19
210.3 Climber	Haddonfield,NJ	99 M	11:23.03
211.Joseph Anello	Woodbury,NJ	26 M	11:24.13
212.Justin Duff	Philadelphia,PA	31 M	11:25.20
213.Molly Northrop	Philadelphia,PA	39 F	11:25.96
214.Jim Stabilito	Scottsdale,AZ	41 M	11:26.39
215.Dennis Heyman	Drexel Hill,PA	31 M	11:26.65
216.Luke Kelly	Philadelphia,PA	32 M	11:27.21
217.Carl Bierbach	Pennsauken,NJ	24 M	11:27.88
218.Sandra Newman	Philadelphia,PA	34 F	11:27.96
219.Andrew Wolf	Philadelphia,PA	30 M	11:28.96
220.Freddie Urbano	Ewing,NJ	42 M	11:29.35

221.Heidi Fuller	Marlton,NJ	43 F	11:29.38
222.4 Climber	Haddonfield,NJ	99 M	11:29.69
223.Michael Day	Oley,PA	22 M	11:30.05
224.Orla Reese	Radnor,PA	51 M	11:30.44
225.Jean Marie Seal	Westampton,NJ	40 F	11:30.47
226.Robert Gardler	Philadelphia,PA	42 M	11:30.69
227.Julian Ortman	Philadelphia,PA	15 M	11:31.82
228.Michael Dieterle	Berwyn,PA	38 M	11:31.90
229.Deborah Lake	Robbinsville,NJ	39 F	11:32.14
230.Mike Carr	Warrington,PA	60 M	11:33.31
231.William Tambussi	Haddon Heights,NJ	27 M	11:33.32
232.Karin Zeller	Ivyland,PA	34 F	11:35.98
233.Jacqueline Finkelste	Spring City,PA	31 F	11:37.31
234.Rhonda Yee	Philadelphia,PA	35 F	11:38.29
235.Christopher White	Bar Harbor,ME	41 M	11:38.87
236.Byrne Remphrey	Parkesburg,PA	34 M	11:38.96
237.Jim Godby	Gilbertsville,PA	51 M	11:39.25
238.Candace Cocron	Doylestown,PA	21 F	11:39.43
239.Kimberly Fusco	Collingswood,NJ	35 F	11:41.25
240.Kimberly Studebaker	Plymouth Meetin,PA	30 F	11:46.65
241.Gregg Crannage	Ewing,NJ	33 M	11:47.89
242.Robert Gurtcheff	Philadelphia,PA	36 M	11:48.64
243.John Myers	Marlton,NJ	30 M	11:49.13
244.Jimmy Klauder	Lower Gwynedd,PA	14 M	11:50.01
245.Marcel Franklin	Philadelphia,PA	30 F	11:50.35
246.Chantay Wiley	Philadelphia,PA	50 F	11:51.46
247.Jim Heisler	Riverton,NJ	25 M	11:51.75
248.Donna Aromando	Lumberton,NJ	49 F	11:52.23
249.Eric Pluckhorn	Moorestown,NJ	44 M	11:52.49
250.Diana Otero	Devon,PA	38 F	11:53.50
251.Stacy Remphrey	Parkesburg,PA	33 F	11:54.09
252.Ryan Miller	Bechtelsville,PA	23 M	11:54.12

253.Mike Mclane	Philadelphia,PA	27 M	11:56.33
254.Rodman Messenger	Philadelphia,PA	34 M	11:59.17
255.Marley Golato	Philadelphia,PA	15 F	11:59.29
256.Dean Patterson	Drexel Hill,PA	44 M	11:59.63
257.Sally Wilson	Doylestown,PA	44 F	12:00.81
258.John Derham	Philadelphia,PA	51 M	12:01.42
259.Tom Clark	Warrington,PA	55 M	12:01.65
260.Alonzo Smith	Bala Cynwyd,PA	51 M	12:02.07
261.Kristen O'grady	Langhorne,PA	41 F	12:05.16
262.Christopher Fath	Philadelphia,PA	33 M	12:05.18
263.Dan Carr	Chalfont,PA	36 M	12:06.04
264.Christina Rooney	Horsham,PA	26 F	12:06.38
265.Bonnie Gildea	Reading,PA	33 F	12:07.08
266.Wilfredo Ruiz	Philadelphia,PA	32 M	12:10.03
267.Andrea Byrne	Philadelphia,PA	28 F	12:12.02
268.Conor Gourley	Wayne,PA	12 M	12:13.54
269.Zachary Mateja	King Of Prussia,PA	22 M	12:14.60
270.Justin Jedwabney	Groton,CT	29 M	12:18.87
271.Richard Fath	Philadelphia,PA	26 M	12:19.15
272.Paul Bradbury	Blue Bell,PA	41 M	12:20.01
273.2 Climber	Haddonfield,NJ	99 M	12:20.44
274.Paul Benz	Jeffersonville,PA	39 M	12:20.59
275.Mike May	Cherry Hill,NJ	30 M	12:20.62
276.Lou Day	Oley,PA	42 M	12:21.40
277.Susan Leo	Aston,PA	46 F	12:23.87
278.Eric Fraint	Cherry Hill,NJ	55 M	12:26.61
279.Kevin Grooms	Philadelphia,PA	37 M	12:27.29
280.Rick Molz	Bensalem,PA	56 M	12:27.51
281.Jeff Mirabello	Haddonfield,NJ	28 M	12:27.78
282.Maria Spada	North Brunswick,NJ	28 F	12:30.78
283.Devaney Camburn	Philadelphia,PA	29 F	12:30.97
284.Steven Picerno	Ewing,NJ	41 M	12:31.20

285.Keunwoo Lee	King Of Prussia,PA	38 M	12:32.48
286.Chris Abate	Philadelphia,PA	32 M	12:32.89
287.Amanda Jacobi	Philadelphia,PA	29 F	12:32.97
288.Timothy Williams	Feasterville,PA	28 M	12:33.21
289.Ashley Bruce	Piscataway,NJ	27 F	12:33.33
290.Constance Meizinger	Doylestown,PA	53 F	12:35.92
291.Dai'jah Diggs	Thorofare,NJ	14 F	12:36.71
292.Sam Myers	Lafayette Hill,PA	11 M	12:38.07
293.Luke Kulikowski	Plymouth Meetin,PA	29 M	12:39.75
294.Nate Moyer	Philadelphia,PA	31 M	12:40.30
295.Elizabeth Melervey	Feasterville,PA	25 F	12:40.80
296.Caitlin Coates	Springfield,PA	24 F	12:43.26
297.Stephen Mines	Cherry Hill,NJ	31 M	12:43.60
298.Abbie Santana	Philadelphia,PA	31 F	12:45.64
299.Olivia Climber	Philly Fire Pea,	99 M	12:45.94
300.Erin Dry	Quakertown,PA	30 F	12:48.55
301.Denise Farrell	Phila,PA	56 F	12:48.82
302.Sarah Fanning	Philadelphia,PA	25 F	12:50.32
303.Rocco Maiorano	Horsham,PA	31 M	12:51.24
304.Cheryl Gilmore	Breinigsville,PA	29 F	12:51.45
305.Joe Biondo	Philadelphia,PA	31 M	12:52.37
306.Jim Carr	Doylestown,PA	64 M	12:52.48
307.Megan Lupo	New Hope,PA	46 F	12:53.29
308.Julie Alber	Philadelphia,PA	30 F	12:58.37
309.Jeffrey Hammond	Philadelphia,PA	41 M	13:01.18
310.Martha Samulewicz-do	Havertown,PA	41 F	13:01.51
311.Shun Klinger	Philadelphia,PA	22 M	13:04.04
312.Kelee Whalon	Lansdale,PA	49 F	13:04.63
313.Jonathan Smith	Philadelphia,PA	27 M	13:05.20
314.Timothy Weaver	New Hope,PA	49 M	13:05.53
315.Brett Darchuk	Plymouth Meetin,PA	33 M	13:05.79
316.Samantha Brown	Schwenksville,PA	19 F	13:06.53

317.Becky Perkins	Mount Laurel,NJ	33 F	13:10.52
318.Noelle Samulewicz	Havertown,PA	36 F	13:11.24
319.Michael O'rourke	Philadelphia,PA	30 M	13:11.25
320.Jackie Weaver	Lancaster,PA	45 F	13:11.38
321.Dan Carr Sr.	Telford,PA	60 M	13:13.02
322.Trish Maxson	Doylestown,PA	52 F	13:15.37
323.Joe Dunn	Haddonfield,NJ	25 M	13:16.05
324.Mark Pomager	Plymouth Mtng,PA	35 M	13:16.37
325.Jennifer Brandt	Philadelphia,PA	36 F	13:17.84
326.Kevin Hoarn	Ewing,NJ	34 M	13:17.98
327.Kevin Rooney	Horsham,PA	26 M	13:18.46
328.Tom Henry	King Of Prussia,PA	26 M	13:19.28
329.Johnathan Kennedy	Jeffersonville,PA	18 M	13:19.96
330.Elaine Dorley	Collegeville,PA	43 F	13:20.10
331.Vince Mulray	Philadelphia,PA	50 M	13:21.46
332.Joan Ellis	Collegeville,PA	44 F	13:21.70
333.Matt Stahley	Schnecksville,PA	36 M	13:22.79
334.Mark Mohlin	Pennsauken,NJ	32 M	13:23.22
335.Krystin Hale	Souderton,PA	21 F	13:23.66
336.Hank Rutkowski	Trenton,NJ	33 M	13:24.24
337.Jennifer Zullo	Maple Shade,NJ	27 F	13:25.38
338.Ruth Dulaney	Allentown,PA	39 F	13:27.97
339.Steve Brown	Kennett Square,PA	50 M	13:28.93
340.John Princiotta	Cherry Hill,NJ	23 M	13:29.61
341.Kelly Young	Drexel Hill,PA	26 F	13:29.64
342.Nicholas Muscente	Titusville,NJ	42 M	13:30.82
343.Joseph Jedwabny	Sewell,NJ	24 M	13:31.02
344.Kara Stahley	Schnecksville,PA	37 F	13:31.04
345.Verna Defonseka	Ocean,NJ	39 F	13:31.62
346.Phi Dang	Philadelphia,PA	27 M	13:31.64

347.Brittany Farnsworth	Chester Springs,PA	26 F	13:31.92
348.Cherisse Sammartino	Pennsville,NJ	22 F	13:33.57
349.Douglas Bozarth	Westville,NJ	38 M	13:34.51
350.Tony Cifelli	Trenton,NJ	46 M	13:36.02
351.Maryann Pease	Drexel Hill,PA	47 F	13:37.60
352.Joanne Linneman	Philadelphia,PA	56 F	13:37.64
353.Jessica Justice	Philadelphia,PA	29 F	13:39.86
354.Jaime Cheng	Philadelphia,PA	33 F	13:39.92
355.Gwenevere Johnson	Dover,DE	45 F	13:41.24
356.Not Registered	,	99 M	0:00.00
357.Tia Gray	Philadelphia,PA	50 F	13:42.47
358.Maryann Defrancesco	Ewing,NJ	47 F	13:45.31
359.Third Climber	Haddonfield,NJ	99 M	13:46.40
360.Sabra Kurth	,	49 F	13:50.11
361.Gwendolyn Stephens	Philadelphia,PA	27 F	13:52.15
362.Pat Dulaney	Allentown,PA	41 M	13:56.59
363.John Cancelliere	Philadelphia,PA	43 M	13:56.95
364.Karen Lavoie	Warrington,PA	54 F	13:57.41
365.Denise Picerno	Trenton,NJ	37 F	14:01.28
366.Ronnie Milbar	Huntingdon Vall,PA	29 F	14:03.82
367.Greg Bullough	Doylestown,PA	51 M	14:05.36
368.Glenn Large	Downingtown,PA	36 M	14:05.72
369.Brian Pease	Philadelphia,PA	38 M	14:06.96
370.Michael Fanning	Philadelphia,PA	34 M	14:08.21
371.Sam Trotman	Haddonfield,NJ	51 M	14:11.30
372.Suzanne Cartlidge	Woodstown,NJ	46 F	14:11.71
373.Henry Ford Iv	Delran,NJ	16 M	14:11.82
374.Greta Roser	East Berlin,PA	30 F	14:12.58
375.Jason Thompson	Springfield,PA	37 M	14:13.03
376.Nancy Cop	Medford,NJ	51 F	14:14.68
377.Ron Clearfield	Richboro,PA	53 M	14:15.59

378.Ryan Gallatig	Philadelphia,PA	32 M	14:18.64
379.Randi Plevy	Pennington,NJ	46 F	14:20.91
380.Jim Gallelli	Philadelphia,PA	47	M 14:21.93
381.Tom Little	Turnersville,NJ	28 M	14:22.19
382.Ryan Albertson	Holland,PA	32 M	14:24.28
383.Robyn Cartlidge	Woodstown,NJ	23 F	14:24.79
384.George Royers	Merchantville,NJ	22 M	14:25.59
385.Tom Hasson	Phila,PA	58 M	14:27.02
386.Megan Plummer	Ewing,NJ	40 F	14:28.45
387.Francis Costello	Philadelphia,PA	24 M	14:29.18
388.Michelle Rose	Philadelphia,PA	43 F	14:30.10
389.Tara Linney	Philadelphia,PA	27 F	14:30.93
390.Greg Hammond	Baltimore,MD	40 M	14:31.46
391.Jeffrey Seamans	Eagleville,PA	25M	14:31.60
392.Amanda Loomis	Somerdale,NJ	25 F	14:34.61
393.Theodore Paulakis	Conshohocken,PA	29 M	14:34.77
394.Azeez Scott	Cheltenham,PA	12 M	14:34.95
395.Kelly Barlow	Palmyra,NJ	38 F	14:35.92
396.Michael Lobecker	Fallsington,PA	32 M	14:36.59
397.John Clark	Pennsauken,NJ	29 M	14:37.08
398.Sean Conklin	Ewing,NJ	42 M	14:38.29
399.Benjamin Jakus	Philadelphia,PA	27 M	14:39.18
400.Jason Burton	Jeffersonville,PA	39 M	14:39.63
401.Robert Cole	Rancocas,NJ	23 M	14:40.40
402.David Koehler	Yardley,PA	43 M	14:41.04
403.Daniel Brofft	Cherry Hill,NJ	41 M	14:42.22
404.Alvin Munson	Philadelphia,PA	53 M	14:42.74
405.Michelle Long	Philadelphia,PA	27 F	14:42.83
406.Tracie Comuso	Philadelphia,PA	28 F	14:43.65
407.Ryan Barlow	Philadelphia,PA	27 M	14:43.82
408.Abe Awad	Philadelphia,PA	30 M	14:45.69

409.Jason Smith	Philadelphia,PA	26 M	14:46.05
410.Wanda Jenkins	Philadelphia,PA	40 F	14:47.97
411.Philip Gutis	New Hope,PA	49 M	14:48.62
412.Eric Burke	Philadelphia,PA	26 M	14:48.71
413.Not Registered	,	99 M	0:00.00
414.Hilda Bradshaw	Philadelphia,PA	33 F	14:49.92
415.Kevin Guirate	Jeffersonville,PA	33 M	14:50.79
416.Sharon Adelstein	Blue Bell,PA	40 F	14:51.27
417.Theresa Thoma	Holland,PA	34 F	14:51.44
418.Maura Koehler	Yardley,PA	43 F	14:51.85
419.Katie Hammer	,PA	29 F	14:52.26
420.Bill Stockage	Phila,PA	42 M	14:53.02
421.Kayla Le	Philadelphia,PA	23 F	14:53.57
422.Eida Green	Lansdale,PA	33 F	14:59.49
423.Kris Greaves	Philadelphia,PA	31 M	15:00.20
424.Beth Clearfield	Richboro,PA	45 F	15:00.55
425.Katherine Bloost	Philadelphia,PA	34 F	15:02.15
426.Krystina Faillace	Philadelphia,PA	26 F	15:03.22
427.Lisa Gechman	Philadelphia,PA	33 F	15:05.07
428.Jan Terry	Thorndale,PA	39 F	15:08.38
429.Beverly Prisco	Morton,PA	52 F	15:10.22
430.Maria Schaller	Philadelphia,PA	64 F	15:10.54
431.Amanda Bukata	Conshohocken,PA	29 F	15:13.39
432.Katie Kelly	Jeffersonville,PA	17 F	15:14.86
433.Joe Gerace	Cherry Hill,NJ	40 M	15:14.99
434.Michael Voegele	Philadelphia,PA	34 M	15:15.46
435.Yalanda Jenkins	Philadelphia,PA	40 F	15:15.65
436.Jamie Carey	Trevose,PA	27 F	15:16.27
437.John Lyons	Aldan,PA	58 M	15:16.44
438.Laura Nagle	Philadelphia,PA	32 F	15:17.87
439.Bryan Ames	Rancocas,NJ	24 M	15:17.98

440.Amy Myers	Marlton,NJ	33 F	15:18.29
441.Cathy Picerno	Ewing,NJ	43 F	15:20.14
442.Janette Repsch	Philadelphia,PA	27 F	15:23.05
443.Brian Mcdade	Bloomfield,NJ	32 M	15:26.22
444.David Mills	Philadelphia,PA	25 M	15:26.38
445.Nicholas Scardino	Audubon,NJ	42 M	15:29.99
446.Kerry Wheeler	Philadelphia,PA	26 F	15:30.01
447.Joe Royle	Levittown,PA	31 M	15:30.18
448.Thomas Milewski	West Collingswo,NJ	34 M	15:30.92
449.Peter Giuliano	Bellmawr,NJ	39 M	15:31.73
450.Mary Gonzalez	Philadelphia,PA	43 F	15:32.98
451.Samantha Clearfield	Richboro,PA	19 F	15:33.86
452.Jamie Galasso	Philadelphia,PA	27 F	15:34.78
453.James Aleski	South Amboy,NJ	36 M	15:35.15
454.David Gechman	Philadelphia,PA	35 M	15:36.80
455.Lindsay Guge	Philadelphia,PA	24 F	15:37.37
456.Brian Poliafico	Haddonfield,NJ	36 M	15:38.34
457.Rosa Rodriguez	Philadelphia,PA	45 F	15:41.90
458.Ryan Daughton	North Brunswick,NJ	27 M	15:45.29
459.Timothy Moore	Lansdowne,PA	24 M	15:45.86
460.Gigi Boudwin	Palmyra,NJ	43 F	15:47.72
461.Ramesh Vaidya	Chester Springs,PA	51 M	15:50.51
462.John O'neill	Philadelphia,PA	47 M	15:51.04
463.Jorge Santana	Philadelphia,PA	32 M	15:51.58
464.Corinne Hefter	Southampton,PA	30 F	15:56.28
465.Leighkaren Labay	Feasterville,PA	42 F	16:04.37
466.Adam Phillips	Philadelphia,PA	24 M	16:06.26
467.Danielle Lathrop	Secane,PA	31 F	16:07.13
468.Michael Miller	Haddonfield,NJ	39 M	16:08.81
469.Craig Messick	Aston,PA	35 M	16:09.19
470.Justin Squibb	Pennsauken,NJ	27 M	16:09.26
471.Beverly Carter	Philadelphia,PA	29 F	16:10.07

472.Stephen Kinky	Maple Shade,NJ	24 M	16:10.14
473.Katelyn Thompson	Millville,NJ	14 F	16:11.24
474.Curtis Patrick	Temple,PA	34 M	16:16.32
475.Stacey Crannage	West Trenton,NJ	28 F	16:17.01
476.George Kronbar	Philadelphia,PA	28 M	16:17.58
477.Butch Brees	Haddonfield,NJ	66 M	16:18.87
478.Terrence Delahanty	Ewing,NJ	33 M	16:20.28
479.Cristina Mcdonald	Langhorne,PA	48 F	16:23.63
480.Tom Mcgovern	Toms River,N	J30 M	16:24.08
481.Paul Hartstein	Audubon,NJ	26 M	16:25.90
482.Zachary Houck	Oaklyn,NJ	25 M	16:26.74
483.Isabel Gourley	Wayne,PA	13 F	16:30.56
484.Jennifer Ryan	Morrisville,PA	27 F	16:32.02
485.Matt Baron	Philadelphia,PA	38 M	16:37.37
486.Marie Schueren	Upper Chicheste,PA	46 F	16:39.88
487.John Schueren	Upper Chicheste,PA	44 M	16:40.00
488.Angela Gilmore	Pennsburg,PA	31 F	16:40.65
489.Norman Schmidt	Philadelphia,PA	56 M	16:41.96
490.Alicia Carroll	Pennington,NJ	24 F	16:45.66
491.Nancy Zuk	Philadelphia,PA	51 F	16:45.83
492.Dana Green	Ambler,PA	30 F	16:46.04
493.Caryn Gourley	Wayne,PA	48 F	16:47.28
494.James Smith	Ambler,PA	54 M	16:48.59
495.Marty Marcussen	West Deptford,NJ	37 M	16:50.35
496.Ivene Echels	Philadelphia,PA	32 F	16:52.26
497.Christopher Kolbe	Cherry Hill,NJ	19 M	16:52.74
498.Alain Joinville	Philadelphia,PA	33 M	16:53.43
499.Olivia Myers	Philadelphia,PA	31 F	16:57.86
500.Christina Moore	Yardley,PA	23 F	16:58.03
501.Amanee Scott-stephan	Philadelphia,PA	33 F	17:00.38
502.Ronald Murr	Springfield,PA	46 M	17:03.38
503.Jose Rivera	Pennsauken,NJ	36 M	17:07.06

504.Kevin Ferko	Warminster,PA	33 M	17:07.30
505.Kenneth Zborowski	Philadelphia,PA	46 M	17:08.77
506.Climber Fourth	,	99 M	17:11.75
507.Patrick Giordano	Haddon Heights,NJ	54 M	17:15.67
508.Donald Carmody	Haddonfield,NJ	22 M	17:21.63
509.Joanna Elkes	Philadelphia,PA	22 F	17:22.43
510.Sean Ward	Haddon Heights,NJ	32 M	17:23.46
511.Cheryl Serdaru	Newtown,PA	52 F	17:30.35
512.Jennifer Bigwood	Berlin,NJ	31 F	17:32.11
513.John Schmidt	Haddon Heights,NJ	20 M	17:36.94
514.Jason Witkowski	Moorestown,NJ	16 M	17:39.74
515.Sharyn Diggs	West Deptford,NJ	34 F	17:41.01
516.Sarah Finnegan	Plymouth Meetin,PA	32 F	17:41.82
517.Philip Cook	Voorhees,NJ	30 M	17:41.97
518.Vanessa Veasley	Ardmore,PA	30 F	17:42.48
519.Jason Kolbe	Cherry Hill,NJ	21 M	17:45.48
520.Andrew Stowell	Mount Laurel,NJ	22 M	17:52.55
521.Reed Costello	Audubon,NJ	40 M	17:52.82
522.Rex Rostrom	Sewell,NJ	38 M	17:55.50
523.Paul Toroni	Philadelphia,PA	26 M	17:58.73
524.Laurenn Strabone	Philadelphia,PA	42 F	18:00.47
525.Kendra Johnson	Oley,PA	22 F	18:00.90
526.Kelly Witt	Milltown,NJ	32 F	18:06.53
527.Tara Rhoads	Bala Cynwyd,PA	24 F	18:08.12
528.John Lysaght	West Deptford,NJ	52 M	18:10.54
529.Deb Stratton	Lititz,PA	56 F	18:12.56
530.Kristen Meitzler	Royersford,PA	35 F	18:16.15
531.Brian Coughlin	Philadelphia,PA	39 M	18:16.43
532.Sara Eyster Pa	Furnace,PA	46 F	18:21.06
533.Rasheed Bellamy	Clementon,NJ	30 M	18:22.84
534.Brian Ball	Westmont,NJ	36 M	18:25.93
535.Meredith Crowley	West Chester,PA	38 F	18:27.51

536.Tina DeanWest	Chester,PA	33 F	18:28.18
537.John Smaldore	Haddon Heights,NJ	44 M	18:28.99
538.Gilberto Ramirez	Yardley,PA	37 M	18:30.25
539.Julio Adorno	Philadelphia,PA	30 M	18:31.56
540.John Bergstrasser	Jeffersonville,PA	53 M	18:34.74
541.Joshua Bennett	Haddon Township,NJ	18 M	18:46.93
542.Michele Hayes	West Chester,PA	36 F	18:51.36
543.Jerry Kershaw	Philadelphia,PA	45 M	18:55.71
544.Melinda Houvig	Wayne,PA	33 F	18:59.64
545.Crissta Worman	Reading,PA	39 F	19:02.49
546.Elisa Palmarini	Palmyra,NJ	27 F	19:03.60
547.Rochelle Smith	Philadelphia,PA	47 F	19:15.35
548.Anthony Creamer	Philadelphia,PA	55 M	19:22.38
549.Katelynn Hodgens	Newtown,PA	26 F	19:25.47
550.Ronald Smith	Marlton,NJ	59 M	19:30.79
551.Chip Pildis	Laurel Springs,NJ	46 M	19:35.24
552.Lyndsey Mccusker	West Berlin,NJ	28 F	19:37.10
553.Harry Scharle	Haddon Heights,NJ	48 M	19:37.82
554.James Dunham	Hawthorne,NJ	35 M	19:50.3
555.Swathi Sambhani	Wayne,PA	35 F	19:50.32
556.Katelyn Smith	Philadelphia,PA	24 F	19:51.59
557.Carolyn Philhower	Morrisville,PA	35 F	19:53.41
558.Sharon Bruckart	Reading,PA	46 F	19:54.89
559.Jennifer Dunham	Hawthorne,NJ	33 F	20:02.23
560.Donna Orsatti	Sinking Spring,PA	39 F	20:03.86
561.Mya Mcconnell	Baltimore,MD	29 F	20:07.64
562.Chris Labb	Philadelphia,PA	36 M	20:14.51
563.Kelli Schulthess	Bernville,PA	43 F	20:16.91
564.Cheryl Echols	Bryn Athyn,PA	51 F	20:17.97
565.Emily Baron	Philadelphia,PA	48 F	20:27.25
566.Ashley Osgood	Gilbert,AZ	13 F	20:28.17
567.Danielle Treloar	Jeffersonville,PA	30 F	20:30.17

568.Lynn Ewell	Lafayette Hill,PA	38 F	20:34.22
569.Danielle Roberts	Lawrenceville,NJ	30 F	20:35.98
570.Tabitha Patrick	Temple,PA	30 F	20:36.11
571.Jennifer Royle	Levittown,PA	31 F	20:36.83
572.Kristian Hamilton	Philadelphia,PA	22 M	20:37.46
573.Gary Cop	Medford,NJ	57 M	20:43.82
574.Melissa Lebowitz	Deptford,NJ	40 F	20:45.32
575.Cathy Williams	Warminster,PA	55 F	20:56.19
576.Jesse Blake	Philadelphia,PA	24 M	21:04.31
577.Ann Marie Frankel	Bala Cynwyd,PA	42 F	21:11.72
578.Lisa Hasson	Philadelphia,PA	28 F	21:11.96
579.Lanette Waddell	Philadelphia,PA	46 F	21:13.97
580.Jennifer Snow	Delran,NJ	23 F	21:17.67
581.Mike Bortnowski	Cherry Hill,NJ	22 M	21:23.86
582.Melissa Elmore	Philadelphia,PA	28 F	21:28.98
583.Rita Rambo	Plymouth Meetin,PA	28 F	21:34.72
584.Samantha Iraca	Lambertville,NJ	39 F	21:45.49
585.Rebecca Gallant	Maple Shade,NJ	30 F	22:19.46
586.Heather Selzer	Annandale,VA	33 F	22:30.04
587.Eileen Moulin	Newtown,PA	42 F	22:37.65
588.Karen Hayman	Churchville,PA	47 F	22:41.82
589.**Nora McCloskey**	Bristol,PA	25 F	22:44.55
590.Randy Waddell	Philadelphia,PA	44 M	22:47.54
591.Nancy Debasio	Norristown,PA	50 F	22:48.73
592.**Danielle Turner**	Riverside,NJ	22 F	22:50.88
593.Randolph Waddell	Philadelphia,PA	15 M	23:00.14
594.Brittany Williams	Bala Cynwyd,PA	25 F	23:17.24
595.William Daywalt	King Of Prussia,PA	42 M	23:24.49
596.Nicole Dubrow	Voorhees,NJ	40 F	23:38.41
597.Rudy Thomas	Moorestown,NJ	46 M	24:03.67
598.Catherine Carroll	Philadelphia,PA	51 F	24:07.66
599.Karl Bispels	Philadelphia,PA	37 M	24:11.49

600.Jennifer Truex	Philadelphia,PA	36 F	24:12.94
601.Holly Lockwood	Marlton,NJ	53 F	24:14.92
602.Alfred Ditore	Cherry Hill,NJ	51 M	24:25.70
603.Philip Drangula	Roebling,NJ	31 M	24:27.85
604.Jeanine Wilson	Philadelphia,PA	45 F	24:45.51
605.Maria Accardi	Somerdale,NJ	63 F	25:11.92
606.Phillip Stowell	Mount Laurel,NJ	65 M	25:19.49
607.Margaret Patton	Collingswood,NJ	45 F	25:24.08
608.Brian Appleman	Cherry Hill,NJ	49 M	25:26.55
609.Melannie Diaz	Pennsauken,NJ	35 F	25:53.81
610.Kevin Quinn	Chesterfield,NJ	39 M	25:54.49
611.Phyllis Hilly	Philadelphia,PA	61 F	26:06.95
612.Scott Morse	Oaklyn,NJ	32 M	26:11.65
613.Jeff Riley	Haddon Township,NJ	30 M	26:13.80
614.Elizabeth Mullin	Philadelphia,PA	23 F	26:34.78
615.Suyen Lee	King Of Prussia,PA	38 F	26:53.50
616.Janice Little	Philadelphia,PA	54 F	27:05.93
617.Timothy Mcgeady	Cherry Hill,NJ	38 M	27:44.10
618.Andres Torres	Philadelphia,PA	33 M	28:27.47
619.Judy Cheng	Pemberton,NJ	73 F	28:41.67
620.Renee Sylvester	New Castle,DE	49 F 2	9:21.62
621.Jennifer Suker	Perkasie,PA	41 F	29:24.45
622.Jeanine Radziszewski	Philadelphia,PA	36 F	29:31.50
623.Lisa Belfield	Aldan,PA	41 F	29:33.49
624.Bernadette Jervis	Atco,NJ	43 F	31:34.14
625.Erik Jervis	Audubon,NJ	19 M	32:14.95
626.Tiffanie Mcfadden	Pine Hill,NJ	35 F	32:36.53
627.Amy Robinson	Phila,PA	34 F	32:41.08
628.Kathryn Omalley	Philadelphia,PA	52 F	32:55.70
629.Jason Miles	Sicklerville,NJ	33 M	33:18.65
630.Angelina Robinson	Philadelphia,PA	43 F	34:03.60
631.Keara Kilpatrick	Ewing,NJ	36 F	35:59.84

632.Zaimarie Leriche	Philadelphia,PA	32	F	36:42.89
633.Christa Levengood	Kutztown,PA	36	F	42:41.16
634.Leigh Pires	Brooklyn,NY	33	F	44:09.85
635.Alyson Witkowski	Voorhees,NJ	31	F	44:21.56
636.Dayna Thompson	Millville,NJ	34	F	45:10.65
637.Sandy Gallagher	Williamstown,NJ	35	F	45:36.37
638.Victoria Mckoy	Dover,DE	64	F	46:48.19

Many thanks to the 71 teams who participated and raised money!

1406 FINANCIAL	5 members
A STAPLES SOUL	6 members
ACH DIVISION 61	2 members
AZEEZ'S CLIMBERS	5 members
BCFD	1 member
BEACH BUMS	8 members
BELL	2 members
BLANK STAIRS	8 members
BLOOMFIELD FIRE DEPARTMENT	1 member
BREATH FOR BECKY	8 members
BRIANA & THE BOYS	9 members
BURT'S BUDDIES	6 members
CHA BLUE DEVILS	5 members
CHERRY HILL FIRE DEPARTMENT	17 members
CINNAMINSON FIRE DEPARTMENT	4 members
CINTAS STEPPING MANIACS	12 members
CLIMB FOR A CURE	10 members
CROSSFIT PRIME	15 members
CROSSFIT LOVE	9 members
DAYNE'S GANG	9 members
EAST FRANKLIN	2 member
EXCELLENCE TO THE TOP	8 members
FAST & FIERCE	6 members
FEEL THE BURN	12 members
FITNESS WORKS PHILADELPHIA	7 members

434

GIT R DONE	3 members
GRANNIE ANNIE'S GIRLIES	4 members
HADDON HEIGHTS FIRE DEPARTMENT	6 members
HADDONFIELD FIRE	12 members
HEAVY BREATHERS	3 members
HIGH STEPPERS	2 members
INGENIX	8 members
JEFFERSON FIRE	7 members
JUST BREATHE	3 members
KING OF PRUSSIA FIRE	7 members
LOOKING UP	3 members
MAMA CASS'S CLIMBERS	2 members
MARCH FOR MARY ELLEN	11 members
MISSION OPS	5 members
MISSION STAIRPOSSIBLE	6 members
MOORESTOWN FIRE DEPARTMENT	6 members
NAT'S GIRLS	4 members
NOVACARE REHABILITATION	8 members
OAKLYN FIRE DEPARTMENT	1 member
PENNSAUKEN FIRE DEPARTMENT	6 members
PHILLY FIRE	38 members
PHILADELPHIA POLICE	14 members
RISING UP FOR THE CAUSE-FORTALEZA-TEA	4 members
RV 2011 TOUR	4 members
SERENITY STEPERS	4 members
SKY'S THE LIMIT	1 member
SOCIAL CLIMBERS	8 members
STAIR CHALLENGERS	3 members
STAIRMASTERS	3 members
STEADY AS A ROCK	6 members
STEP IT UP!	3 members
STEP UP FOR FRANK	34 members
SUNGARD	3 members

TEAM A&W	2 members
TEAM BABC CLIMBERS	7 members
TEAM FEZ	3 members
TEAM SMILEY	7 members
TEAM STAB	18 members
TEMPLE MED	6 members
THE FIGHTING IRISH	4 members
THE SWEATBANDS	4 members
UPENN NROTC MARINE OPTIONS	5 members
YOUR PART-TIME CONTROLLER	3 members
WE B CLIMB'N	3 members
WESTMONT FIRE COMPANY	2 members
WILLINGBORO FIRE DEPARTMENT	1 member

Philadelphia America Lung Association Fight For Air 2012

First Responder Team Results

PLACE (#) TEAM				TOTAL
1 PHILLY FIRE TEAM 2				**0:33:17**
9.Christopher Fath	Philadelphia,PA	33 M	7:41.00	
18.Justin Duff	Philadelphia,PA	31 M	8:01.00	
21.Michael O'rourke	Philadelphia,PA	30 M	8:05.00	
88.Climber Fourth		99 M	9:29.00	
2 PHILLY FIRE TEAM 1				**0:34:14**
12.Benjamin Jakus	Philadelphia,PA	27 M	7:54.00	
28.Eric Burke	Philadelphia,PA	26 M	8:18.00	
49.Ryan Gallatig	Philadelphia,PA	32 M	8:50.00	
67.Francis Costello	Philadelphia,PA	24 M	9:11.00	
3 PHILADELPHIA POLICE				**0:35:22**
27.Charles Ruchalski	Philadelphia,PA	38 M	8:18.00	
36.John Shields	Philadelphia,PA	25 M	8:36.00	
54.Dianne San Luis	Philadelphia,PA	32M	8:53.00	
91.Joseph Lynch	Philadelphia,PA	52 M	9:32.00	
4 CHERRY HILL FIRE DEPT TEAM 2				**0:38:28**
53.Climber Second		99 M	8:53.00	
58.Climber Third		99 M	9:02.00	
106.Climber First		99 M	9:45.00	
171.Climber Fourth		99 M	10:46.00	
5 PHILLY FIRE PEAK HUMAN				**0:38:44**
31.Will Climber	Philly Fire Pea	99 M	8:23.00	
43.Dick Climber	Philly Fire Pea	99 M	8:43.00	
52.Brian Climber	Philly Fire Pea	99 M	8:50.00	
300.Olivia Climber	Philly Fire Pea	99 M	12:45.00	
6 CHERRY HILL FIRE DEPT TEAM 1				**0:38:54**

60.Climber Fourth		99 M	9:05.00
72.Climber First		99 M	9:15.00
104.Climber Second		99 M	9:44.00
173.Climber Third		99 M	10:48.00

7 HADDONFIELD FIRE CO TEAM 1   **0:38:58**

33.2 Climber	Haddonfield,NJ	99 M	8:25.00
40.1 Climber	Haddonfield,NJ	99	8:40.00
153.4 Climber	Haddonfield,NJ	99 M	10:28.00
210.3 Climber	Haddonfield,NJ	99 M	11:23.00

8 BLOOMFIELD FIRE DEPT.   **0:39:36**

59.Third Climber		99 M	9:03.00
110.Fourth Climber		99 M	9:51.00
137.Second Climber		99	10:18.00
145.First Climber		99 M	10:23.00

9 UPPER MERION POLICE   **0:41:50**

13.John Wright	King Of PrussiaPA	32 M	7:54.00
116.Susan Bednar	JeffersonvillePA	33 F	9:56.00
237.Jim Godby	Gilbertsville,PA	51 M	11:39.00
273.Paul Bradbury	Blue Bell,PA	41 M	12:20.00

10   WILLINGBORO FIRE DEPT   **0:43:14**

117.Reed Costello	Audubon,NJ	40 M	9:57.00
172.Jason Carty Mount Holly,NJ		34 M	10:48.00
190.James Rydarowski	Eastampton,NJ	29 M	11:07.00
208.Brian Gardner	Lumberton,NJ	40 M	11:20.00

11   HADDONFIELD FIRE CO TEAM 2   **0:47:52**

135.1 Climber	Haddonfield	99 M	10:15.00
222.4 Climber	Haddonfield,NJ	99 M	11:29.00
274.2 Climber	Haddonfield,NJ	99 M	12:20.00
360.Third Climber	Haddonfield,NJ	99 M	13:46.00

12   SPRINGFIELD DELCO EMS   **1:01:11**

297.Caitlin Coates	Springfield,PA	24 F	12:43.00
376.Jason Thompson	Springfield,PA	37 M	14:13.00
504.Ronald Murr	Springfield,PA	46 M	17:03.00
508.Climber Fourth		99 M	17:11.00

American Lung Association Stratosphere Tower Climb
108 Floors (equivalent), 1455 Steps
February 6, 2011

Top 10 Men

Kevin Crossman	Snohomish	27 M	7:26
Javier Santiago	Mexico, D.F.	39 M	7:33
Rolf Majcen			7:36
Jesse Berg	Chicago	37 M	7:37
Matt Novakovich			8:00
Michael Schramm			8:52
Pj Glassey			8:54
Michael Karlin			9:09
John Ringenbach			9:32
Branden Collinsworth			9:33

Top 10 Women

Erica Schramm			8:58
Kourtney Dexter	Seattle	31 F	9:07
Karla Kent			11:21
Emily Bisaro			11:24
Tara Maras			11:31
Yiviani Arb			11:41
Mary Hodges			13:20
Susan Opas			18:36

3rd Sky Rise Chicago
Willis (Sears) Tower, Chicago
103 Floors, 2109 Steps
February 6, 2011

Top 10 Men

Sproule Love	New York	40 M	13:03
Jesse Berg	Chicago	37 M	13:40
Eric Leninger	Geneva	27 M	13:51
Daniel Ackermann	Hombburg	M5059	13:59
Kevin Crossman	Snohomish	27 M	14:05
Rolf Majcen	Teesdorf Austria	M4049	14:25
John Osborn	Springfield	M3039	14:26
Lawrence Pelo	Denver	M3039	14:30
Brian Crossman	Snohomish	M2029	14:36
Justin Stewart	Springfield	M2029	14:49

Top 10 Women

Cindy Harris	Indianapolis	F4049	14:57
Kristin Frey	Schaumberg	F 27	16:26
Kourtney Dexter	Seattle	F 31	17:02
Sherri Albus	Hoffman Estates	F2029	17:22
Catherine Demet	Lake Forest	F4049	18:08
Veronica Stocker	Los Angeles	F4049	18:57
Carol Sullivan	Glenview	F4049	19:04
Cathy Fritchen	Seattle	F6069	19:27
Sandra Nuez	Mexico City	F3039	19:32
Allison Harris	Northbrook	F4049	19:38

14th Hustle Up The Hancock
Hancock Tower, Chicago
94 Floors, 1632 Steps
February 27, 2011

Top 10 Men

Terry Purcell	Springfield	40 M	10:03.1
Christopher Schmidt	Chicago	36 M	10:04.9
Jesse Berg	Chicago	37 M	10:08.1
Kevin Crossman	Snohomish	27 M	10:18.7
Javier Santiago	Mexico, D.F.	39 M	10:31.5
John Osborn	Rochester	37 M	10:55.7
Eric Leninger	Geneva	27 M	11:10.1
Wesley Naviaux	Chicago	40 M	11:14.6
John Kubacki	Lemont	52 M	11:34.2
Michael Newman	Oak Park	37 M	11:51.9

Top 10 Women

Cindy Harris	Indianapolis	42 F	11:21.0
Sarah Ryerson	Batavia	33 F	12:04.5
Kristin Frey	Schaumburg	26 F	12:33.4
Catherine Demet	Lake Forest	43 F	12:39.5
Sandra NuÑEZ	Mexico City	38 F	13:15.2
Shelby Bernard	Sycamore	29 F	13:25.7
Jessica Merecki	Chicago	37 F	14:19.9
Alissa Ferry	Chicago	27 F	15:07.9
Katy Gentile	Chicago	39 F	16:34.2
Betsy Ballentine	Chicago	25 F	17:20.3

34th Empire State Building Run Up
Empire State Building, New York
86 Floors, 1576 Steps
February 1, 2011

The granddaddy of them all.

Links:

BBC Video on the Empire State Building Run Up

http://news.bbc.co.uk/2/hi/in_depth/8495030.stm

Fascinating facts about the empire state building
http://www.mastersoftrivia.com/blog/2011/05/11-
fascinating-facts-about-the-empire-state-
building/

Top 10 Men

Thomas Dold	Stuttgart, Germany	M 26	10:10
Omar Bekkali	Liège	M 32	11:25
Christian Riedl	Erlangen	M 30	11:29
Tim Van Orden	Bennington, VT	M 42	11:35
Jesse Berg	Chicago, IL	M 38	11:46
Rolf Majcen	Teesdorf	M 44	11:51
Tomas Celko	Žilina	M 26	11:55
Jacob Korsholm	Horsens	M 37	12:02
Tomasz Klisz	Bielsko-Biala	M 29	12:12
Javier Santiago	Mexico D.F.	M 39	12:13

Top 10 Women

Alice McNamara	Melbourne	F 24	13:03
Cristina Bonacina	Pontida	F 35	13:54
Cindy Harris	Indianapolis, IN	F 42	14:03
Suzy Walsham	Singapore	F 37	14:18
Amy Fredericks	Norwalk, CT	F 44	14:27
Marcy Akard	San Francisco, CA	F 33	14:33
Kristin Frey	Schaumburg, IL	F 27	14:47

Shari Klarfeld	Plainview, NY	F 30	14:50
Erika Aklufi	Los Angeles, CA	F 34	14:51
Erica Ruge	Rhinebeck, NY	F 38	14:54

14th Step Up For Kids
AON Center, Chicago
80 Floors, 1643 Steps
January 30, 2011

Top 10 Men

Jesse Berg	Chicago	37 M	9:56
Kevin Crossman	Snohomish	27 M	10:19
Rolf Majcen	Teesdorf	44 M	10:25
John Osborn	Rochester	37 M	10:32
Brian Crossman	Snohomish		10:44
Eric Leninger	Geneva	27 M	11:17
Braden Renshaw			11:25
Jacob Nye			11:26
Wesley Naviaux	Chicago	40 M	11:34
Kevin Burke			12:07

Top 10 Women

Bridget Carlson			12:40
Kristin Frey	Schaumberg	27 F	13:00
Patricia Scott			14:21
Alissa Ferry	Chicago	27 F	14:44
Susan Trick			14:47
Sophia Krause-Levy			14:50
Angela Meltzer			14:54
Allayna Gagnard			15:00
Eliza Weaver			15:01
Emily Kofman			15:09

18th Stair Climb for Los Angeles
US Bank Tower, Los Angeles
75 Floors, 1500 Steps
September 23, 2011

Top 10 Men

Jesse Berg	Chicago	37 M	9:38
Kevin Crossman	Snohomish	27 M	10:04
Wesley Reutimann			10:18
Lawrence Pelo			10:40
Alex Miller			11:16
James Fieberg			12:07
Pj Glassey			12:13
Chris Whitney			12:33
Randy Tran			13:18
Matt Mower			13:23

Top 10 Women

Erika Aklufi	Los Angeles, CA	F 34	10:35
Kourtney Dexter	Los Angeles, CA	F 31	12:25
Sandra Nunez			13:11
Lisa Zeigel			15:21
Misty Rosas			18:48
Imelda Briseno Monraz			22:08

CHAPTER THIRTEEN

International Ranking Organizations

OK. So how do you determine who is the world's best stair climber? Two International Ranking Organizations have set out to try.: TowerRunning's World Cup and the Vertical World Circuit

The World Cup of Stair Climbing

The World Cup of Stair Climbing is the older of the 2 International Organizations that rate and rank Stair Climbing events and stair climbers. It is sponsored by TowerRunning.com

Through the generosity of its two principals, Michael Reicehtzeder and Sebastian Wurster, I'm able to include here, in their own words, the history of Towerunning.com and its World Cup.

This section on the evolution of Towerrunning.com was provided by Michael Reicehtzeder.

The story of Towerrunning.com

My first encounter with organized sports was back in 1984 when in my hometown Vienna the inaugural Vienna City Marathon was held. My two brothers and me took the challenge, trained as we thought it right and finished some minutes before the 4:15 deadline.

Since then this marathon has become a family fixture and we hope to extend our finishing streak to 29 in April ! Besides marathon in these last nearly three decades I tried and enjoyed all the various facets of running, from 100m sprints within an Everybody Decathlon to 24 hour races. Always having trained according to feeling and without plan my 11 sub3 marathon finishes are the greatest success of my "running career".

The thing I loved most were mountain runs, besides the nature feeling going up fascinated me. Back in 1997 then fate struck when I competed in my first stair race.

It was in Vienna at the Donauturm at an event held yearly since 1992. Initially this Donauturm Treppenlauf for me was just a particularly challenging race.

As it was very well organized and offered many goodies I did it again and after my third participation my interest in this special kind of race awoke.

In 1999 the Internet just started to spread and I tried to find other stair races on the web.

I had a small personal homepage then and just for fun I published there a list of all the races I found. This very first compilation included just **ten** races – among them two in the US – the Empire State Building Run Up in New York and the Bop To The Top in Indianapolis !

Meanwhile I had realized that stairs are the most effective way to make altitude and reaching for the top is somehow a basic human desire and stair races fascinated me more and more.

2001 was the year when the domain **towerrunning.com** came alive and in the following decade the site slowly grew and grew. In this time I have met very interesting personalities, runners and race organizers, most virtual but many of them personally too.

I think that I can say that with all the collected inputs provided from many sources the site has developed into the source of information regarding the sport of Towerrunning.

Of course I still regularly compete myself and I'm most proud of finishing on 5th position in the inaugural Mount Everest Stair Marathon in Radebeul, Germany in 2005.

The last big push on the website was – together with its developer Sebastian Wurther– the introduction of the **Towerrunning World Cup** in 2009.

This worldwide ranking of stair racers motivates athletes to travel and spread the sport.

In 2011 the World Cup united 170 races in 25 countries culminating with an official final event in Bogota, Colombia !

This section was written by Sebastian Wurster.

Towerrunning World Cup 2012

For some it's pure horror, for others a special challenge: **Tower Running - the vertical trend sport**, where towers, skyscrapers and outdoor stairs are to be climbed. Worldwide, about 200 Stair Climbing events are held regularly with more than 100,000 participants in its spell. While most of the participants are amateur runners, who climb for the fitness reason - very often combined with a charity aspect, there is a growing group of elite runners. For them the race itself is becoming increasingly important - the idea of championships and titles lies in the very nature of sport. Until 2008 no official ranking for comparing the elite stairs runners existed. This circumstance has changed by the 2009 inaugural Tower Running World Cup.

The **Towerrunning World Cup** is an **international ranking system** for the Stair Climbing sport, organized by Tower Running Office Vienna - the governing World Association for the Stair Climbing sport - under the leadership of President Michael Reichetzeder (AUT) and Sports Director Sebastian Wurster (GER). The main goal of the ranking is the objective determination of the best athletes throughout the season. A mathematically balanced scoring system, the consideration of many different distances from sprint races over the classes in the International skyscrapers to the Stairs Marathons, and the differentiated evaluation of all event modes (individual time trail, mass start, tournament systems, multi climbs, etc.) provide a fair and reasonable **recognition of many facets of the Towerruning sport**. The World Cup ranking is currently the only scoring system for stair climbers, which evaluates almost all Towerrunning events worldwide and especially also considers smaller events with local participants. On the other hand a central pillar of the ranking is a selection consisting of the 18 most spectacular events - such as the prestigious Empire State Building Run Up or the races in the metropolises of the Far East in Taipei and Singapore - chosen because of world class participants fields and the internationality of the runners. These so-called **"Masters Races"** get a higher weight for the ranking.

The Towerrunning World Cup was won three times in a row by **Thomas Dold** (GER) since its introduction in 2009. As the defending champion in the women's ranking **Cristina Bonacina** (ITA) started into the 2012 season. The system also includes a World Cup Nations ranking, which was won by the German team last year. All three decisions in 2011 were tight and have fallen in the lat week of the season or at the traditional final race "Carrera Ascenso" in Bogota, Columbia. Also in 2012 a thrilling and spectacular season is guaranteed, when the battle for the coveted World Cup trophy will be opened again and tens of thousands of runners around the world will again accept the unique challenge "Towerrunning".

Towerrunning World Club - The Story behind...

Official Towerrunning events are held since 1978, when the Empire State Building run Up and the CN Tower Climb took place for the first time. However, it took more than 30 years until a World Cup ranking evaluating the performance of the athletes through the entire season was installed. Also for me as the developer of the World Cup system it was a long journey to the publication of the first rankings on February 7th 2009.

Generally I am interested in many sports (from the viewer's perspective) and also like to watch TV broadcasts of minority sports such as snooker, darts or golf. Nevertheless my access to the Towerrunning sport was completely different.

During my school time I was quite strong performing student so in the exams I usually scored very good grades without spending too much learning time. For this reason, I was often under-challenged and bored at school.

Therefore, I regularly chose the school hours for other more interesting activities. During my elementary school years one of these activities was to prepare a list of the pupils, who had arrived at the fastest in the classroom upstairs after the lunch break.

Some classmates, who took notice of the list, found the whole thing interesting, so quickly there was a small circle of pupils sprinting upstairs at the sounding of the gong after the break. I then relatively soon used the term "Treppenrennen" (=Stair race) for these small sprints and the issue of a weekly, monthly and annual ranking came on.

I tried several different scoring systems (in the beginning changing almost monthly) - sometimes there were only 3-2-1 points for the first three, sometimes up to 50 points were awarded using a complex schema and then again a system with only 10 points for a win was used.

I never achieved good grades in physical education and in general I would characterize myself as a rather weak athlete - but sometimes I also won one of our stair races and also the monthly overall ranking.

Even after moving to the High School I continued to prepare the stair running lists, but there my classmates unfortunately were hardly interested in the rankings, so I lack of competition between the 5th and 10th Class and won my more or less private overall ranking every year.

On the other hand, the disinterest of the others gave me the opportunity to try out several changes of the scoring scheme and to improve the system by introducing penalties, bonus points, and a virtual team ranking.

Then in the 10th Class at once a group; of three classmates seriously started to challenge me in the month ranking. This circumstance has motivated me so much that I not only tried to achieve as much victories and points as possible, but handed attractively designed computer printouts showing the distribution of points and the current standings to my classmates every day.

When it came to the final race of that month and four runners had a chance to win, including me, there was even a training run and a single time qualifying to determine the "starting grid" for the final. Of course the times were stopped by hand. I actually won against the other much more athletic students, not only in the qualifying, but also in the final race and thus in the overall ranking. This unfortunately discouraged the competitors so that the next month no classmate was interested in the ranking anymore.

I spent the three final school years on another High School and of course I also continued the stair running rankings there. Remarkably the interest of my new classmates was immediately aroused. This led me to a magnificent display of new ideas such as a round-robin system, a league system with relegation and promotion or a knock-out tournament with an "official" draw of the pairings. In the final year, we even combined a league system in the beginning with a knock out tournament for the final rounds. I declared the whole system then as the "ICC" ("International Classmates Championships") of Stair Climbing. Actually at the end of my school days in 2006, for me the theme "Stair Climbing" could have found an end, since I moved to the University and had to spend a lot of hours of learning for the exams.

Exactly in this year 2006 Thomas Dold (Germany) won for the first time the legendary Empire State Building Run Up, which as issued in the German media. So I first took notice of the fact that the sport "Stair Running" really exists and even International competitions are held. Fascinated by this discovery, I searched the Internet for everything I could find on staircase running sport.

Quickly I came on the Towerrunning-website of Michael Reichetzeder (then still in the old, more like a private homepage looking design). Of particular interest to me was to find an official scoring system and to answer the question who actually was the best Stair Climbing athlete in the world. I found a lot of things about this sport, but no world ranking, points system or something comparable. The surprise at this fact, my interest in statistics and the increasing media coverage of the Stair Climbing sport led me to concern myself with the development of a ranking system. From the beginning I used the working title "Towerrunning World Cup" for this project.

With all the different modes, which I trued during my school days, I was aware of a crucial difference to the "real" Stair Climbing scene: While in our classmates championships again and again the same small circle of runners competing for the points, in the Towerrunning sport the athletes rarely have the opportunity to directly race against each other. While at that time almost 100 races existed, there was hardly a runner who started more than 5 times in a season.

After some calculations and statistics during the 2007 season, finally I had found a suitable mode for the Stair Climbing elite. The races had to be divided into those with an International participants field ("Masters Races") and on the other hand the smaller, local races ("Trial Races"). This must be expressed for the ranking by using a different weighting factor. For the points breakdown I based my system on other World Cups, especially those used for winter sports (where usually points are awarded to the best 30 athletes of each event), but I did not want to easily take over any existing system. So I decided to create the 80 points system, which is still in use today.

In 2008 I then performed the ranking (only for male athletes and nations, not for female athletes) throughout the entire season as an internal test for the now well-established regulations. At this point I still had not contacted any official, runners or other representatives of the Towerunning sport to talk about the World Cup idea so it was still a "private pleasure."

When in the summer of 2008 it became apparent that the intermediate standings confirmed my subjective view of the achievements of different elite stairs runners, I contacted Thomas Dold to inform him about my new ranking system. Unfortunately, in contrast to some other suggestions regarding the "Stair Climbing-marketing" I made to him, he showed no recognizable interest in the World Cup project.

Nevertheless, I continued to calculate the rankings until the end of the season. The secret of the previously unpublished 2008 World Cup rankings will now be uncovered for the first time. After 39 considered races Thomas Dold was in the lead with 800 points, well ahead of Matthias Jahn (GER, 504 points) and Jesse Berg (USA, 440 points). Germany won the nation ranking with 1660 points ahead of the USA (1635 points) and Austria (1034 points)

Since I wanted to perform the ranking in 2009 again - but this time on a official and public basis, I sent my plans the 2008 rankings to Michael Reicehtzeder, who I could identify as the only officially recognized authority of the Stair Climbing scene, on January 18th 2009. My plans there immediately aroused interest and only 12 days later - just in time for the Empire State Building Run Up - the regulations for the inaugural World Cup season were determined. In the first ranking published on February 7th 2009 the name of the leader was Thomas Dold.

The extensive feedback of stair runners from all over the world, my increasing insight into the Towerrunning scene and numerous telephone conversations with Michale Reichetzeder helped me to refine the system, to further optimize the statistics and graphics and to realize new ideas such as the first continental Towerrunning championships (Towerrunning European Championships in Frankfurt).

This is the story of how the Towerrunning athletes got their World Cup system and I became the Sports Director of Towerruning Office Vienna, without ever having taken part in any race listed at towerrunning.com. Of course I've tried the stairwells of different skyscrapers when visiting Towerrunning events besides the official competition and was already totally out of breath after just a few floors.

So when calculating the World Cup rankings I regularly have a feeling of admiration for each of the therein listed athletes who truly have lost much sweat to accumulate the points I am comfortably awarding with just a few clicks sitting in front of my computer.

How the World Cup system influenced the Towerrunning sport

A comparison of the season 2008 (before the World Cup system has been officially introduced) and the three World Cup seasons 2009, 2010 and 2011 reveals some interesting developments.

	2008	2009	2010	2011
Towerunning Events	109	138	164	170
Races in the USA	40	69	87	92
Countries with at least one event	20	22	23	26
Considered World Cup Races	39*	115	127	134**
Races with factor 1.0 or higher	39*	30	51	59
Masters Races	4*	12	14	16
Male runners with 6 or more races	2	18	29	34
Female runners with 6 ore more races	0	3	7	9
Participating nations	22	35	45	55

* data of the unofficial World Cup test

** one additional race was considered for the 2012 ranking

Vertical World Circuit

I want to mention the Vertical World Circuit, although I haven't done a lot of research on it (I will do more for the 2013 edition of this book.)

It's a group, much like TowerRunning, that has established a ranking system for stair climbers.

The Vertical Word Circuit ranks, and counts, many of the same climbs that Towerrunning does, and like Towerrunning, has a year end ranking system.

Here are the links on the organization for you to check out for yourselves.

verticalrunning.org

skyrunning.com

For 2012, the Vertical World Circuit consists of 8 main races:

New York (Empire State Building) February 1st

Basel, Switzerland, February 20th

London, March 3rd

Taipei, Taiwan, June 5th

Berlin, Germany, June 12th

Milan, Italy, September 25th

Singapore, November 20th

San Paolo, Postponed

and 4 Trial Races

Chicago, February 27th

Austria, Vienna, October 1st

Vietnam, Ho Chi Minh City, October 30th

Bogota, Columbia December 8th

Vertical World Circuit Ranking

In a seven to nine race calendar, athletes count the four best results obtained in the main VWC races and one VWC Trial (4 + 1). In the event of a tie, the athlete with the best result in the final race will be awarded the title.

Ranking points system

Each race will assign points based on the winning men's/women's results according to the following breakdown: 100-88-78-72-68-66-64-62-60-58-56-54-52-50 down to 2 points to the 30th position for men and the same system for women down to 10th position. The ranking points in the final race will be increased by 20% for all Vertical World Circuit competitors.

(*) Ranking points valid for 2012

CHAPTER FOURTEEN

Records and Rankings

Rankings (thanks to TowerRunning) and Stair Climbing Records

2011 World Cup Leaders (TowerRunning)

Runners climb skyscrapers, towers and outdoor staircases. The main concern of the elite runners is to be faster than the others - most of us climb stairs for fitness reasons very often combined with a charity aspect and we like race atmosphere. The idea of this World Cup is to create a ranking for elite stair racers taking into account that for obvious reasons there are not many possibilities of direct competition.

2011 World Cup Top 10 Men

Name	Country	World Cup Points
Thomas Dold	GER	1000
Jesse Berg	USA	838
Tomas Celko	SVK	814
Piotr Lobodzinski	POL	804
Omar Bekkali	BEL	724
Matthias Jahn	GER	692
Fabio Ruga	ITA	680
Pavel Holek	CZE	638
Justin Stewart	USA	627
Kevin Crossman	USA	619

2011 World Cup Top 10 Women

Name	Country	World Cup Points
Cristina Bonacina	ITA	840
Cindy Harris	USA	780
Kristin Frey	USA	774
Kourtney Dexter	USA	700
Kerstin Sewczyk	GER	649
Julia Evangelist	AUT	614
Valentina Belotti	ITA	550
Melissa Moon	NZL	497
Sandra Nunez Castillo	MEX	403
Marie Fee-Breyer	GER	382

Top 50 Stair Climbers Of All Time
Men and Women

According to TowerRunning.com, these are the top 50 Stair Climbers of all time.

Based on performances in an age/gender group from year 1987 to present for the Empire State Building Run Up (NYC) and from year 2002 to present for the Willis (Sears) Tower (Sears Tower) race (ST) and from year 2003 to present for the US Bank Tower Race (LA) and from 2005 to present for the Taipei 101 race (TP). These races are chosen because they are major events and get a good International turnout.

Highest rankings go to the athletes with the most points. 3 points for first place finishes, 2 points for second place, 1 point for third place. If two or more athletes are tied, then the faster time. Overall win among male or female counts as an additional win (3 points).

Name	1st-2nd-3rd	Home	Total Points
1. Cindy Harris	32-3-0	Indiana	102 points
2. Thomas Dold	16-1-2	Germany,	62 points
3. Piero Dettin	16-3-0	Italy,	54 points
4. Chico Scimone	15-0-0	Italy,	45 points
5. Terry Purcell	13-1-1	Australia	42 points
6. Paul Crake	12-0-0	Australia	42 points
7. Syd Arak	10-4-2	Indiana	40 points
8. Andrea Mayr	9-0-0	Austria	36 points
9. Hal Carlson	8-4-3	Illinois	35 points
10. Tim Van Orden	10-1-1	Vermont	33 points
11. Jesse Berg	7-4-3	Illinois	32 points
12. Joseph Kenny	7-3-4	Indiana	31 points
13. Suzanne Walsham	7-2-0	Singapore	29 points
14. Albert Puma	6-5-1	New York	29 points
15. Mary DeNitto	8-2-0	New York	28 points
16. Stacy Creamer	8-1-1	New York	27 points
17. Salomon Salha	9-0-0	Venezuela	27 points
18. Rudolf Reitberger	6-3-1	Austria	26 points
19. Sproule Love	6-4-0	New York	26 points

20. Henry Wigglesworth	8-1-0,	Wash, DC	26 points
21. Joanne Keaton	8-1-0	Indiana	26 points
22. Marco DeGasperi	3-3-1	Italy	25 points
23. Bridget Carlson	6-3-1	Illinois	25 points
24. Kurt Konig	7-0-0	Germany	21 points
25. Bill Kanarek	5-3-0	Pennsylvania	21 points
26. Evelyn Davis	7-0-0	New Jersey	21 points
27. Beth Gray	4-2-4	Illinois	20 points
28. Bob Feuling	4-3-1	California	19 points
29. Eric Leninger	4-3-0	Illinois	18 points
30. Geoff Case	6-0-0	Australia	18 points
31. Belinda Soszyn	6-0-0	Australia	18 points
32. Fiona Bayly	3-3-2	New York	17 points
33. Veronica Stocker	3-3-2		17 points
34. Mark Trahanovsky	3-3-1	California	16 points
35. Marybeth Zajac	4-1-1	Illinois	15 points
36. Amy Fredericks	1-5-1	Connecticut	14 points
37. Ginette Bedard	4-1-0	New York	14 points
38. Gloria Schiffler	2-4-0	Illinois	14 points
39. Theresa Uhrig	4-0-1	California	13 points
40. Diana Greenwood	3-1-2		13 points
41. Melissa Moon	3-0-1	New Zealand	13 points
42. Stuart Calderwood	2-2-2	New York	13 points
43. Emmy Stocker	1-5-0	Connecticut	13 points
44. Sandra Nunez	3-1-1	Mexico	12 points
45. Carmelo Gallodoro	2-3-0	Italy	12 points
46. Inge Granzow	4-0-0	California	12 points
47. Tommy Coleman	2-2-1	California	11 points
48. Kathryn Froelich	3-1-0	Illinois	11 points
49. Kourtney Dexter	3-1-0	Washington	11 points
50. Matthias Jahn	2-1-2	Germany	10 points

Top Ranked United States Stair Climbers

According to TowerRunning.com, these are the top United States Stair climbers it currently ranks. Note the Legend:

WC 20xx 18, **WC 20xx 11** denotes the final placing in the Towerrunning **World Cup 20xx.**

For instance, WC 2012 8 indicates an 8th place finish in the 2011 World Cup Standing.

Men

Name	World Cup Year/Placement
Jesse Berg	WC 2009 8,WC 2010 4
Jon Blackburn	
Matthew Byrne	WC 2010 30
José Camacho	WC 2009 25
Hal Carlson	WC 2010 28
Kevin Crossman	WC 2010 10
Rickey Gates	WC 2009 17
P.J. Glassey.	WC 2010 31 XGym
Joseph Kenny	
Eric Leninger	WC 2009 12 WC 2010 14
Ken Myers	
John Osborn	WC 2010 21
Terry Purcell	WC 2009 11
Braden Renshaw	WC 2010 25
Zach Schade	
Christopher Schmidt	WC 2009 13
Dave Shafron	WC 2009 25
Chris Solarz	WC 2010 33
Love Sproule	
David Snyder	
Jusin Stewart	
David Tromp	WC 2009 22 WC 2010 23
Julian Torres	

| Mark Trahanovsky | WC 2009 27 WC 2010 22 West Coast Labels |
| Tim VanOrden | WC 2010 7 |

Women

Name	World Cup Year/Placement
Erika Aklufi	WC 2010 14
Marcy Akard	WC 2009 19 WC 2010 26
Fiona Bayly	
Lorie Black	WC 2009 14
Michelle Blessing	WC 2009 9 WC 2010 33
Jennifer Carder	WC 2009 6
Bridget Carlson	WC 2009 7 WC 2010 19
Stacey Creamer	WC 2010 24
Christy Crnkovic	WC 2009 29
Emily Curley	WC 2009 26
Catherine Demet	WC 2009 21 WC 2010 23
Kourtney Dexter	WC 2010 16
Kacie Fischer	WC 2010 8
Amy Fredericks	WC 2010 13
Kristin Frey	WC 2010 3
Kathryn Froehlich	
Caroline Gaynor	WC 2010 20
Melissa Gehl	WC 2010 15
Gretch Grindle Hurlbutt	WC 2010 12
Cindy Harris	WC 2009 4 WC 2010 9
Emily Kindlon	WC 2009 18
Lilian Kroner	WC 2009 24
Nancy Lamb	WC 2010 28

Stair Climb Records for Men and Women

Empire State Building Run Up, New York (1,576 Steps)

Men: Paul Crake, 9:33, 2003

Women: Andrea Mayr, 11:23, 2006

Willis (Sears Tower Climb. Chicago (2,109 Steps)

Men: Sproule Love, 13:03, 2011

Women: Cindy Harris, 14:57, 2011

US Bank Tower Los Angeles (1,500 Steps)

Men: Terry Purcell, 9:32, 2009

      Tim Van Orden, 9:32, 2009

Women: Ericka Allofi, 10:35, 2011

Taipei 101, Taiwan (2,046 Steps)

Men: Paul Crake, 10:29, 2006

Women: Andrea Mayr, 12:38, 2007

Hustle Up The Hancock, Chicago (94 Floors)

Men: Terry Purcell, 9:37, 2007

Women: Cindy Harris, 10:51, 2008

Bop To The Top, Indianapolis

Men:

Women: Cindy Harris, 4:26, 2001

CHAPTER FIFTEEN

Older Stair Climbers

A special tribute to the older Stair Climbers that I've been able to uncover. Some, like Shirley Lansing and Ginette Bedard, appear in the spotlight section.

Here's a list of the oldest finishing climbers in the 95 Stair Climbs I have covered.

I was hoping to have some interviews with these guys, but only managed one, with Shirley Lansing. Many thanks to Shirley for her contributions.

Oldest Male Finishers in 2011 (in Age order)

Michael Feely(55),11:03 CFF Boston (46 floors)

Mark Matson(55),5:59 ALA Columbus (24 floors)

Jerry Rioux(56),8:24:83 ALA Atlanta (32 floors)

David McCommon(57),12:58:63 ALA North Charleston (Stadium)

Michael Passeero(59),14:40:59 ALA Stamford (34 floors)

Dan Brown(60),2:51:00 ALA Palm Beach (29 floors)

John Garcia(60),4:29 ALA Orlando (25 floors)

Phil Hammonds(60),7:30 ALA Birmingham (Tower)

Douglas Heintz(60),22:04 CFF San Antonio (58 floors)

Herm Kreiley(60),4:02 ALA Fort Myers (30 floors)

Frank Nicolosi(60),10:52 ALA Miami (55 floors)

Ken Raggio(60),7:58 3rd Big D Climb, Dallas (52

Luis Altimiarano Shehab(60),10:34 ALA Las Vegas (108 floors)

D.E. Brower(62),7:04 CFF Oklahoma City (36 floors)

D.E. Brower(62),7:04 ALA Oklahoma City (29 floors)

David Allard(63),8:26:50 CFF Albany (42 floors)

Denis McKevitt(63),4:07:22 ALA Greenville (39 floors)

Ed Rhodes(63),21:32 ALA Little Rock (39 floors)

Stephen Cross(64),10:03:50 ALA Dallas (53 floors)

James Dohn(64),17:52 ALA Los Angeles (62 floors)

Robby Robertson(64),33:30:53 ALA Fort Worth (30 floors)

James Bromitt(65),13:10 CFF Los Angeles (51 floors)

Peter Kennedy(65),13:01 2nd Climb to the Top, Boston (61

George Sumner(65),7:51:30 ALA Salt Lake (23 floors)

Butch Brees(66),16:18:87 ALA Philadelphia (50 floors)

William Buchanan(66),17:55 ALA Wichita (34 floors)

Larry Cerny(66),11:45 ALA Milwaukee (47 floors)

Larry Sykes(66),30:43:70 ALA Jackson (Stadium)

James Elder(67),8:04 ALA Minneapolis (30 floors)

Mike Merritt(67),4:03 ALA Bennington (Tower)

Paul Lanier(67),6:11 2nd Power up the Tower, Winstom-Salem (30

William Blanchard(68),6:41 ALA Indianapolis (30 floors)

George Burnham(68),9:28 ALA Reno (36 floors)

Bill Coyne(68),9:12 ALA St. Louis (42 floors)

Forrest Cramer(68),9:30 ALA Springfield MA (24 floors)

Robert Trozzo(68),1:15:15 ALA Pittsburg (38 floors)

Jim Bryce(69),8:15:46 ALA Austin (30 floors)

George Burnham(69),15:26 CFF Seattle (56 floors)

George Burnham(69),15:29:22 ALA Phoenix (53 floors)

George Burnham(69).6;56 ALA Anchorage (35 floors)

Bill Clayter(69),12:09 1st Race to the Top, Charlotte (49

George Dorsey(69),20:45 ALA Des Moines (17 floors)

Richard Karberg(69),26:46 ALA Cleveland (42 floors)

Dale Murray(69),12:00 ALA Springfield IL (30 floors)

James Nasby(69),8:36 ALA Chicago (45 floors)

Bob McKenna(70),9:45 ALA Jacksonville (42 floors)

Frank Nicolosi(70),7:40 ALA Tampa (42 floors)

John Popp(70),13:59:70 9th Tackle The Tower, Cleveland (38

Tony Cavender(71),26:27 ALA Houston (48 floors)

John Chalupa(71),8:56 ALA Hartford (34 floors)

Carl Chase(71),6:35:94 ALA Columbia (40 floors)

David Emmanuel(71),5:51 ALA San Diego (31 floors)

Jim McIntosh(72),16:02 ALA Tulsa (50 floors)

Piero Dettin(73),18:55 34th Empire State Building Run Up (86

Hess Dyas(73),12:01, 5th Trek up the Tower Omaha (40

Ed Parker(73),13:21 CFF Milwaukee (47 floors)

Piero Dettin(74),23:16 3rd Sky Rise Chicago (103

Bill Haggerty(74),17:48 ALA Detroit (70 floors)

Robert Grouche(76),44:28:15 2nd Step-Up for the Up Center, Norfolk (100

Tom Kutrosky(76),8:19 18th Stair Climb for Los Angeles (75

Mike Mollo(76),7:22 ALA Providence (28 floors)

Kenneth Ryan(78),12:41 ALA Denver (56 floors)

John Schultz(78),16:14 CFF Philadelphia (53 floors)

Herb Rozansky(80),38:12, MS New York Climb To The Top

John Troy(80),36:28 ALA Boston (41 floors)

Tony Yacek(81),32:08 ALA San Francisco (52 floors)

Charles Coleman(82),10:47 ALA Oakbrook Terrace (31 floors)

Bob Terry(83),14:36 28th Bop To The Top, Indianapolis (36 floors)

James Devenney(86),40:14 14th Hustle UpThe Hancock, Chiago (94 floors)

Anders Jacobsen(86),14:59 ALS Seattle (51 floors)

Anders Jacobsen(86),25:25 25th Big Climb Seattle (69 floors)

Oldest Female Finishers in 2011 (in Age order)

Bridget Morin(41),20:06 ALA Detroit (70 floors)

Janet Dobson(51),25:58:65 2nd Step-Up for the Up Center, Norfolk (100 floors)

Mary Beth Forbes(53),22:38 2nd Climb to the Top, Boston (61 floors)

Amy Powell(54),13:25 CFF Boston (46 floors)

Cathy Sewell(54),17:07 ALA Birmingham (Tower)

Rhonda Rhoades(55),14:09:38 ALA Atlanta (32 floors)

Hannah Kirschenfeld(58),6:24:33 ALA Columbia (40 floors)

Gloria Blankinship(59),9:38 ALA Oklahoma City (29 floors)

Gloria Blankinship(59),9:38 CFF Oklahoma City (36 floors)

Joanne Stanley(59),14:25 1st Race to the Top, Charlotte (49 floors)

Cathy Crawford(60),5:42 ALA Ft. Myers (30 floors)

Cheri Donohoe(60),11:12 ALA Tampa (42 floors)

Charlene Heintz(60),23:09 CFF San Antonio (58 floors)

Cindy Hollo(60),16:10 ALA Cleveland (42 floors)

Susan Istre(60),15:15 3rd Big D Climb, Dallas (52 floors)

Carol Kirkland(60),5:19 ALA Orlando (25 floors)

Mirella Ruiz(60),13:32:00 ALA Miami (56 floors)

Tracy Vosburgh(60),5:38:00 ALA Palm Beach (29 floors)

Rosalind Giddens(61),15:17:15 ALA North Charleston (Stadium)

Susan Opas(61),18:36 ALA Las Vegas (108 floors)

Sandy Pearson(61),14:37 CFF Seattle (56 floors)

Ann Reding(61),10:05:90 ALA Stamford (34 floors)

Barbara Vanderhoff(61),6:31 ALA Springfield MA (24 floors)

Patti Kastle(62),15:12 ALA Tulsa (50 floors)

Sharon Roche(62),7:50 ALA Columbus (24 floors)

Nydia Caruso(63),9:51 ALA Providence (28 floors)

Carol Dvorchak(63),10:57 ALA Pittsburgh (38 floors)

Gail Jacobs(63),8:22:50 ALA Austin (30 floors)

Candie Martikainen(63),10:44 ALA Hartford (34 floors)

Suzanne Nason(63),15:41 CFF Milwaukee (47 floors)

Linda Reppucci(63),18:45 ALA Boston (41 floors)

Otilia Sanchez(63),20:14 ALA Houston (48 floors)

Devora Krischer(64),25:07:46 ALA Pheonix (53 floors)

Kandy Lee(64),7:35 ALA San Diego (31 floors)

Maria Schaller(64),17:06 CFF Philadelphia (53 floors)

Jill Sunday(64),7:21 ALA Anchorage (35 floors)

Patricia Wedgeworth(64),14:35:41 ALA Dallas (53 floors)

Loretta Durbin(65),13:37 ALA Springfield IL (30 floors)

Valerie Gardner(65),14:16 2nd Power up the Tower, Winstom-Salem (30 floors)

Jane Byrnes(66),25:14 ALA Wichita (34 floors)

Mili Ghose(66),10:09:61 ALA Ft. Worth (30 floors)

Rita Hellich(66),11:36 ALA St. Louis (42 floors)

Laura Sutherland(66),12:15 ALA Milwaukee (47 floors)

Carole Eshenbaugh(67),13:53:32 ALA Greenville (39 floors)

Ilonka Herber(67),10:36 28th Bop To The Top, Indianapolis (36 floors)

Lucinda Huggins(67),12:16:30 CFF Albany (42 floors)

Edythe Meller(67),33:03 ALA Des Moines (17 floors)

Judith Kostman(68),27:42, MS New York Climb To The Top

Barbara Burnett(68),22:42 CFF Los Angeles (61 floors)

Jane Forrest(68),4:29 ALA Bennington (Tower)

Carole Lambert(68),35:36 ALA Los Angeles (62 floors)

Martha Mayer(68),7:44 ALA Minneapolis (30 floors)

Virginia Craig(69),10:20 ALA Reno (36 floors)

Jaon Kramer(69),23:32 18th Stair Climb for Los Angeles (75 floors)

Sue Elliott(70),21:21 ALA Seattle (51 floors)

Gloria Barnes(70),24:55 ALA Jacksonville (42 floors)

Linda Clausel(70),40:01:80 ALA Jackson (Stadium)

Dioane Teece(71),10:11:60 ALA Salt Lake (23 floors)

Gail Bruffee(72),22:06 14th Hustle UpThe Hancock, Chicago (94 floors)

Judy Cheng(73),28:41:67 ALA Philadelphia (50 floors)

Judy Hess(73),17:45 5th Trek up the Tower, Omaha (40 floors)

Charlotte Prozan(74),29:21 ALA San Francisco (52 floors)

Hallie Simmins(74),23:49 ALA Little Rock (39 floors)

Jean Toth(74),9:39:10 9th Tackle The Tower, Cleveland (38 floors)

Ginette Bedard(77),22:15 34th Empire State Building Run Up (86 floors)

Cathi Watson(77),18:24 ALA Chicago (45 floors)

Joanne Keaton(78),10:46 ALA Indianapolis (30 floors)

Joanne Keaton(78),8:49 ALA Oakbrook Terrace (31 floors)

Shirley Lansing(81),36:49 25th Big Climb Seattle (69 floors)

Marilyn Olen(83),20:47 ALA Denver (56 floors)

Gloria Schiffler(83),1:00:33 3rd Sky Rise Chicago (103 floors)

Links, Blogs and Videos

Here are links to every major Stair Climber, News Story, Blog, Website or Video referenced in this book.

Cities

Bennington Battle Monument Opens After years 'iron steps'
http://www.vpr.net/news_detail/85105/after-30-years-bennington-battle-monument-opens-ir/

Bennington Monument 2010 Climb
http://youtu.be/HAwnDbdjk0w

Bennington Monument Tower Climb 2011
http://youtu.be/0a_HoBokFIg

Bisbee Arizona 1000---2008
http://youtu.be/U8yCkBOxQws

Bisbee Arizona 1000 - The Course October 17, 2008
http://youtu.be/MvA5JTAc5ew

Boston---Race up Boston Stair Climb
http://youtu.be/eftA30B0FXM

Chicago Cystic Fibrosis Foundation Climb For Life Chicago 2011
http://youtu.be/0fkXNKiyh-A

http://youtu.be/Xv26mGY2SIM

Chicago Willis (Sears) Tower Stair Climb 2009
http://youtu.be/4da5ljOlHKs

Chicago Willis (Sears) Tower Stair Climb 2011
http://youtu.be/30FYvYRoSNc

Chicago Stairs, Speed And Suffering: The Elite Runners of Willis Sears) Tower (November 17, 2010)
http://news.medill.northwestern.edu/chicago/news.aspx?id=173165&print=1

Chicago Sears Tower Climb: The Tortoise And The Stair
http://www.outsideonline.com/fitness/endurance-training/The-Tortoise-and-the-Stair.html

Culver City California Stairs 4.0
http://youtu.be/d_AyXi1ew6I

Culver City California Stairs
http://youtu.be/SLxfTgWFbVU

Culver City California Stairs
http://youtu.be/6kHEqPUhs9I

Cleveland---Tackle The Tower Practice Day
http://youtu.be/H_2Tb-R-nZA

Denver American Lung Association Climb 2011
http://denver.cbslocal.com/2011/02/27/anthem-fight-for-air-climb-raises-434000/

Denver American Lung Association Climb 2011
http://www.kdvr.com/news/kdvr-thousands-climb-denver-stairs-to-fight-lung-cancer-20110227,0,5392133.story

Denver American Lung Association Climb 2011
http://www.afhill.com/gothedistance/2011/02/fight-for-air-stair-climb-race-report/

Denver American Lung Association Climb 2011
http://youtu.be/khBZad-M9sw

Fort Myers American Lung Association Climb 2011
http://youtu.be/oiEzegXP-NY

Hollywood California Area Steps
http://franklinhills.org/stairwaywalk.pdf

Los Angeles American Lung Association (AON) Stair Climb
http://youtu.be/DOCqCB0-rkw

Los Angeles American Lung Association (AON) Stair Climb 2010 Results
http://youtu.be/oGCWP8Tsln0

Los Angeles American Lung Association (AON) Stair Climb 2011
http://youtu.be/rdm1ExurxDg

Los Angeles American Lung Association (AON) Stair Climb 2011
http://youtu.be/GmLmI3MAl9g

Los Angeles Stair Climb for Los Angeles (YMCA Climb) 2009 Pre Race Prep
http://youtu.be/5HaoJxTVJp4

Los Angeles Stair Climb for Los Angeles (YMCA Climb) 2009
http://youtu.be/mhZvwvc_PVE

Los Angeles Stair Climb for Los Angeles (YMCA Climb) 2011
http://youtu.be/bpCAh5g-bpU

Los Angeles Stair Climb for Los Angeles (YMCA Climb) 2011
http://youtu.be/rnpbWsqTl-Y

Las Vegas American Lung Association Stratosphere climb 2009
http://www.lasvegassun.com/news/2009/feb/21/climbers-scale-strat-one-step-time/

Las Vegas American Lung Association Stratosphere Climb 2011
http://youtu.be/G5497C5XeXA

London: The Rise of Vertical Rush in London (February 2010)
http://www.thisislondon.co.uk/lifestyle/article-23808444-the-rise-of-vertical-rush.do

London: Vertical Running Hits London
http://www.itnsource.com/shotlist/RTV/2010/02/09/RTV449410/?v=1&a=0

Milwaukee Stair Climb US Bank Building 2011
http://youtu.be/MFVHhyw1M-U

Fascinating facts about the empire state building
http://www.mastersoftrivia.com/blog/2011/05/11-fascinating-facts-about-the-empire-state-building/

New York Racer Wins Empire State Building Crown (1994)
http://articles.latimes.com/1994-02-18/news/mn-24469_1_empire-state-building

New York Empire State Building Run up was in 1978
http://www.youtube.com/VYrRu640k68

New York Empire State Building Run Up 2001
http://youtu.be/8dqGhln8bDQ

New York Empire State Building Run Up 2002
http://runningtimes.com/Article.aspx?ArticleID=6284

A Race To The top 2004
http://web.jrn.columbia.edu/studentwork/deadline/2004/empire-parekh.asp

New York Empire State Building Run Up 2007
http://www.speakuponline.it/articolo/the-race-to-the-top

New York Empire State Building Run Up 2009
http://youtu.be/s1ndXZtDxlU

New York Empire State Building Run Up 2010
http://www.dailymotion.com/video/xc5a12_empire-state-building-run-up-2010_news

New York Empire State Building Run Up 2011
http://www.nytimes.com/2011/01/31/sports/31staircase.html?pagewanted=all

New York Empire State Building Run Up 2011
http://www.nytimes.com/2011/01/31/sports/31staircase.html?pagewanted=all

New York Fight For Air Climb New York 2011
http://youtu.be/wItjxScsegQ

Athletes Run Up Empire State Building In Annual Race
http://news.bbc.co.uk/2/hi/8495030.stm

New York Firefighters Stair Climb at the 2011 NYC Police & Fire Games
http://youtu.be/UkMuXLLfX0o

New York Empire State Stair Race Draws Pros, Amateurs, And Seniors Up 86 Flights
http://blogs.villagevoice.com/runninscared/2010/02/empire_state_st.php

New York Reporting from the 86th Floor
http://sports.espn.go.com/espnmag/story?id=3232736

New York Empire State Building No Building Too Tall For These StairMasters
http://articles.nydailynews.com/2005-02-01/sports/18286927_1_empire-state-building-run-up-flights-stairs

Philadelphia Fight For Air Climb 2010
http://youtu.be/w1ltQama8Cs

Philadelphia Fight For Air Results 2011
http://www.compuscore.com/cs2011/march/phlstair.htm

Philadelphia Fight For Air Climb 2011
http://youtu.be/ H634MmuGmvs

Philadelphia Fight For Air Climb 2011
http://youtu.be/Kzs85tCZLM4

San Francisco Bank Of America Climb 2010
http://youtu.be/WHYNXptSoDk

Seattle Big Climb Seattle 2010
http://youtu.be/sd3ZVlIawYM

Seattle Big Climb Seattle 2010
http://youtu.be/xTG3c4ByKmE

Seattle Big Climb Seattle 2010
http://youtu.be/ttUaRpCjpMk

Seattle Columbia Tower Stairs
http://vimeo.com/9950093

Seattle Washington Mutual Results 2010
http://youtu.be/U2Kws-gQDtc

Seattle Washington Mutual Stair Climb-2011
http://youtu.be/OQbO6eNo1q4

Seattle Washington---Scott Firefighter Stair Climb 2009 - Columbia Tower - Seattle, WA
http://youtu.be/OAHLfWWmZ4o

Seattle Columbia Center Firefighter Stairclimb (1993)
http://youtu.be/iZP3ZCXZTOE

Seattle Firefighters Prepare For Big Stair Climb 2011
http://youtu.be/PnBwj-HHN_E

Seattle Firefighter Stair Climb 2011
http://youtu.be/KG-yzHBWe-g

Springfield, IL American Lung Association Stair Climb 2012
http://youtu.be/tHQbV70ZUYY

Toronto Stair Climb 2011
http://youtu.be/V8d1s7W6n_M

Vienna Austria Millennium Tower Run Up 2011
http://www.runinternational.eu/race-reports/2011/105-2011/587-2nd-millenium-tower-run-up-2011-vienna

People

Alfred---71 Yr Old Alfred Flying Up 1,237 Stairs in Thailand!
http://youtu.be/hnejXp9ie9c

Erika Aklufi
http://www.triathloninformer.com/undercovered/erika_aklufi.html

Hometown Hero Erika Aklufi
http://susancloke.blogspot.com/2010/07/hometown-hero-erika-aklufi.html

Syd Arak on the Culver City California Stairs
http://youtu.be/mMCVNvtLGBU

Getting schooled on the stairs by Jesse Berg
http://youtu.be/bz1Z1lrh4yI

Ginette Bedard Interview
http://www.maridavis.com/stories_Detail.php?id=8\

Ginette Bedard---Marathon Runner Gets Better With Age
http://articles.nydailynews.com/2008-11-01/sports/17910915_1_paula-radcliffe-year-s-marathon-paul-tergat

Hal Carlson, Fire Chief of Aurora
http://www.aurora-il.org/detail_news.php?newsDateID=519

Barefoot Ted Interviews Stair Climbing Master Kevin Crossman
http://youtu.be/NlfHvdNeFI8

Kevin Crossman's Blog:
http://www.kevinclimbs.com/blog.html

Paul Crake Excelling In His Biggest Challenge
http://www.canberratimes.com.au/news/local/news/general/crake-excelling-in-his-biggest-challenge/2371590.aspx

Paul Crake Conquered An Empire Then Was Told He'd Never Walk Again
http://www.smh.com.au/news/sport/paul-crake-conquered-an-empire-then-was-told-hed-never-walk-again/2007/01/06/1167777323353.html

Kevin Crossman's Website:
http://www.kevinclimbs.com/

Forget the elevator, Snohomish's Kevin Crossman Climbs The Stairs Of Iconic Skyscrapers For Sport
http://www.heraldnet.com/article/20110426/SPORTS/704269971

Kourtney Dexter She Came, She Conquered, She Coughed
http://www.seattlepi.com/lifestyle/health/article/1-300-stairs-She-came-she-conquered-she-coughed-1267937.php

Thomas Dold's Website
http://www.thomasdold.com/en/

Thomas Dold Wikipedia Entry
http://en.wikipedia.org/wiki/Thomas_Dold

Thomas Dold Interview
http://youtu.be/EjQ3UWmLZcY

Thomas Dold Wins The Empire State Building Run Up For A Record 6th Straight Time
http://www.huffingtonpost.com/2011/02/01/thomas-dold-wins-empires_0_n_816958.html

Thomas Dold Too Strong At Berlin Skyrun
http://www.mudsweatandtears.co.uk/2011/06/15/dold-too-strong-at-berlin-skyrun/

Thomas Dold Press Conference For Vietnam Vertical Run
http://youtu.be/5mHBaFvuzhs

Dwane Fernandes: Amputee Takes On Empire State Building
http://blacktown-advocate.whereilive.com.au/news/story/amputee-takes-on-empire-state-building/

Dwayne Fernandes Website
http://www.dwaynefernandes.com.au/

Dwayne Fernandes Press Conference For Vietnam Vertical Run
http://youtu.be/5mHBaFvuzhs

Dwayne Fernandes: Men's Health Interview
http://www.menshealth.com.sg/guy-wisdom/mh-interview-dwayne-fernandes

Trevor Folgering---Explosive Churpees to Improve Stair Climbing Performance
http://youtu.be/QMKaHaKzcwk

Trevor Folgering Blogs
http://optimumlifestylecenter.blogspot.com/
http://stairclimbcanada.blogspot.com/

Trevor Folgering Websites
http://www.trevorfolgering.com
http://www.stairclimbmeetups.com

Kristin Frey Blog
http://kristinfrey.blogspot.com/

PJ Glassey's Websites
http://www.xygm.com
http://www.fightclubseattle.com

PJ Glassey's Book, Cracking Your Calorie Code
http://www.amazon.com/exec/obidos/ASIN/1436345073/ref=nosim/p
ofessorsmileys

PJ Glassy's You Tube Channel
http://www.youtube.com/user/xgym/featured

PJ Glassey---His Stair Training Guide:
http://www.lungusa.org/pledge-events/wa/seattle-climb-
fy12/local/doc/fight-for-air-climb-training-manual.pdf

PJ Glassey's Top 7 Techniques For Stair Climbers
http://youtu.be/oay_hI-4et4

PJ Glassey and the subject of handrails…
http://xgym.com/xtras/stair_training/

PJ Glassey Seattle Personal Trainer Extraordinaire
http://www.dennis-yu.com/seattle-personal-trainer-extraordinare-pj-glassey

Stair Climbing Boot camp 101 Part 1 by PJ Glassey
http://youtu.be/XNHRZKA7Hgc

Stair Climbing Boot camp 101 Part 2 by PJ Glassey
http://youtu.be/GXaA1MhwNTk

PJ Glassey Flight Club Seattle
http://www.flightclubseattle.com

PJ Glassey Racing To The Top
http://renton.patch.com/articles/racing-to-the-top-8

Kristin Frey World Record Stair Runner Kristin Frey On 1035 KISS FM
http://youtu.be/JnW8M19Cfks

Matthias John website:
http://www.matthiasjahn.com/

94 year old Peng Hung-nian
http://www.wantchinatimes.com/news-subclass-
cnt.aspx?id=20110606000017&cid=1104

John Korff's Tips on the Empire State Building Run UP
http://www.themmrf.org/donate-now-take-action/join-an-event/endurance-events/esbru-training-page-11-2011.pdf

Shirley Lansing---Bellevue woman will be oldest female in Sunday's Big Climb http://www.bellevuereporter.com/sports/88438627.html

Shirley Lansing Shirley's Big Climb 2010
http://youtu.be/pZC8AliGx_Q

Shirley Lansing Woman, 80, Makes 69-story Climb Up Columbia Center With Others For Charity
http://seattletimes.nwsource.com/html/localnews/2011406929_lansing22m.html

Shirley Lansing---80 year old stair climber
http://youtu.be/3w-qD8fOXqU

Shirley Lansing---80-year-old woman Is Inspired To "keep marching"
http://bellevue.komonews.com/content/80-year-old-woman-inpired-keep-marching

Shirley Lansing----81 year Old Stair Climber
http://youtu.be/jnyVq5HoDBU

Dustin Maher---Stair Climbing tips by Dustin Maher
http://youtu.be/hTbpYnP83yY

Melissa Moon's Website:
http://www.melissamoon.co.nz/

Melissa Moon's Training Tips:
http://www.melissamoon.co.nz/uploads/media/Melissa_Moon__s_Training_Notes-1.pdf

Melissa Moon: The Wellington Interview
http://www.stuff.co.nz/dominion-post/news/local-papers/the-wellingtonian/3429967/The-Wellingtonian-interview-Melissa-Moon

Melissa Moon To Run Up World's Second Tallest Building
http://www.3news.co.nz/Melissa-Moon-to-run-up-worlds-second-tallest-building/tabid/317/articleID/157158/Default.aspx

Melissa Moon Wins 2010 Empire State Building Run
http://authspot.com/thoughts/nzer-melissa-moon-wins-empire-state-building-run/

Melissa Moon in Vietnam:
http://www.vietnamrun.com/training/download/MelissaMoon8WeekTraining.pdf

Melissa Moon---Kiwi Woman First Up Empire State Building
http://tvnz.co.nz/othersports-news/kiwi-woman-first-up-empire-state-building-3347640

Melissa Moon Press Conference For Vietnam Vertical Run
http://youtu.be/5mHBaFvuzhs

Apolo Ohno
http://blogs.abcnews.com/george/2011/03/taking-on-apolo-ohno-the-empire-state-building-challenge.html

Felicia Perretti Photography
http://www.perrettiphotography.com/.

Climbing To The Top With Terry Purcell
http://vimeo.com/9243397

Fabio Ruga Rules At Vertical Rush
http://www.mudsweatandtears.co.uk/2011/03/03/ruga-rules-at-vertical-rush/

Stan Schwartz Stan's Obligatory Blog
http://www.1134.org/blog

Chico Scimone---94 year old Runner Heads For The Heights
http://mg.co.za/article/2005-01-26-94yearold-runner-heads-for-the-heights

Chico Scimone---Chico And The Run: Empire State Building Hosts Annual Run Up
http://sports.espn.go.com/espn/page2/story?page=darcy/050211&num=0

Chico Scimone---Chico's Tribute Page
http://www.myspace.com/chicoscimone/blog

Jim Smiley's Blogs:
http://ifatblog.com/
http://teamsmileytraining.com

John Smiley's Websites:
http://www.johnsmiley.com
http://www.johnsmiley.com/main/stairs.htm

John Smiley's 7 Flights Up The Steps In My House
http://youtu.be/uaH77zHHul0

Sophorn Smiley: A Distance Runner From a family that's traveled far
http://www.philly.com/philly/columnists/art_carey/20111205_Well_Being__A_distance_runner_from_a_family_that_s_traveled_far.html

Sophorn Smiley's Blogs:
http://la-vida-smiley.blogspot.com/
http://teamsmileytraining.com

David Snyder's Website:
http//www.StairClimbingSport.com

David Snyder--The Zen of Stair Climbing
http://www.dhammawiki.com/index.php?title=Zen_of_stairclimbing

Chris Solarz---Meet the Hedge Fund Manager Who Holds 5 World Records, Including 1 For Beer Drinking
http://articles.businessinsider.com/2011-09-06/wall_street/30128479_1_marathons-wedding-anniversary-subway-challenge

Chris Solarz World Record Stair Climb. 33,000 Feet In 12 Hours
http://youtu.be/b-DeG_N5Twk

Chris Solarz Sets Another World Record
http://citycoach.typepad.com/weblog/2011/06/chris-solarz-sets-another-world-record.html

Chris Solazr---His Record Setting Subway Ride :)
http://youtu.be/EiLEziw8ItE

Chris Solarz---Marathoner To Attempt Stair Climbing Record
https://thephilanews.com/marathoner-to-attempt-stair-climbing-world-record-18055.htm

A Typical Weekend For Chris Solarz--2 Days, 3 Events, 2 Victories
http://citycoach.typepad.com/weblog/2010/03/chris-solarz-pictured-here-with-emily-kindlon-after-they-each-won-run-the-rock-in-2008-had-a-busy-couple-of-days-last-week.html

Justin Stewart's You Tube Channel|
http://www.youtube.com/user/JTStew8001/feed

Justin Stewart Howe Street Stairs Record
http://youtu.be/oFDV0U97dTE

Justin Stewart---Hilton Stair Workout With Justin Stewart
http://youtu.be/3Gy4OEWoI6E

Justin Stewart---Jacobs Ladder Training With Justin Stewart
http://youtu.be/lLrVSMODZOU

Justin Stewart---Stair Climbing Workout With Justin Stewart
http://youtu.be/hrOj4mA1c9s

Justin Stewart---Tabata Bike Workout With Justin Stewart
http://youtu.be/_1o9XNxi4Us

Mark Trahanovsky---He Never Takes The Elevator Up
http://www.ocregister.com/articles/trahanovsky-236309-stair-climb.html

Mark Trahanovsky---7 Climbing Tips From Mark Trahanovsky
http://pittclimb.blogspot.com/2011/02/7-climbing-tips-from-mark-trahanovsky.html

Tim Van Orden's Blog
http://www.runingraw.com/blog

Tim Van Orden's Website
http://www.runningraw.com/

Tim Van Orden's You Tube Channel
http://www.youtube.com/user/runningraw

Tim Van Orden's 2nd Run Up The Bennington Monument Stairs 2011
http://youtu.be/H3rb3WSZc2c

Tim Van Order: Vegan Athlete
http://www.organicathlete.org/vegan-athlete-tim-vanorden

Rich White Pittsburgh man sets 2012 Goal of climbing 15,000 Flights of Stairs
http://www.joplinglobe.com/local/x1750834367/Staired-Straight-Pittsburg-man-sets-2012-goal-of-climbing-15-000-flights-of-stairs

News Links

43 Flights Of Stairs Challenge
http://youtu.be/z5nsqXfX0-A

Does your city have public stairs?
http://www.publicstairs.com/

The Ecstasy Of The Agony
http://mg.co.za/article/2008-07-03-the-ecstasy-of-agony

Firefighters: A Loaded Climb (Firefighters)
http://blogdowntown.com/2010/09/5716-a-loaded-climb

Firefighter breaks Stair Climb record
http://youtu.be/SxTdyuE_7g4

Firefighters climb hotel to honor 9/11 rescuers
http://www.fox5sandiego.com/news/kswb-stair-climb-911,0,7924995.story

First Time On Jacob's Ladder
http://youtu.be/NqW0EhLjSJI

Great Workout, Forget The View
http://www.nytimes.com/2009/02/19/health/nutrition/19fitness.html

Helping A Good Cause, One Step At A Time
http://articles.chicagotribune.com/2009-01-22/news/0901200229_1_stair-climbers-aon-center-john-hancock-center

How To Take On A Tower And Win
http://www.smh.com.au/executive-style/fitness/how-to-take-on-a-tower-and-win-20110329-1cdy4.html

Is Exercise Better Than Prozac?
http://www.westseattleherald.com/2010/11/25/features/exercise-better-prozac

Jacob's Ladder Workout-First Time On the Ladder
http://youtu.be/D2Nn2fQjwZc

Jacob's Ladder Website
http://www.jacobsladderexercise.com/

No thanks, I'll take the stairs
http://www.businessweek.com/premium/content/06_11/b3975115.htm\

Olympic Speed Skaters Hop Up Stairs To Build Their Power
http://youtu.be/CSlthImZWIk

On Your Own: Fitness; You Might Climb the Walls After This Unusual Workout, New York Times 1988 article about Stair Climbing--back when it was a rather unusual activity. It references one of the

founders of the Aerobics movement in the United States, Dr. Kenneth Cooper., and his believe that Stair Climbing offered twice the payback of running.

http://www.nytimes.com/1988/07/04/sports/on-your-own-fitness-you-might-climb-the-walls-after-this-unusual-workout.html?pagewanted=all

The Only Way Is Up
http://www.guardian.co.uk/lifeandstyle/2008/jun/03/healthandwellbeing.features

Reach For The Sky---Towerrunning
http://content.yudu.com/Library/A1rpaz/RunningFreeApril2011/resources/37.htm

The Science Of Stair Climbing
http://www.docstoc.com/docs/66962119/Stair-Climbing

Smart Training for your best Stair Climb
http://stairsracer.blogspot.com/2007/03/smart-training-for-your-best-stair.html

Stair Climbers push their sports skyward
http://jscms.jrn.columbia.edu/cns/2007-02-13/cox-stairclimbers.html

Stair Climbing Video (60 minutes)
http://youtu.be/WNW5dSlQv3U

Stair Climber Workouts
http://blog.workouthealthy.com/cardio/stair-climber-workouts/

Stair Climbing Becomes Popular Urban Sport
http://youtu.be/fjlsU1ffCKo

Stairs are faster than elevators
http://sweatscience.com/tag/stair-climbing/

Staying With It
http://www.goswim.tv/entries/903/staying-with-it.html

Step By Step Stair Climbs Succeed
http://articles.orlandosentinel.com/2007-03-17/news/STAIRRACING_1_stair-climbing-races-are-run-empire-state-building

Intermittent Stair Climbing Improves Fitness
http://www.acefitness.org/healthandfitnesstips/healthandfitnesstips_display.aspx?itemid=124

Stair Climber Takes Flight With Top Tips
http://articles.chicagotribune.com/2005-02-27/features/0502270483_1_stair-climbing-anaerobic-workout

General Links:

Facebook Stair Climbing Group
http://www.facebook.com/groups/309609752400396/

Frankford Gazette
http://frankfordgazette.com

Lasting Crown
http://www.lastingcrown.com

New York Road Runners
http://web2.nyrrc.org

RunningRaw Project
http://runningraw.com/blog/?p=699

Skyrunning
http://skyrunning.com/

Skyscrapers
http://syscrapers.com

SprintStairs.com
www.sprintstairs.com

StairClimbCanada
http://www.StairClimbCanada.com

StairClimbingSport
www.stairclimbingsport.com

StairClimbingSport Events Page
http://www.stairclimbingsport.com/events-and-records/

TowerRunning.com
http://www.TowerRunning.com

TowerRuning.com Race Schedule
http://www.towerrunning.com/english/races.htm

TowerRuning.com News
http://www.towerrunning.com/news.php

Trinity Training Blog
trinitytraining.blogspot.com
trinitytraining.blogspot.com/search/label/stairs

USAStairClimbing
usastairclimbing.com

West Coast Labels
http://youtu.be/0FFb1F19Gsw

Wikipedia Stair Climbing Page

http://en.wikipedia.org/wiki/Stair_climbing

CHAPTER SEVENTEEN

City Information and References

Looking for a Stair Climb near you? This chapter should help.

Cities With 3 Or More Climbs

Boston

Boston has 3 climbs. ALA, Cystic Fibrosis, and the National Multiple Sclerosis Climb.

Chicago

Chicago has 5 climbs. ALA, Cystic Fibrosis, Sky Rise Chicago (benefitting the Rehab Institute of Chicago), the Hustle Up The Hancock (benefitting the Respiratory Health Association), and Step up for Kids (benefitting the Children's Memorial Hospital)

Dallas

Dallas has 3 climbs. ALA, Cystic Fibrosis, and the Big Bop To The Top benefitting the Leukemia Society

Los Angeles

Los Angeles has 3 climbs. ALA, Cystic Fibrosis and the Stair Climb for Los Angeles benefitting the YMCA.

New York

New York has 3 climbs. ALA, Story by Story (benefitting in Motion) and the Empire State Building Climb.

Philadelphia

Philadelphia has 3 climbs. ALA, Cystic Fibrosis, and for the first time in 2011, the Special Olympics Climb

Seattle

Seattle has 3 climbs. ALA, Cystic Fibrosis and Big Climb Seattle, benefitting the Leukemia Society.

Cities With Two climbs

Albany, NY (ALA,CFF)

Cleveland, OH (ALA and the Tackle the Tower, benefitting the Ronald McDonald House of Cleveland)

Columbus, OH (ALA,CFF)

Fort Worth, TX (ALA,CFF)

Indianapolis, IN (ALA, Bop To The Top benefitting Riley's Hospital for Children

Milwaukee, WI (ALA,CFF)

Minneapolis, MN (ALA,CFF)

Oklahoma City, OK (ALA,CFF)

Orlando, FL (ALA,CFF)

San Francisco, CA (ALA,CFF)

Cities With One Climb

Albuquerque, NM (ALA)

Anchorage, AK (ALA)

Atlanta, GA (ALA)

Austin, TX (ALA)

Bennington, VT (ALA)

Birmingham, AL (ALA)

Buffalo, NY (ALA)

Charlotte, NC (Levine Children's Hospital)

Cincinnati, OH (ALA)

Columbia, SC (ALA)

Denver, CO (ALA)

Des Moines, IA (ALA)

Detroit, MI (ALA)

Fort Meyers, FL (ALA)

Ft. Lauderdale, FL (ALA)

Greenville, SC (ALA)

Hartford, CT (ALA)

Hershey, PA (ALA)

Houston, TX (ALA)

Jackson, MS (ALA)

Jacksonville, FL (ALA)

Kansas City, MO (ALA)

Las Vegas, NV (ALA)

Little Rock, AR (ALA)

Miami, FL (ALA)

Mobile, AL (CFF)

New Haven, CT (ALA)

Norfolk, VA (Step up for the Up Center)

North Charleston, SC (ALA)

Oakbrook Terrace, IL (ALA)

Omaha, NE (Trek Up the Tower, benefitting WELCOM)

Palm Beach, FL (ALA)

Phoenix, AZ (ALA)

Pittsburgh, PA (ALA)

Providence, RI (ALA)

Raleigh, NC (CFF)

Reno, NV (ALA)

Sacramento, CA (ALA)

Salt Lake City, UT (ALA)

San Antonio, TX (CFF)

San Diego, CA (ALA)

Springfield, IL (ALA)

Springfield, MA (ALA)

St. Louis, MO (ALA)

Stamford, CT (ALA)

Tampa, FL (ALA)

Tulsa, OK (ALA)

Virginia Beach (MS)

Wichita, KS (ALA)

Willes-Barre, PA (ALA)

Winston-Salem (MS)

CHAPTER EIGHTEEN

Quiz Questions

Were you paying attention?

Quiz

Answers appear on my Web Site

http://www.johnsmiley.com/main/stairs.htm

1. Who set the record for the most stairs climbed in a 12 hour period?

2. What is the name if the author's first Stair Climb event?

3. What year was the Empire State Building's First Stair Climb held?

4. What is the tallest building in the United States?

5. What is the tallest building in the world?

6. What is the new name of Philadelphia's Bell Atlantic Tower?

7. What city holds the most organized Stair Climbs?

8. Who was Chico Scimone?

9. Who was the oldest female to complete a Stair Climb in 2011?

10. Who was the oldest male to complete a Stair Climb in 2011?

11. Who was the youngest female winner of a Stair Climb competition in the Unites States in 2011?

12. Who was the youngest male winner of a Stair Climb competition in the Unites States in 2011?

13. How many calories do you burn by climbing 10 flights of steps?

14. How many steps does it take to reach the Statue of Liberty?

15. How much money did all of the American Lung Association Stair Climbs raise in 2011?

16. At what age did Ginette Bedard, winner of 99 out of 101 New York Road Racer events she has entered, take up running?

17. Who is Jennifer Lynn Thanem?

18. What is the definitive test to diagnose osteoarthritis in the knees

19. What famous Television Doctor endorses Stair Climbing as a daily exercise?

20. What Charitable Organization has hosted Stair Climbs the longest? The American Lung Association or the Cystic Fibrosis Foundation?

CHAPTER NINETEEN

Photo Gallery

Photographs courtesy of Felicia Perretti

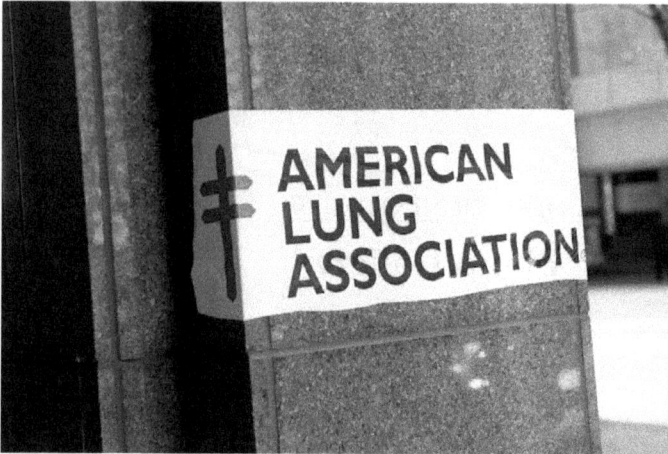

Climb Day!

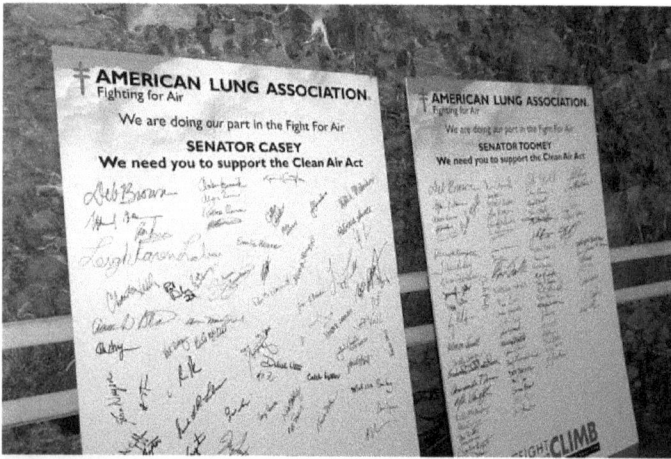

Petitions for clean air

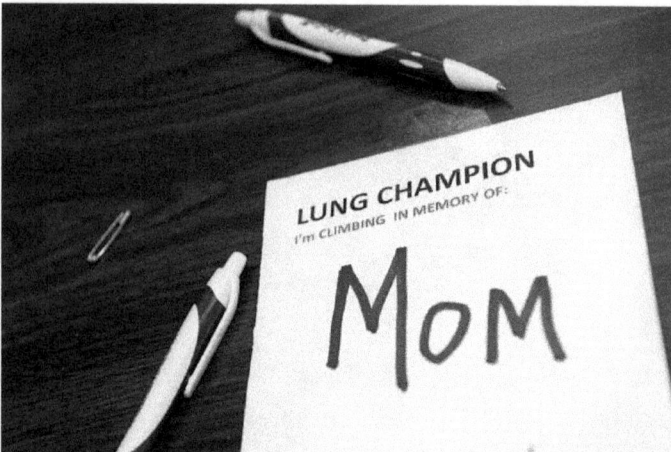

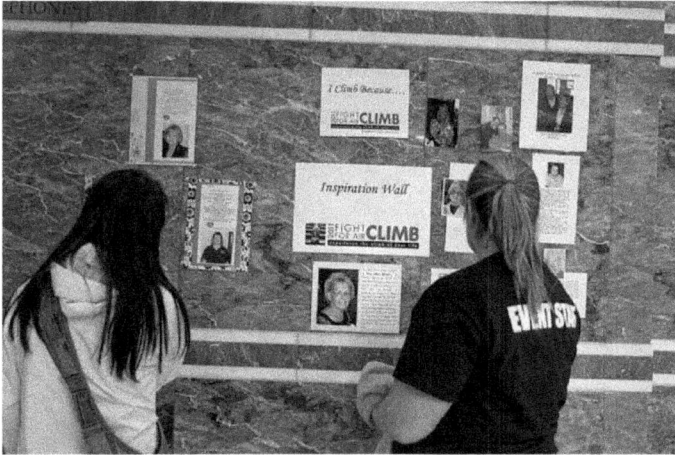

Dedications

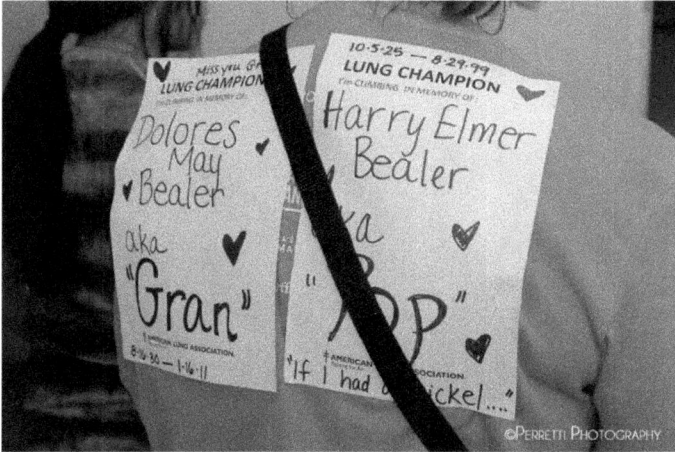

10-5-25 — 8-29-99
LUNG CHAMPION
I'm CLIMBING IN MEMORY OF
Harry Elmer
Bealer
aka
"BP"
"If I had a nickel…"

Miss you Gran
LUNG CHAMPION
CLIMBING IN MEMORY OF:
Dolores
May
Bealer
aka
"Gran"
8-16-30 - 1-16-11

©Perretti Photography

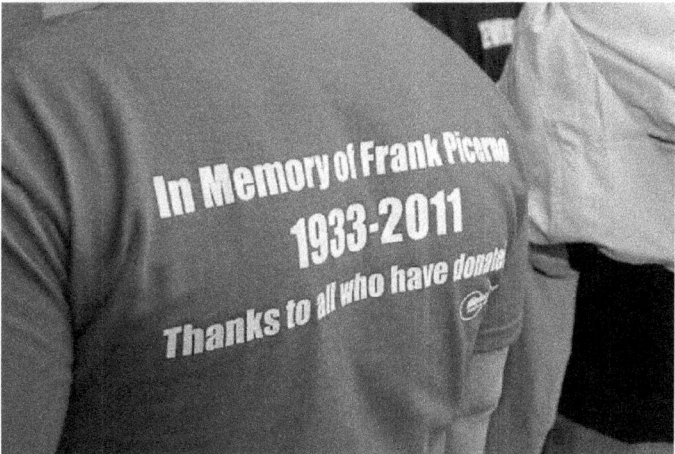

In Memory of Frank Picerno
1933-2011
Thanks to all who have donated

503

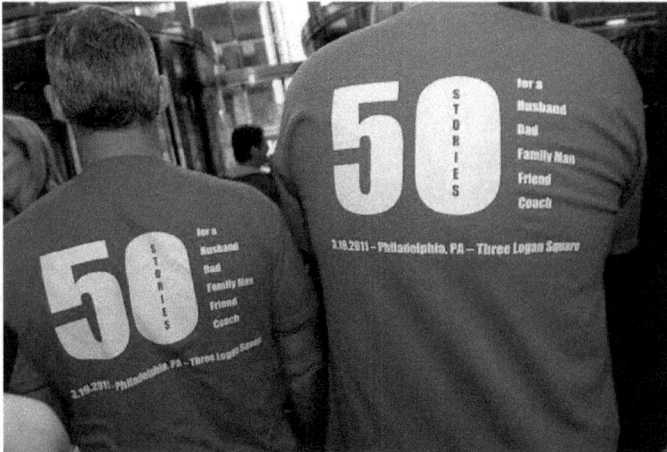

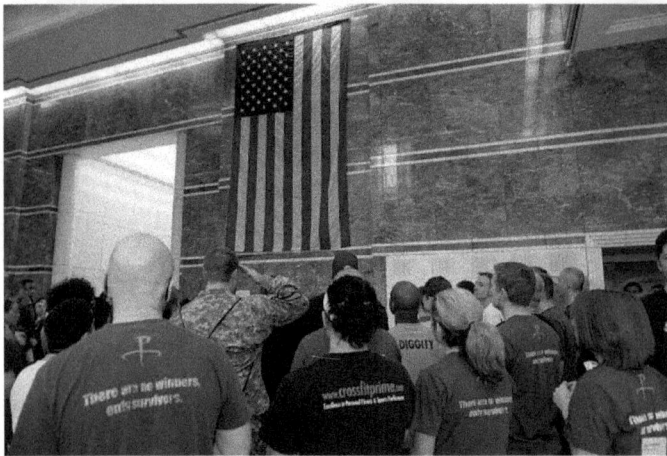

National Anthem

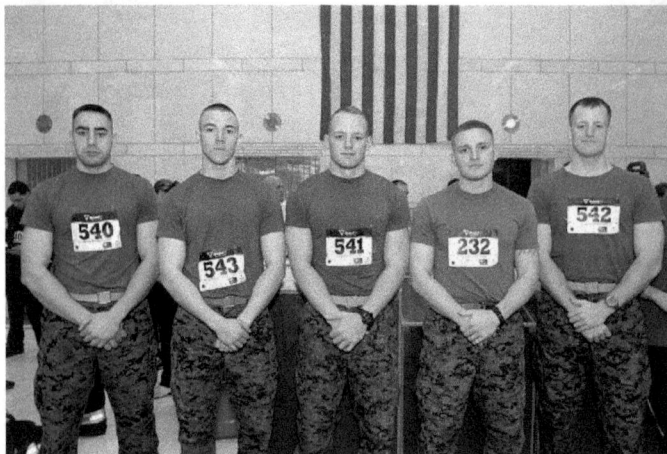

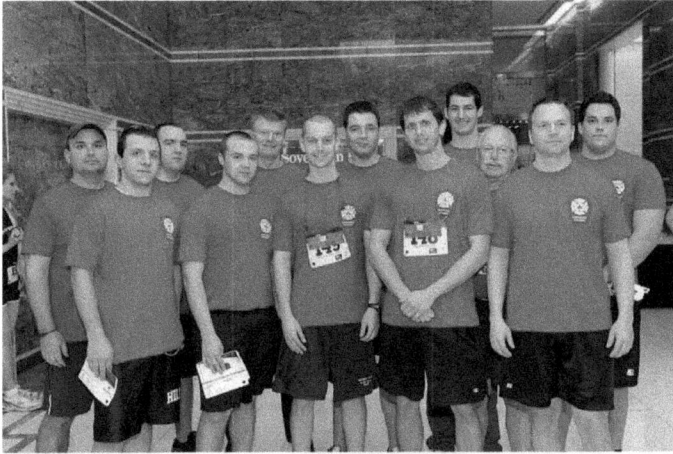

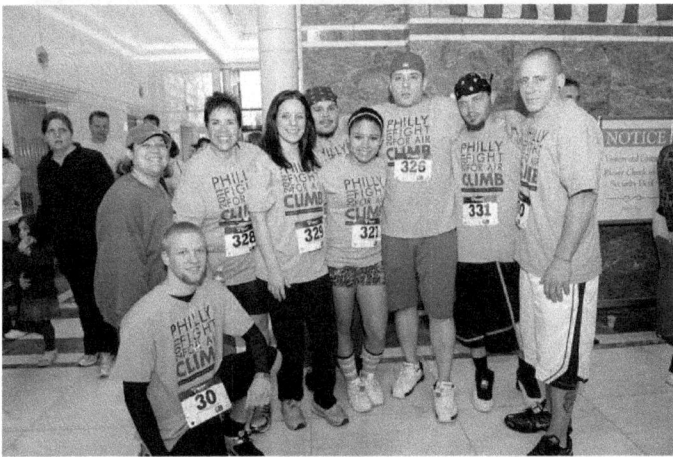

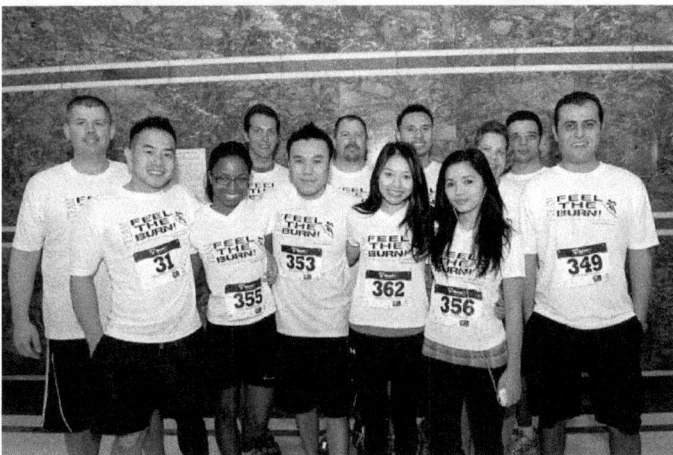

Feel The Burn Team

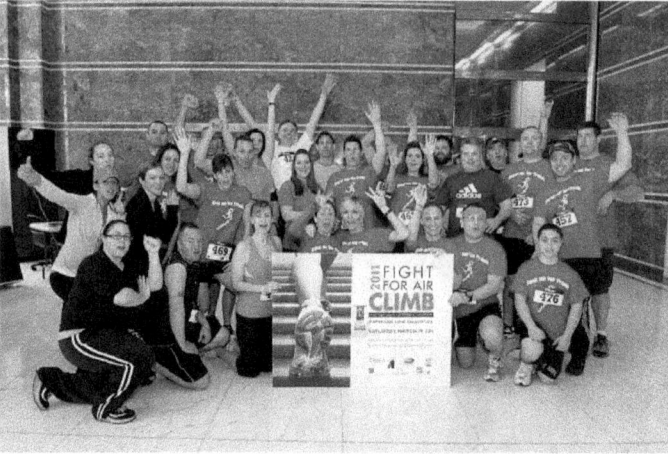
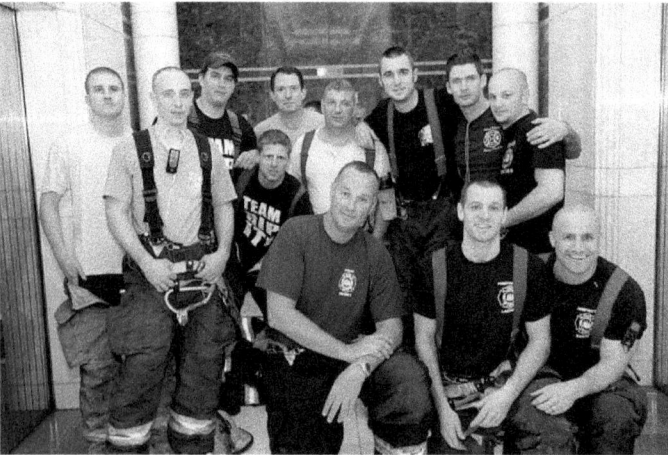
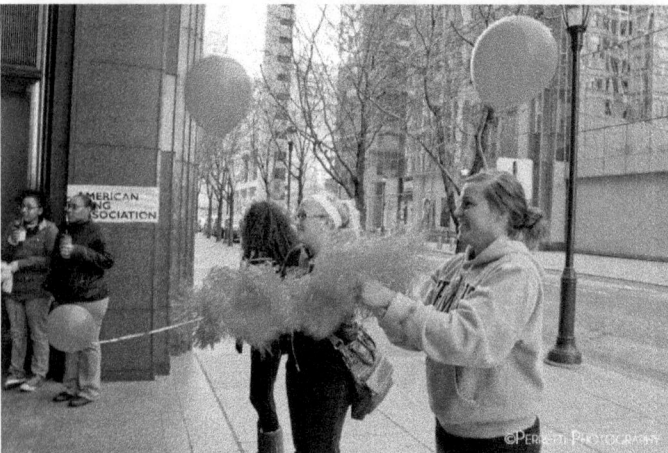

Some of the wonderful volunteers keep things lively

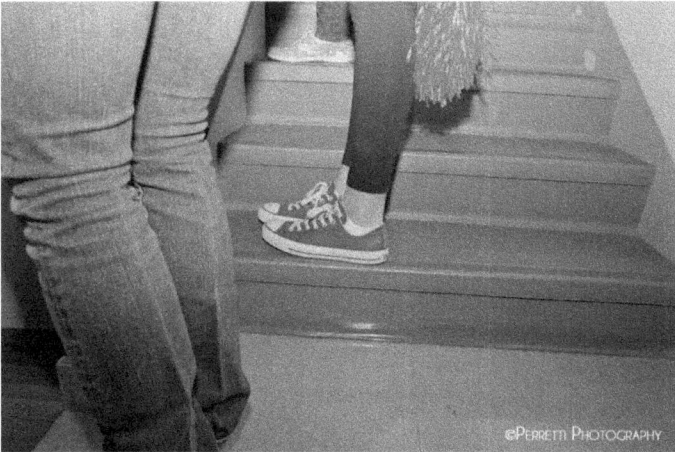

Volunteers on the steps

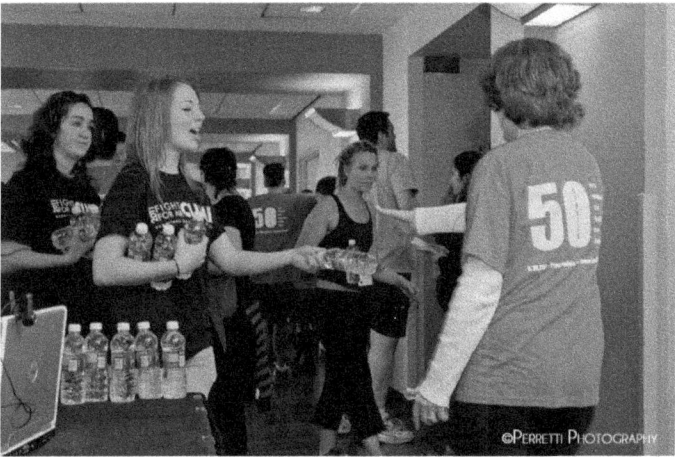

and handing out water bottles at the top

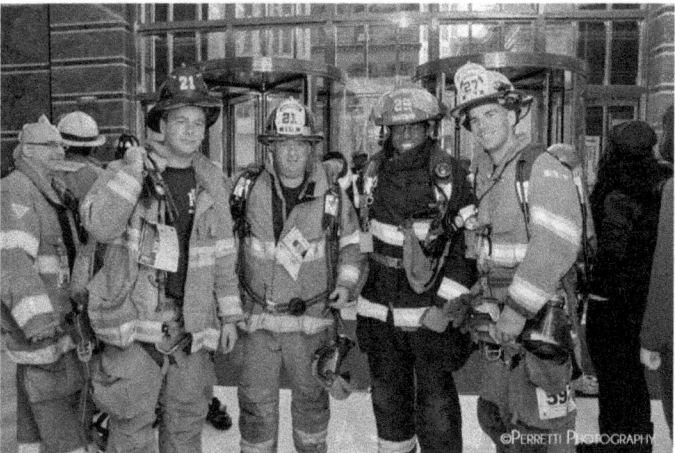

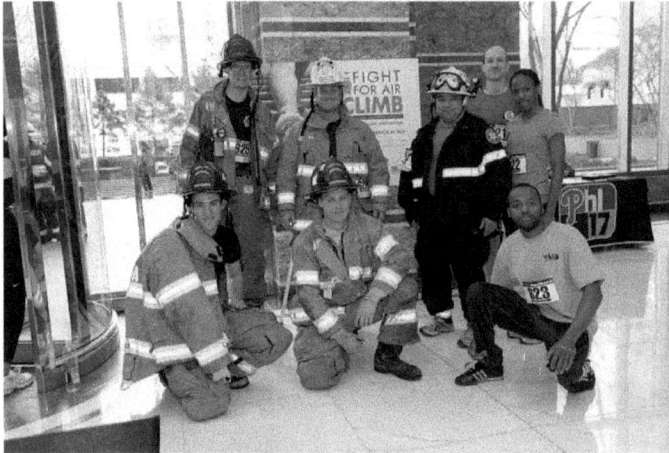

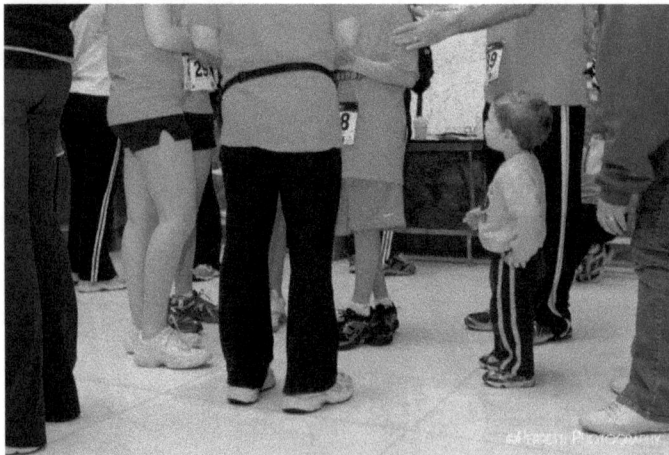

Young team supporter of Burt's Buddies

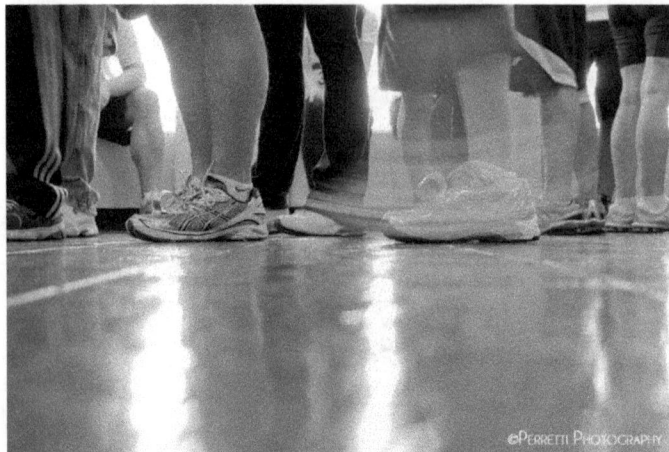

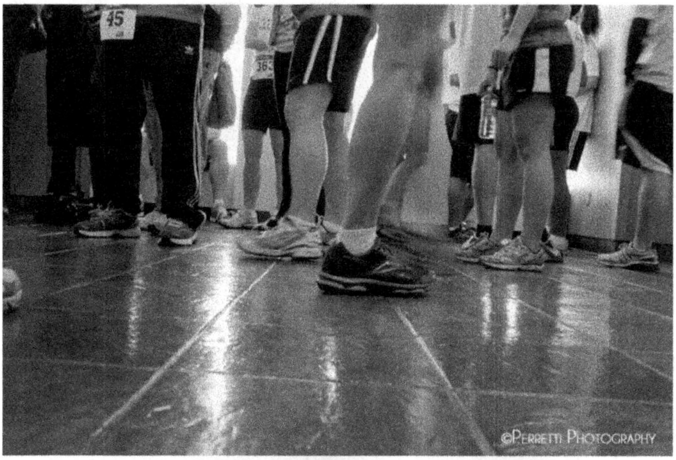
45
©PERRETTI PHOTOGRAPHY

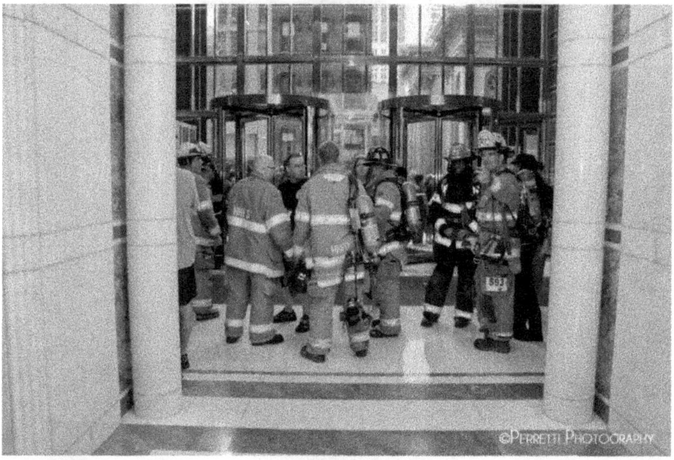
©PERRETTI PHOTOGRAPHY

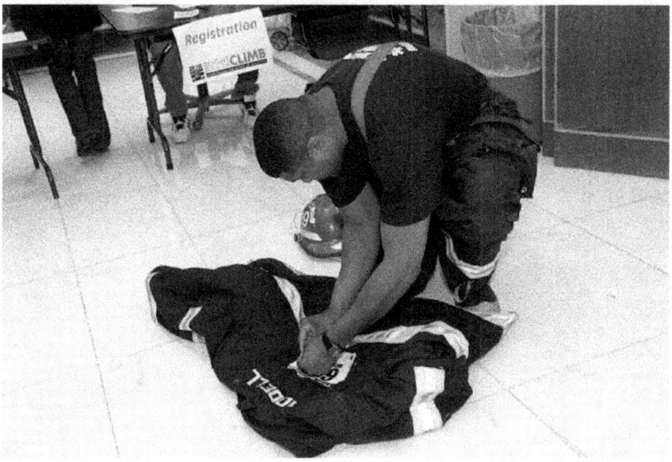
Registration
CLIMB

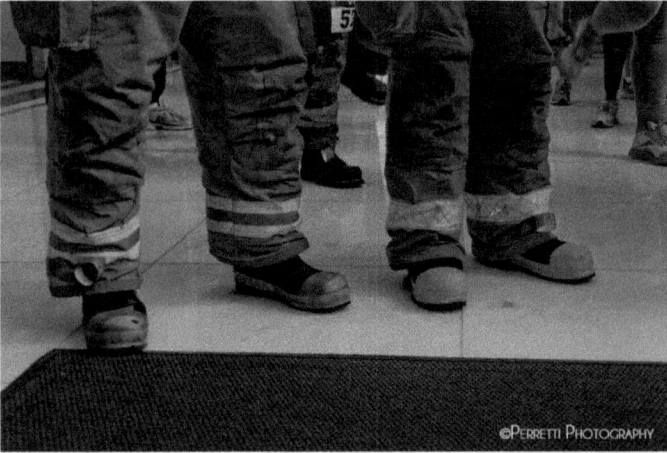

©PERRETTI PHOTOGRAPHY

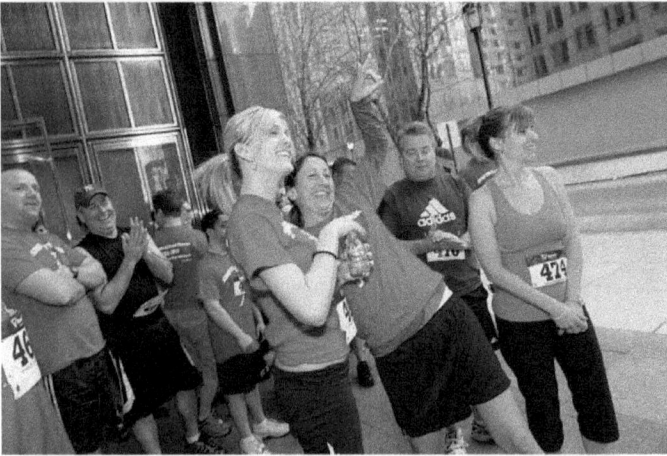

Waiting to go up the stairs. It's a bit chilly.

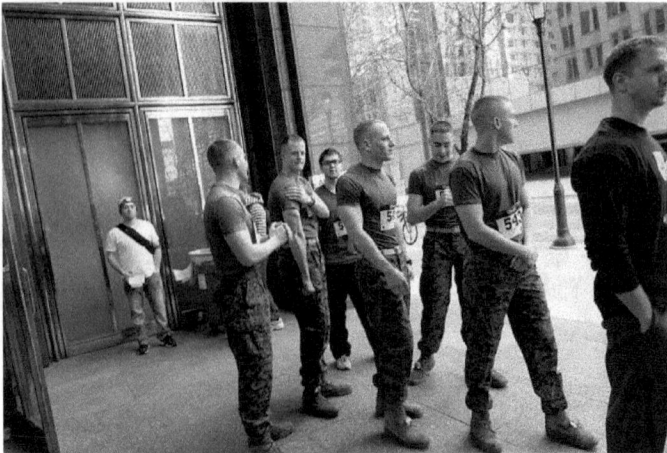

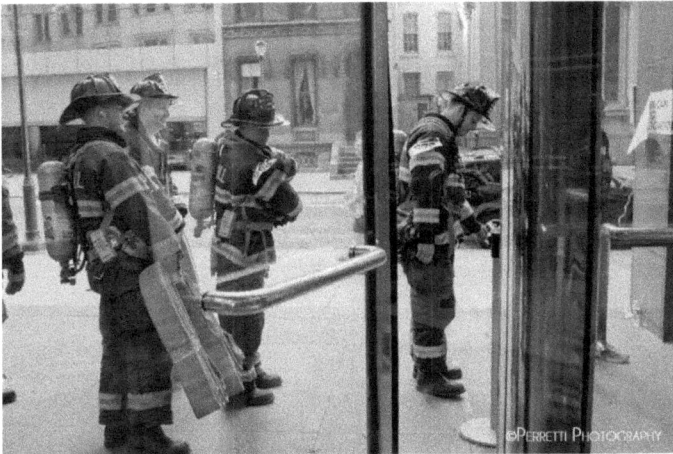

This is what full gear means...

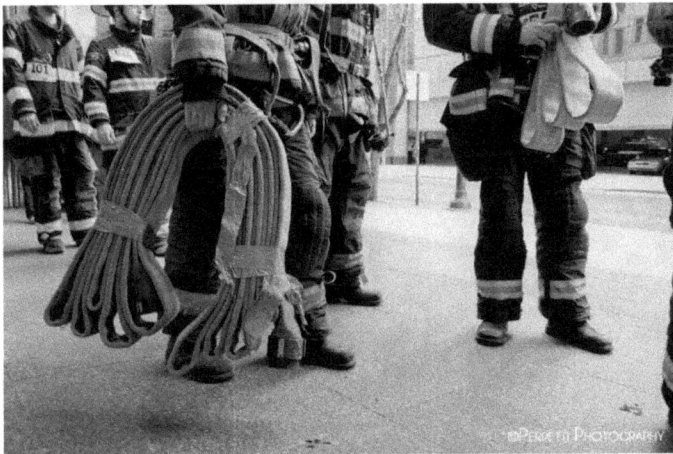

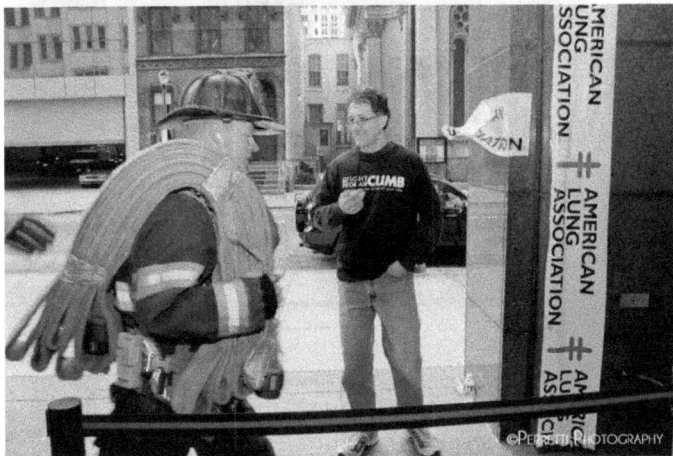

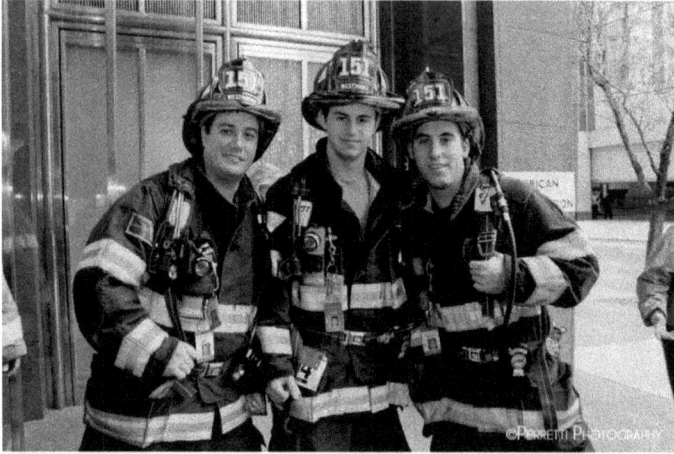

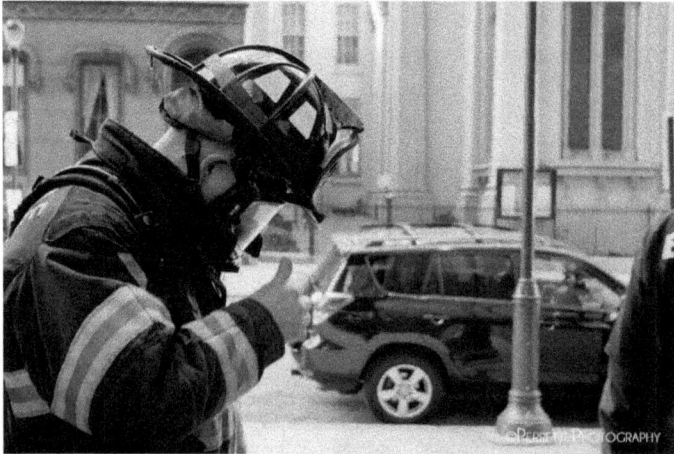

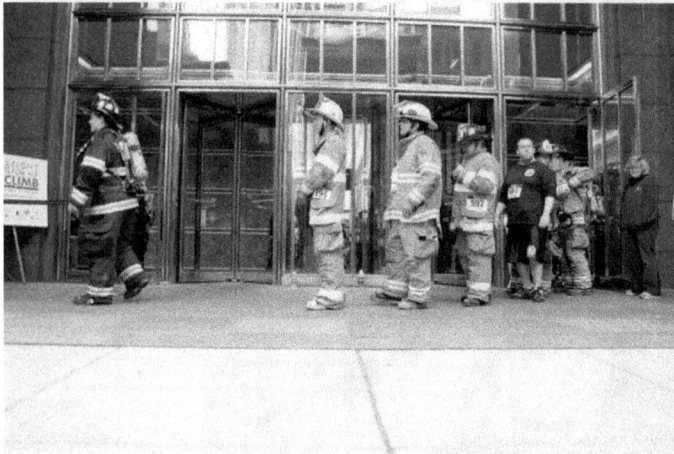

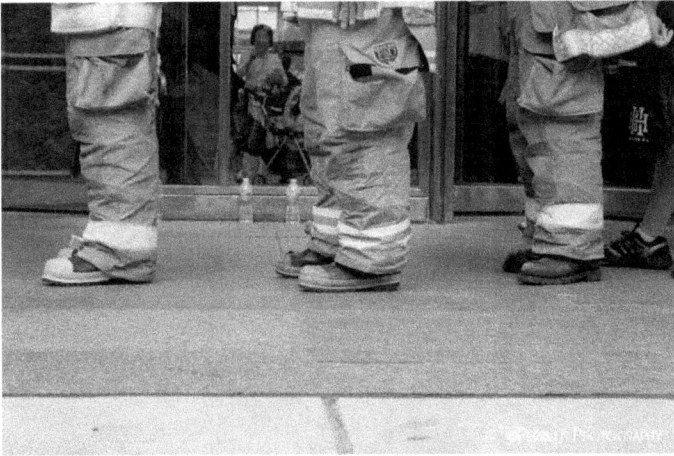

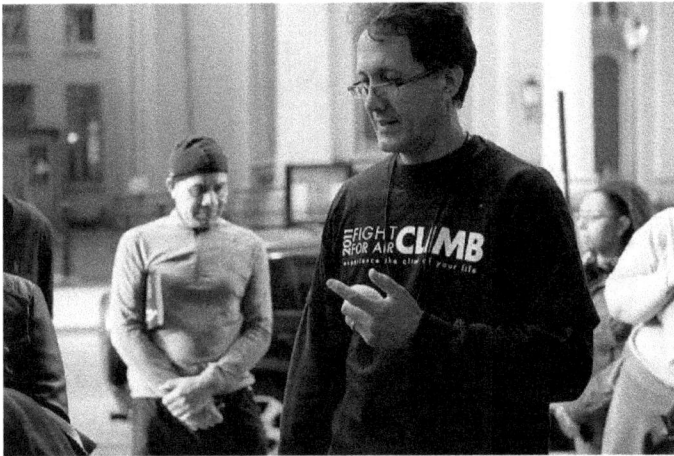

Our timing official ensures a staggered start to the climb....

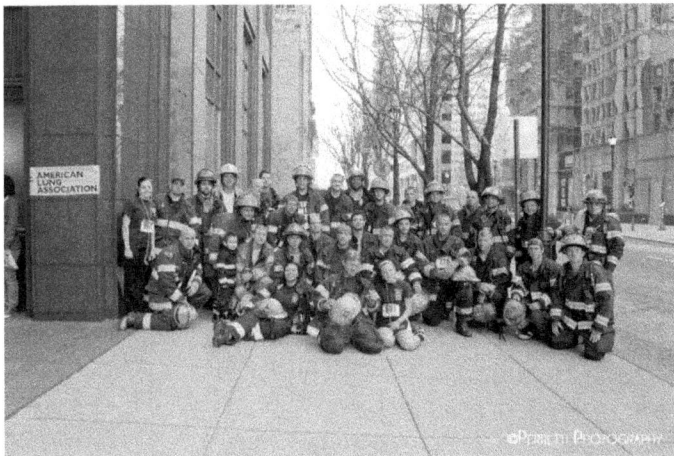

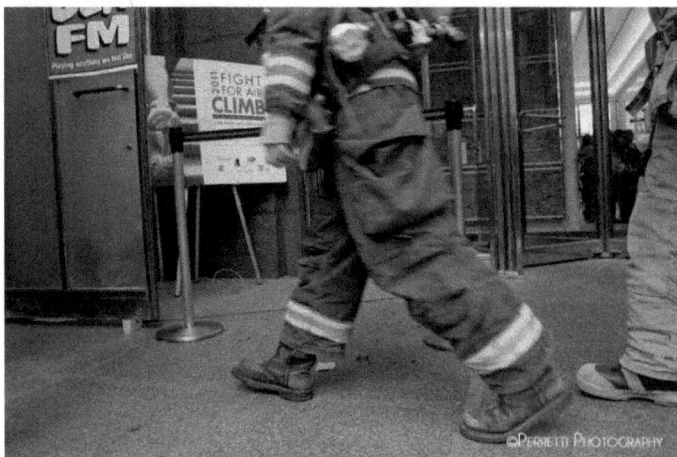

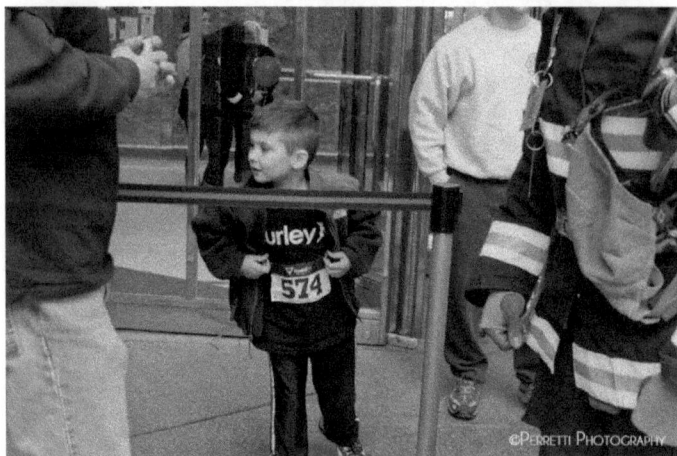

Looking for his buddy...

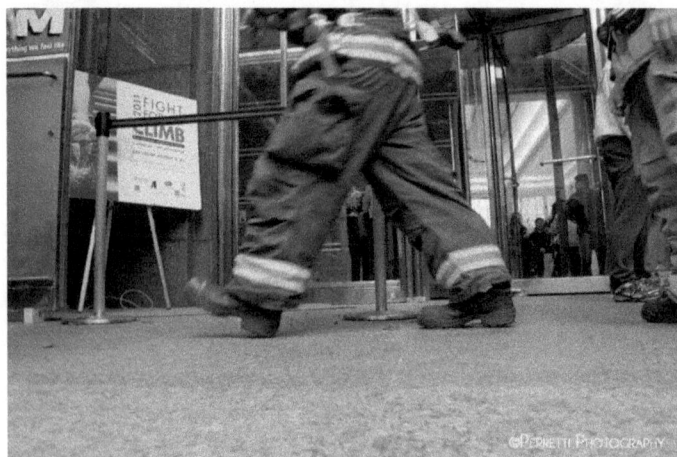

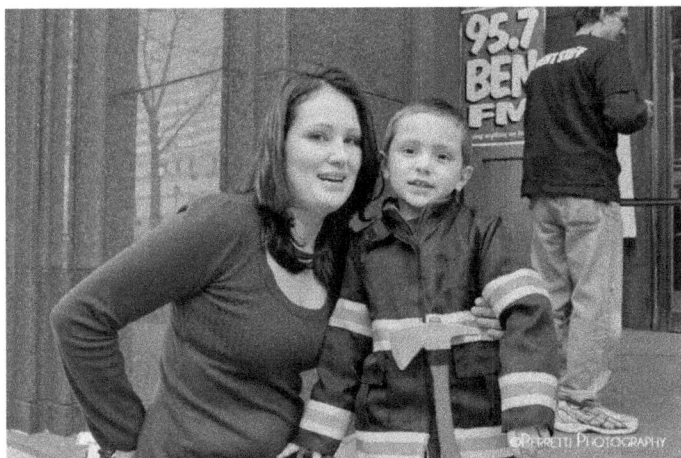
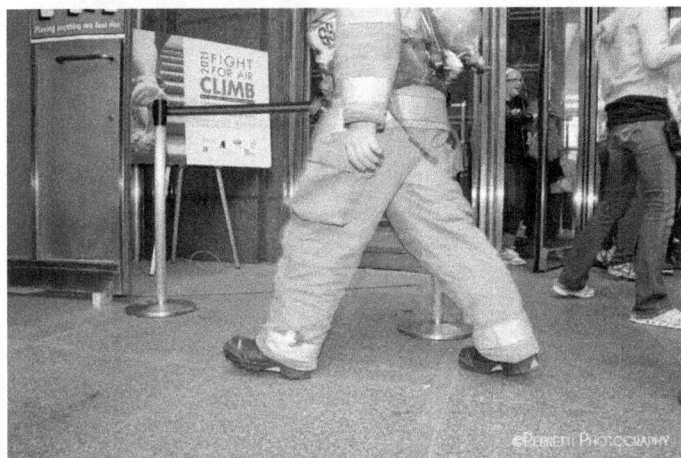
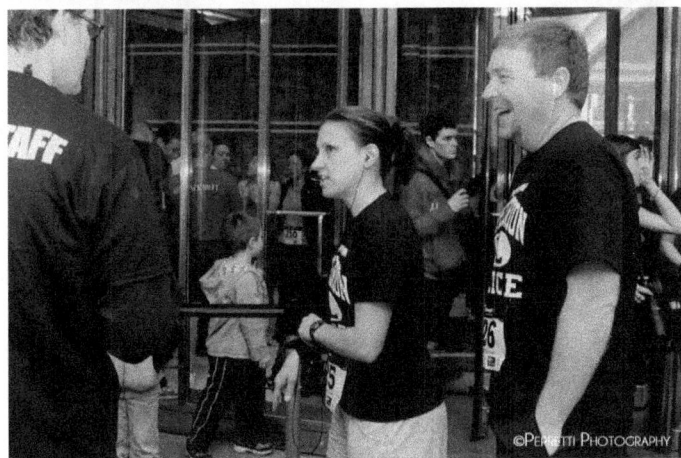

Stop Watch is ready for the trip up the stairs...

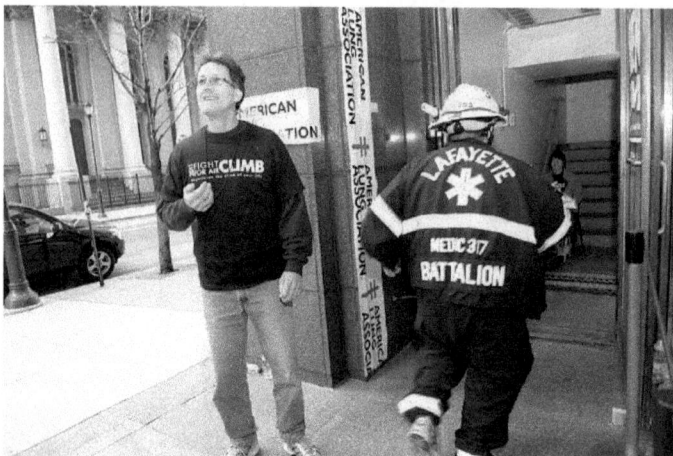

First Responder takes off...

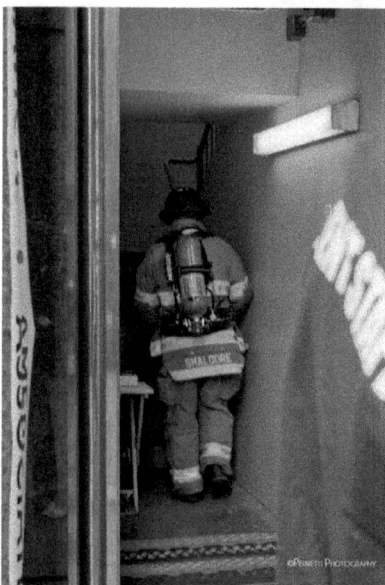

Up the stairs...

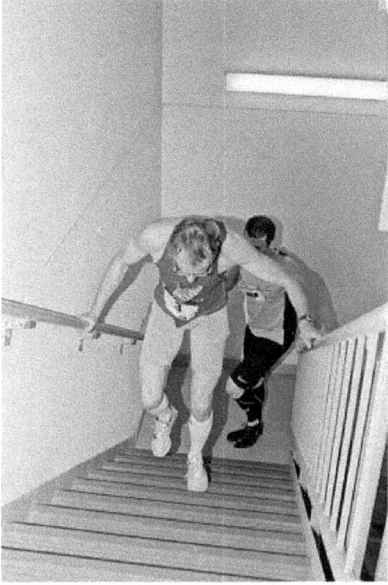

In the stairs, for some, the race is on...

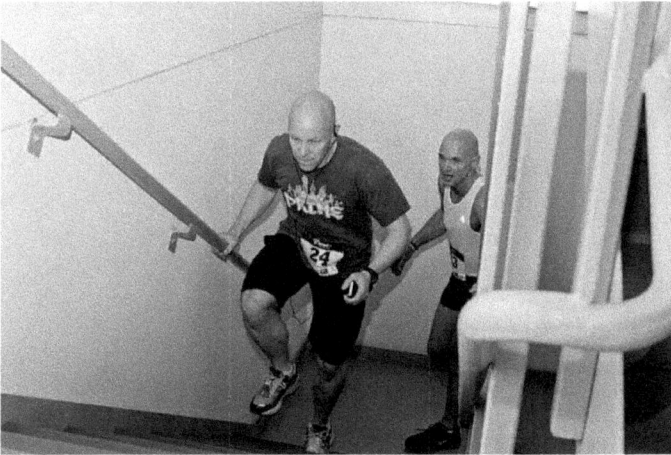

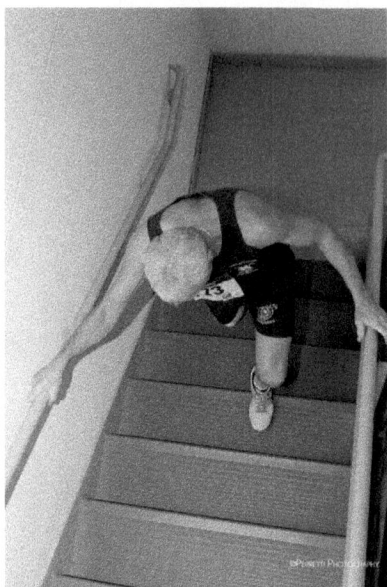

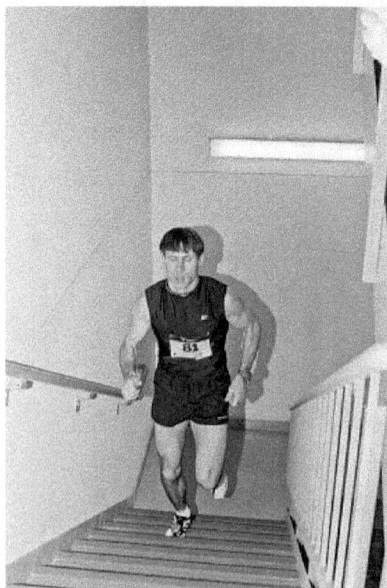

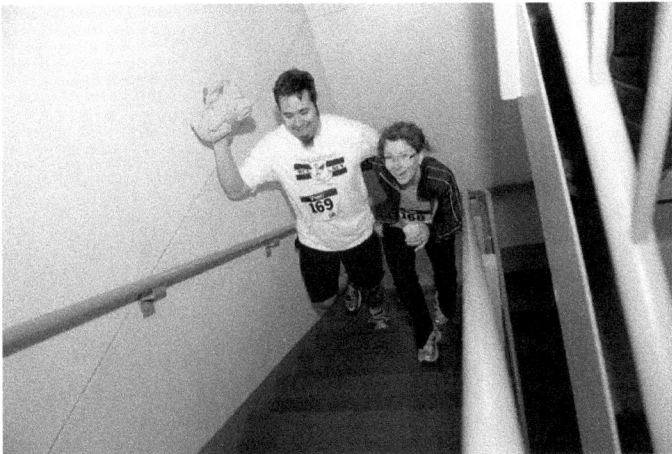

Team work makes the effort easier...

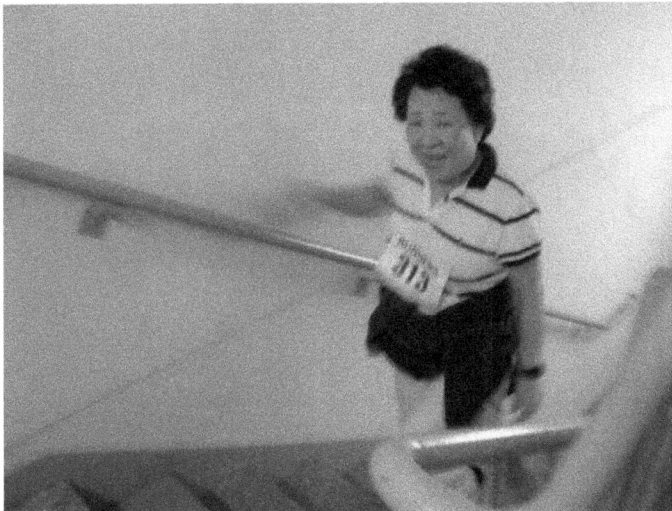

73 year old Judy Cheng in the stairs at the 2011 Philadelphia Fight For Air Climb. She was the oldest finisher in the event and is training for 2012!

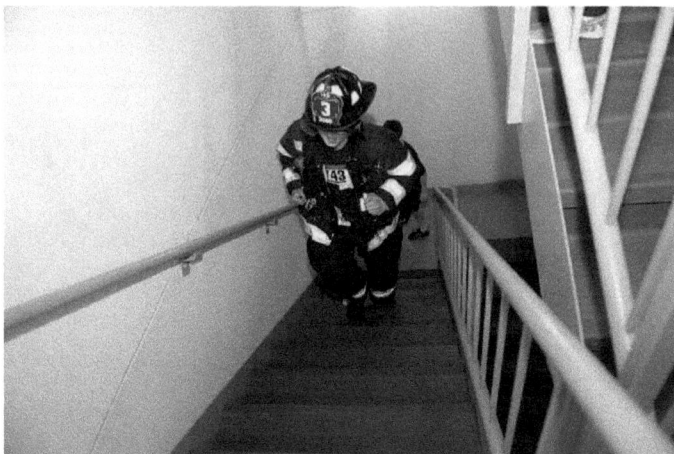

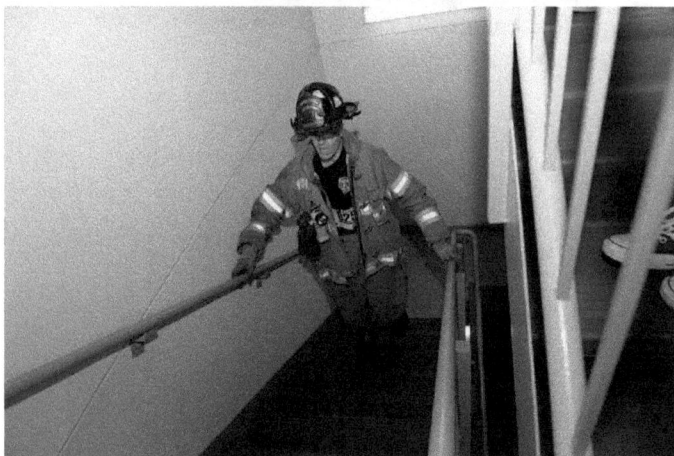

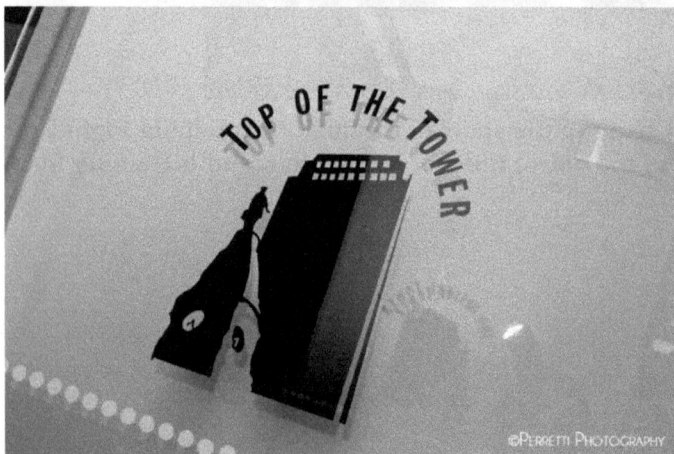

©Perretti Photography

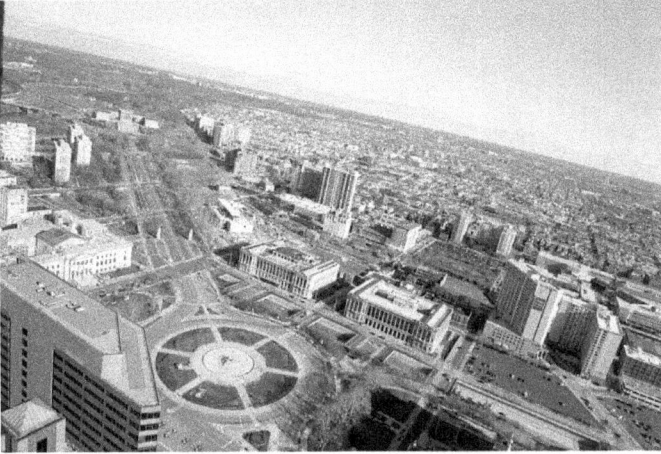

The view is beautiful!

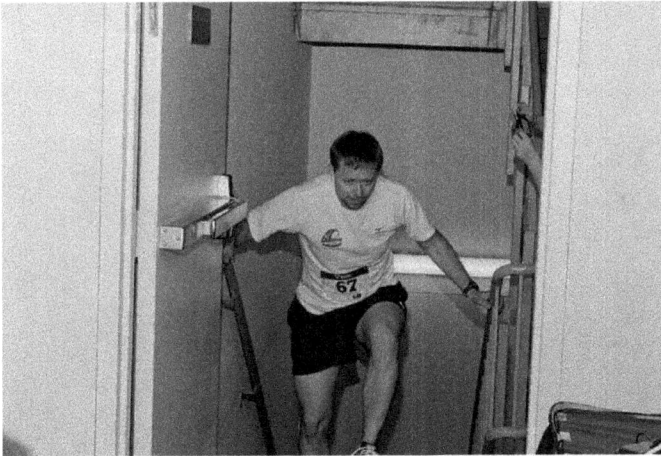

He's at the top!

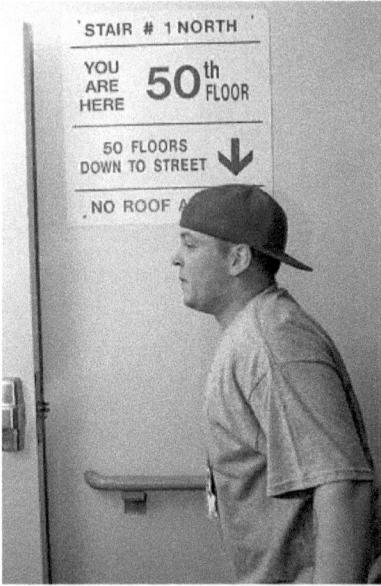

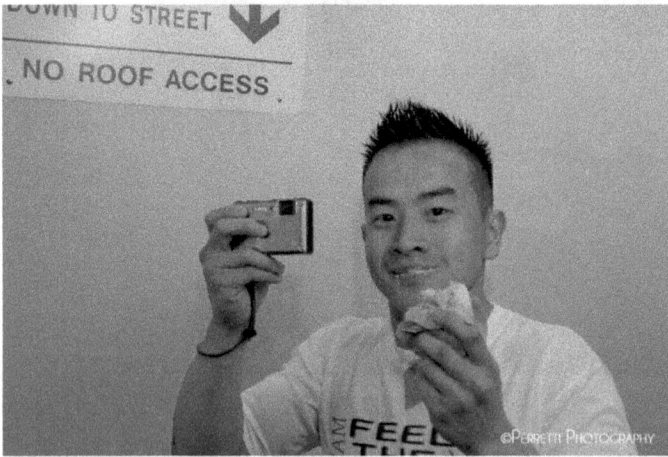

I didn't see donuts at the finish!

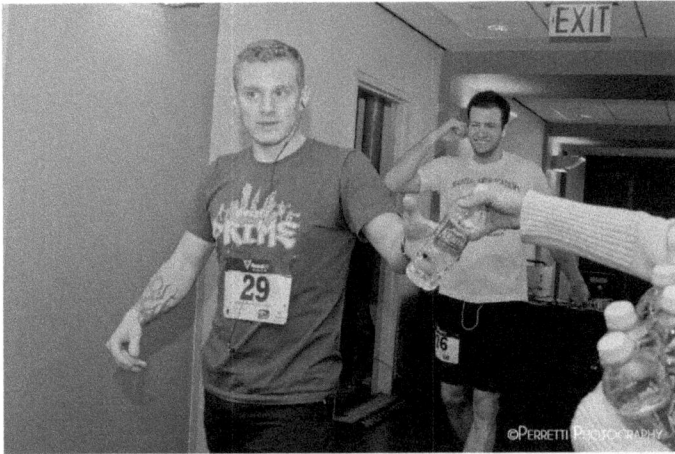

He doesn't look out of breath!

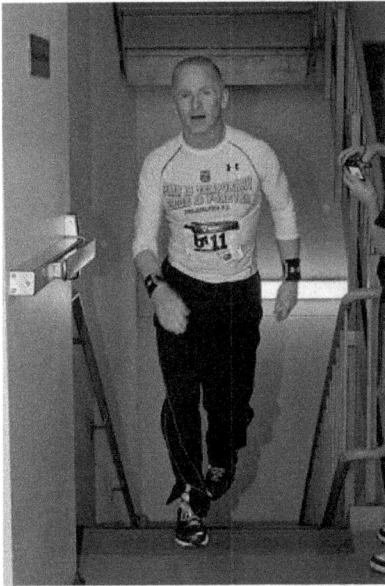

Joe Lynch did the climb twice!

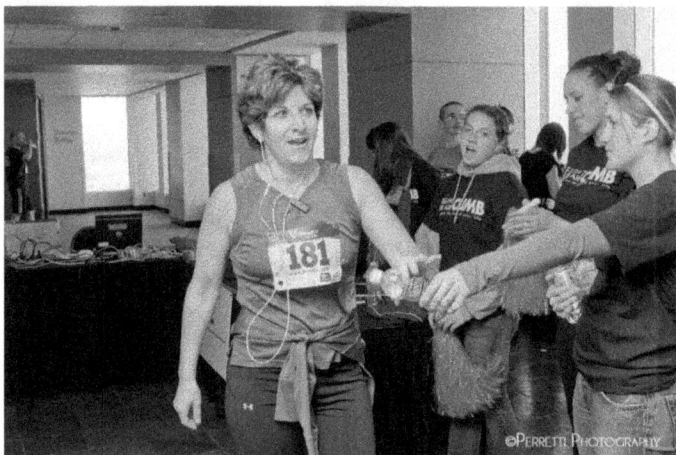

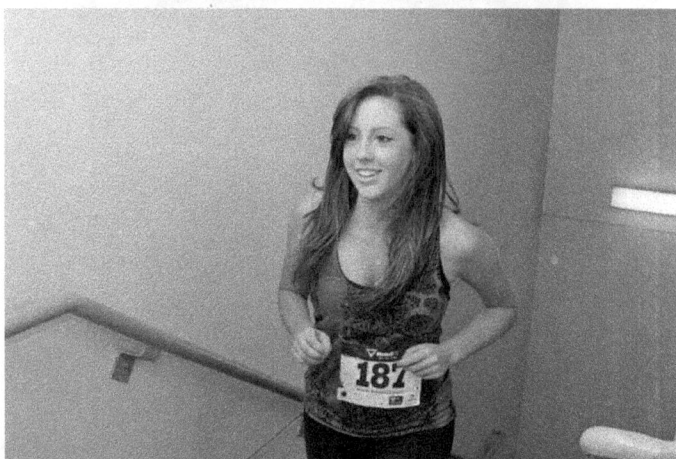

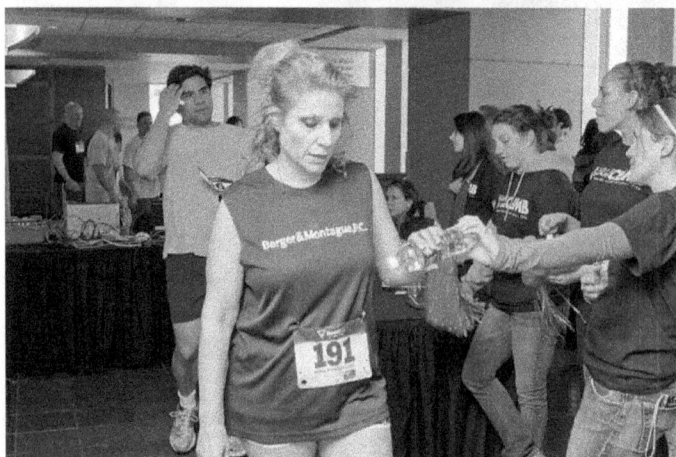

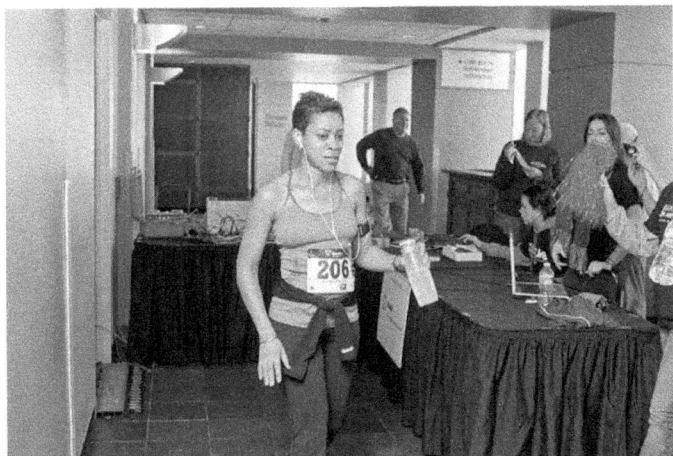

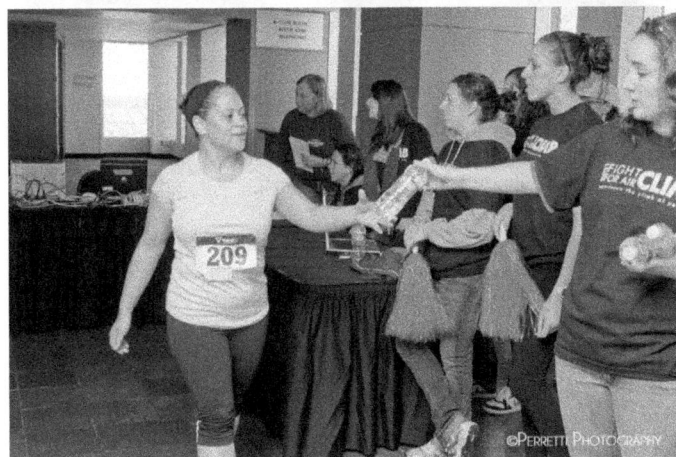

©Perretti Photography

525

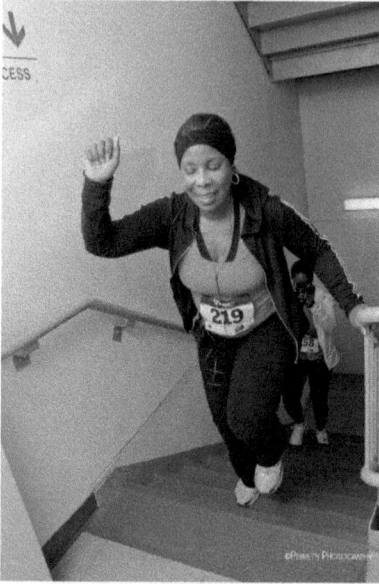

It's a proud accomplishment to reach the top...

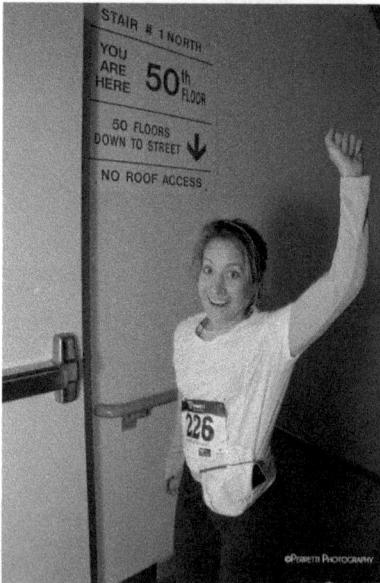

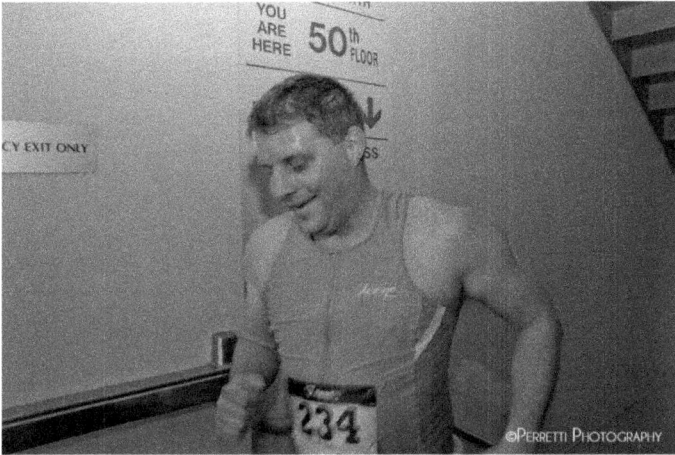
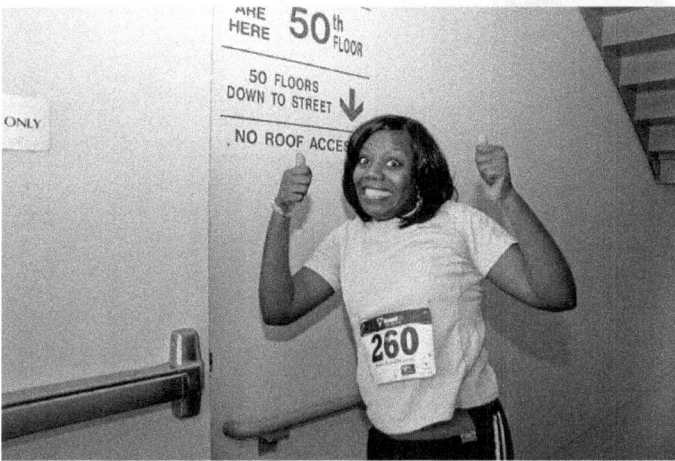
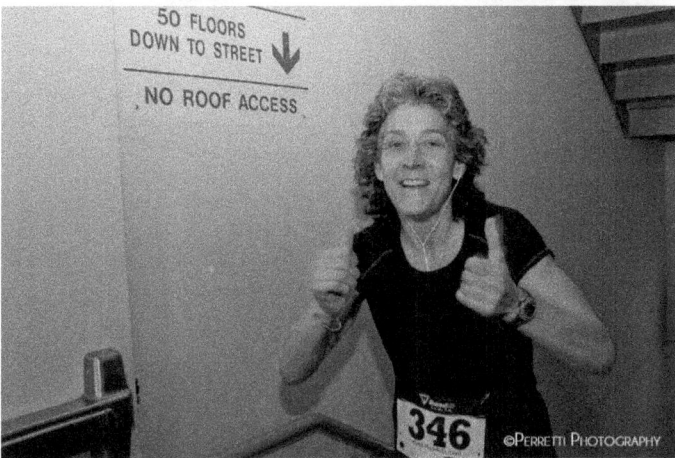

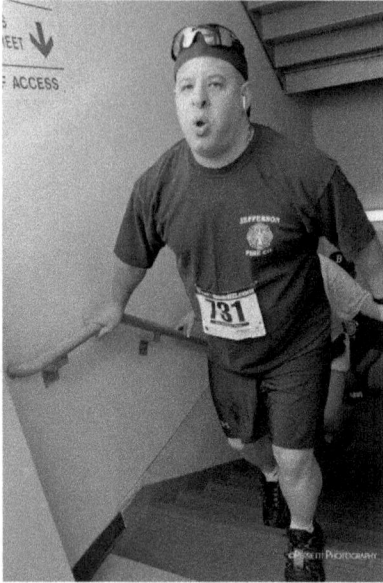

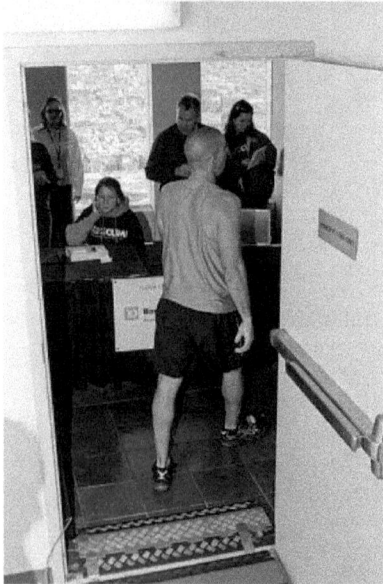

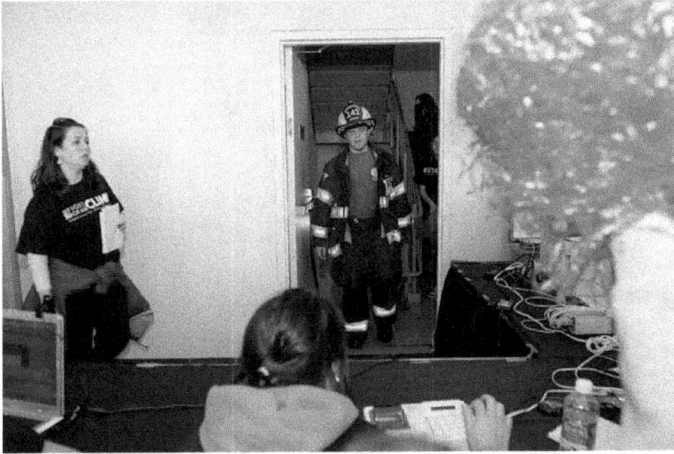

A First Responder reaches the top

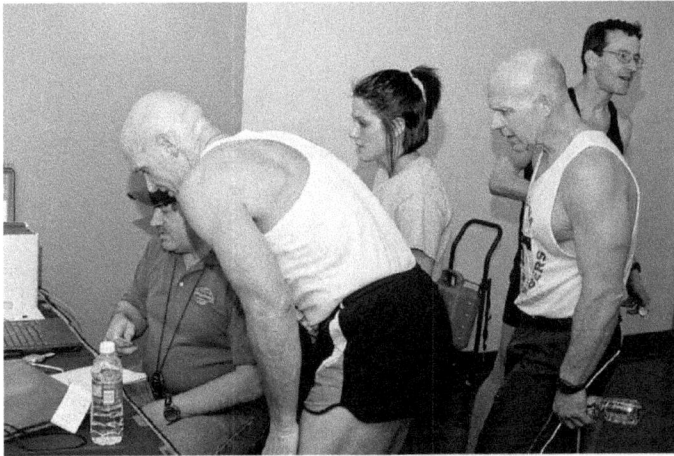

Serious climbers looking for results...

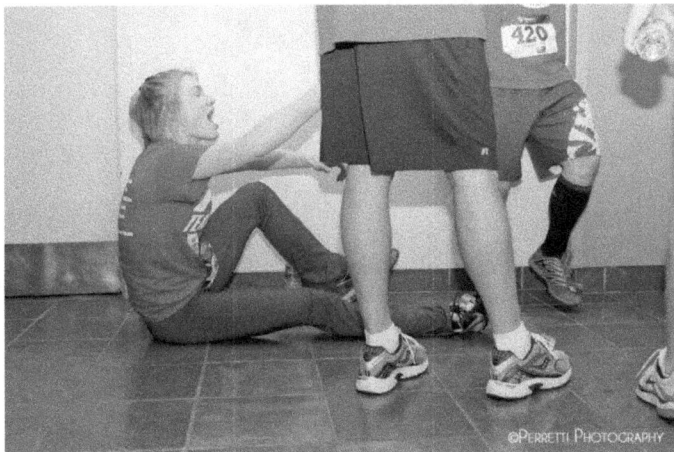

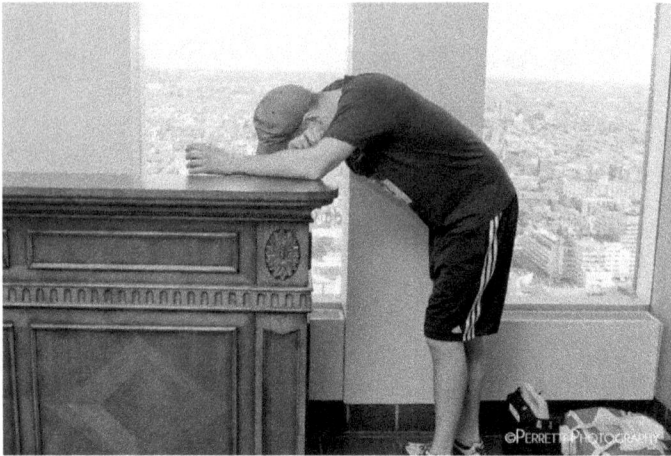

No one said it would be easy...

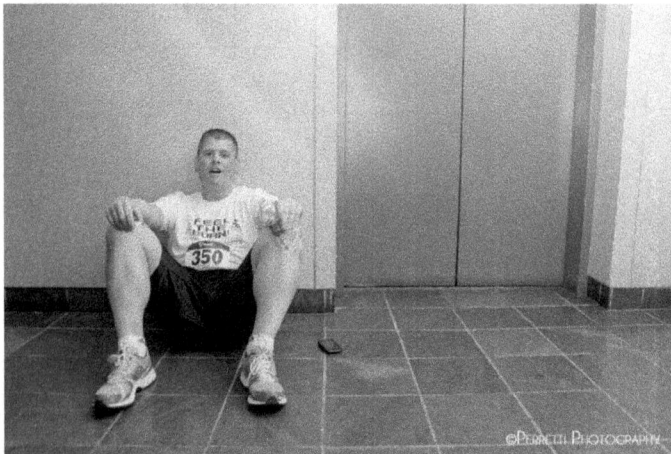

A member of the 'Feel The Burn' team after a job well done

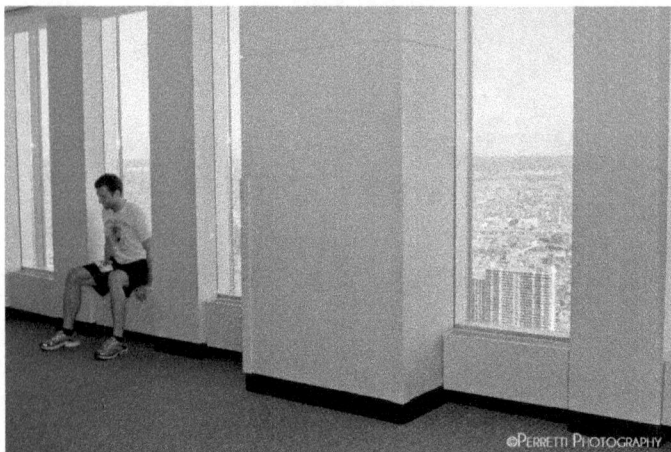

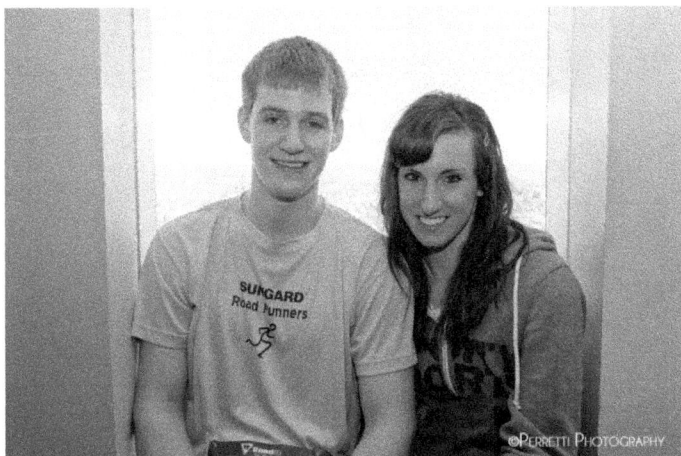

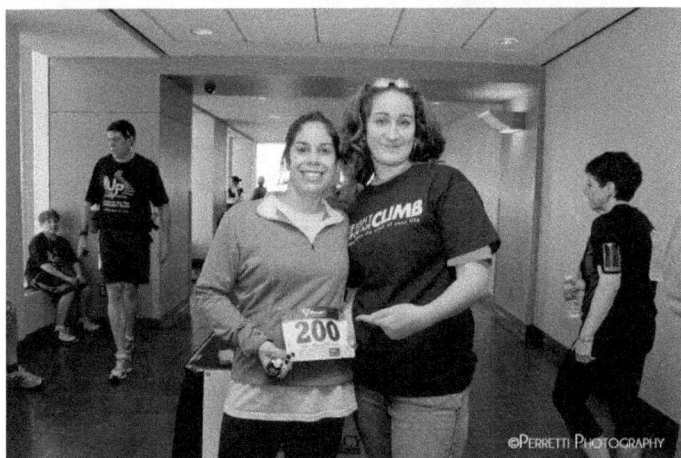

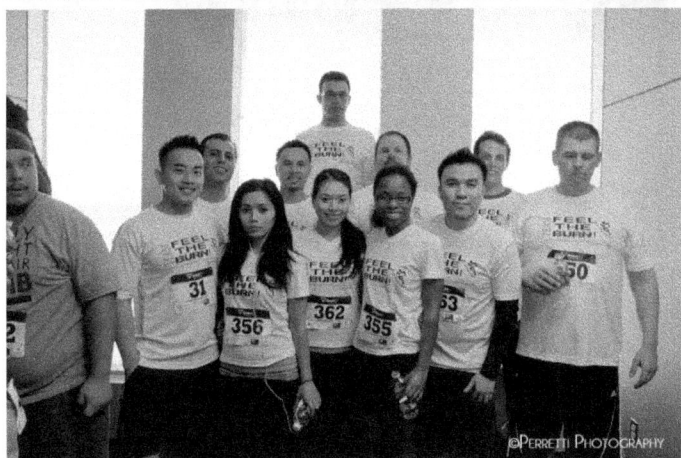

Team Feel The Burn

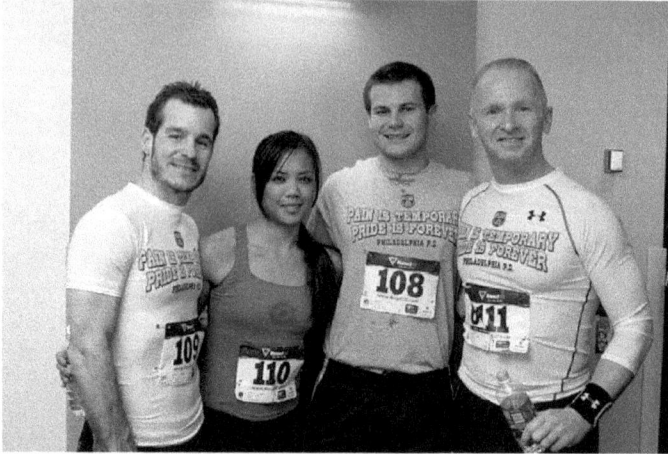

Joe Lynch and team.

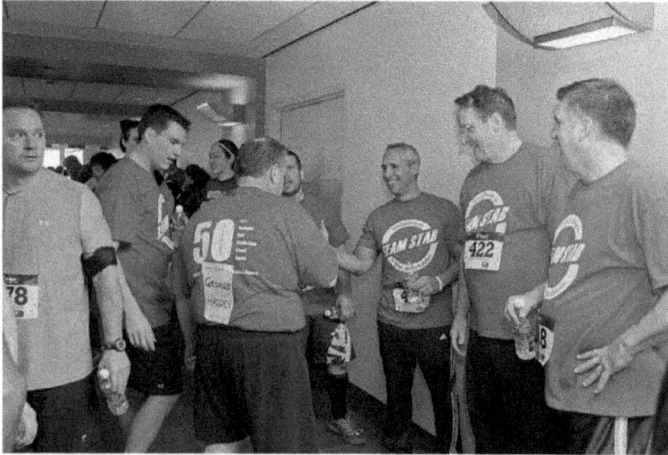

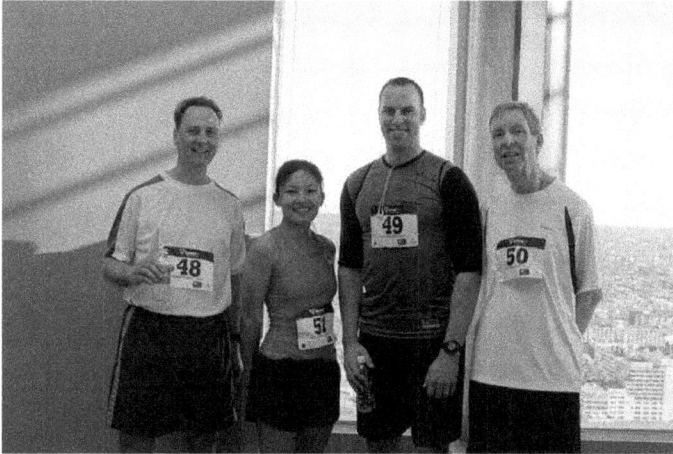

Team Smiley. Bob, Sophorn, Tim and John.

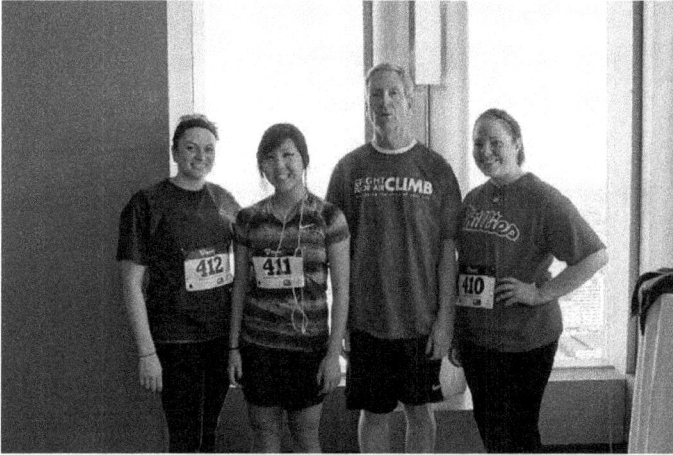

Team Smiley. Danielle, Melissa, John and Nora.

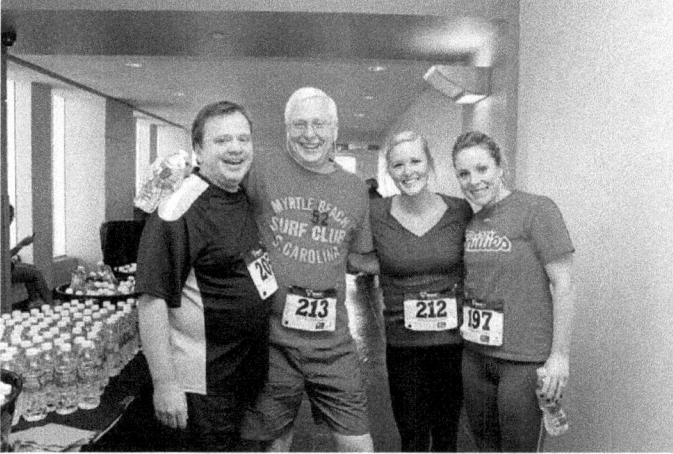

A satisfied team

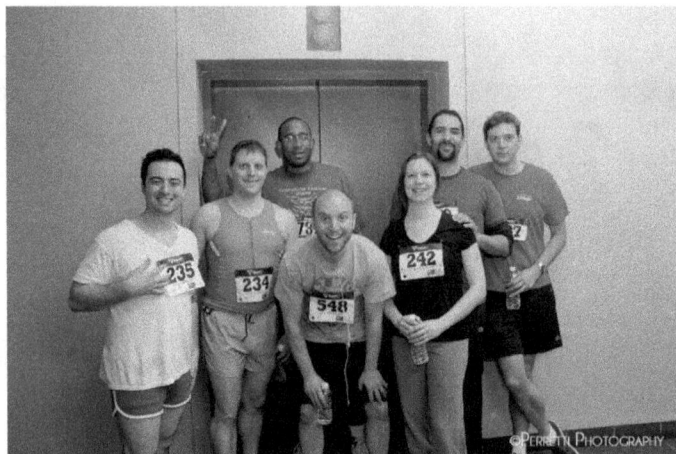

Ready to head down after a job well done...

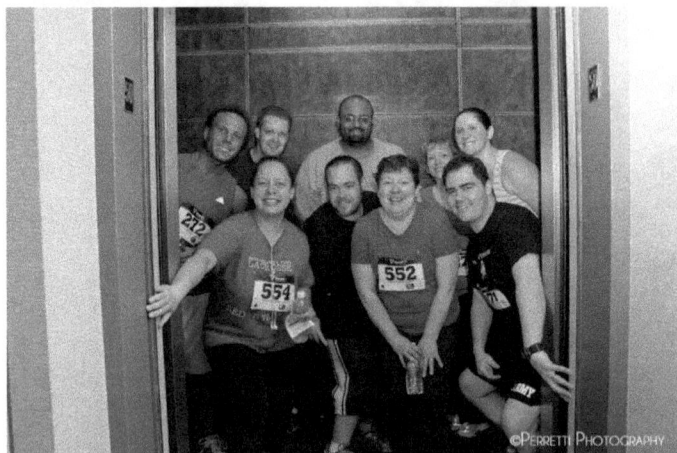

Rob Gurtcheff is holding the door open for the photo

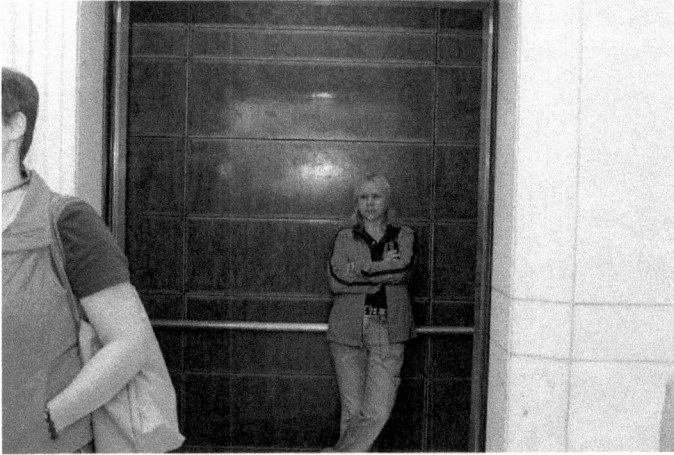

Take us down!

Index

B

C

H

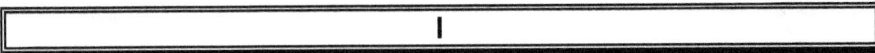

I

J

K

L

M

N

O

P

R

S

558

T

U

V

W

X

Y

Z

www.ingramcontent.com/pod-product-compliance
Lightning Source LLC
Chambersburg PA
CBHW071351290326
41932CB00045B/1421